Progress in Inflammation Research

Series Editor

Prof. Dr. Michael J. Parnham
PLIVA
Research Institute
Prilaz baruna Filipovica 25
10000 Zagreb
Croatia

Published titles:

T Cells in Arthritis, P. Miossec, W. van den Berg, G. Firestein (Editors), 1998
Chemokines and Skin, E. Kownatzki, J. Norgauer (Editors), 1998
Medicinal Fatty Acids, J. Kremer (Editor), 1998
Inducible Enzymes in the Inflammatory Response, D.A. Willoughby, A. Tomlinson (Editors), 1999
Cytokines in Severe Sepsis and Septic Shock, H. Redl, G. Schlag (Editors), 1999
Fatty Acids and Inflammatory Skin Diseases, J.-M. Schröder (Editor), 1999
Immunomodulatory Agents from Plants, H. Wagner (Editor), 1999
Cytokines and Pain, L. Watkins, S. Maier (Editors), 1999
In Vivo *Models of Inflammation*, D. Morgan, L. Marshall (Editors), 1999
Pain and Neurogenic Inflammation, S.D. Brain, P. Moore (Editors), 1999
Anti-Inflammatory Drugs in Asthma, A.P. Sampson, M.K. Church (Editors), 1999
Novel Inhibitors of Leukotrienes, G. Folco, B. Samuelsson, R.C. Murphy (Editors), 1999
Vascular Adhesion Molecules and Inflammation, J.D. Pearson (Editor), 1999
Metalloproteinases as Targets for Anti-Inflammatory Drugs, K.M.K. Bottomley, D. Bradshaw, J.S. Nixon (Editors), 1999
Free Radicals and Inflammation, P.G. Winyard, D.R. Blake, C.H. Evans (Editors), 2000

Forthcoming titles:

New Cytokines as Potential Drugs, S.K. Narula, R. Coffman (Editors), 2000
High-Throughput Screening for Novel Antiinflammatories, M. Kahn (Editor), 2000

Gene Therapy in Inflammatory Diseases

Christopher H. Evans
Paul D. Robbins

Editors

Springer Basel AG

Editors

Prof. Christopher H. Evans
Center for Molecular Orthopaedics
Harvard Medical School
221 Longwood Avenue, Room BL 152
Boston, MA 02115
USA

Prof. Paul D. Robbins
University of Pittsburgh School of Medicine
W1246, Biological Sciences Tower
Pittsburgh, PA 15261
USA

A CIP catalogue record for this book is available from the Library of Congress, Washington D.C., USA

Deutsche Bibliothek Cataloging-in-Publication Data
Gene therapy in inflammatory diseases / ed. by Christopher H.
Evans ; Paul D. Robbins. - Basel ; Boston ; Berlin : Birkhäuser, 2000
(Progress in inflammation research)
ISBN 978-3-0348-9584-2 ISBN 978-3-0348-8478-5 (eBook)
DOI 10.1007/978-3-0348-8478-5

The publisher and editor can give no guarantee for the information on drug dosage and administration contained in this publication. The respective user must check its accuracy by consulting other sources of reference in each individual case.

The use of registered names, trademarks etc. in this publication, even if not identified as such, does not imply that they are exempt from the relevant protective laws and regulations or free for general use.

Originally published by Birkhäuser Verlag Basel, Switzerland in 2000
Softcover reprint of the hardcover 1st edition 2000
Printed on acid-free paper produced from chlorine-free pulp. TCF ∞
Cover design: Markus Etterich, Basel
Cover illustration: Simon Watkins, Center for Biological Imaging, Harvard Medical School, Boston

ISBN 978-3-0348-9584-2

9 8 7 6 5 4 3 2 1

Contents

List of contributors ... vii

Preface ... xi

Christopher H. Evans and Paul D. Robbins
Gene therapy for inflammatory diseases – basic concepts ... 1

Sergei S. Makarov
Gene therapy for rheumatoid arthritis: preclinical studies ... 13

Thomas Pap, Ulf Müller-Ladner, Klaus M. Hummel, Renate E. Gay and Steffen Gay
Cartilage erosion in rheumatoid arthritis: studies in SCID mouse model ... 35

Thomas S. Muzzonigro, Richard Kang, Julio Reinecke, Peter Wehling, Mary C. Wasko and James H. Herndon
Gene therapy for rheumatoid arthritis: clinical studies ... 53

Alistair J. Ramsay, Simon P. Hogan, Paul S. Foster and Yelin Xiong
Cytokine gene therapy of allergic airways inflammation ... 65

Philip C. Fox and Brian C. O'Connell
Gene therapy for inflammatory diseases of the salivary glands ... 83

Huang-Ge Zhang, Martin Fleck, Hui-Chen Hsu, Carl K. Edwards III, David T. Curiel, Tong Zhou and John D. Mountz
Gene therapy for management of lupus: correction of Fas and Fas ligand-induced apoptosis in murine disease – therapeutic rationale and strategies ... 95

Michael K. Shaw, Richard DalCanto and C. Garrison Fathman
Gene therapy for multiple sclerosis 119

Nick Giannoukakis, Massimo Trucco and Paul D. Robbins
Gene therapy for type I diabetes mellitus 133

Jonathan S. Bromberg, Lisa A. DeBruyne, Randall S. Sung and Lihui Qin
Gene transfer to facilitate transplantation 163

Alexis Paul Godillot, Michael Madaio, David B. Weiner and William V. Williams
DNA vaccination as an anti-inflammatory strategy 205

Masayuki Miyata, Yukio Sato and Reiji Kasukawa
Naked DNA as a gene delivery vehicle in inflammatory diseases 231

Steven C. Ghivizzani, Eric R. Lechman, Daniel Jaffurs, Zhibao Mi, Richard Kang, Thomas S. Muzzonigro, Christopher H. Evans and Paul D. Robbins
Animal models of arthritis generated by gene transfer 241

Index 256

List of contributors

Jonathan S. Bromberg, Departments of Surgery and Gene Therapy and Molecular Medicine, Mt. Sinai School of Medicine, One Gustave L. Levy Place, Box 1496, New York, NY 10029-6574, USA; e-mail: jon_bromberg@smtplink.mssm.edu

David T. Curiel, Gene Therapy Program, University of Alabama at Birmingham, 1824 6th Avenue South, WTI 620, Birmingham, AL 35294, USA; e-mail: david.curiel@ccc.uab.edu

Richard DalCanto, Stanford University School of Medicine, Division of Immunology and Rheumatology, Stanford, CA 94305-5111, USA

Lisa A. DeBruyne, Parke-Davis Warner Lambert, Ann Arbor, MI 48109-0331, USA

Carl K. Edwards III, Amgen, Inc., One Amgen Center Drive, Thousand Oaks, CA 91320-1789, USA; e-mail: carle@amgen.com

Christopher H. Evans, Center for Molecular Orthopaedics, Harvard Medical School, 221 Longwood Avenue, Room BL 152, Boston, MA 02115, USA; e-mail: cevans@vms.cis.pitt.edu

Martin Fleck, University of Regensburg Medical Center, Department of Internal Medicine, 93042 Regensburg, Germany; e-mail: martin.fleck@klinik.uni-regensburg.de

Paul S. Foster, Division of Biochemistry and Molecular Biology, The John Curtin School of Medical Research, Australian National University, Canberra ACT 0200, Australia

Philip C. Fox, Amarillo Biosciences, Inc., 6509 Seven Locks Road, Cabin John, MD 20818, USA; e-mail: pcfox@amarbio.com

C. Garrison Fathman, Stanford University School of Medicine, Division of Immunology and Rheumatology, Stanford, CA 94305-5111, USA

Renate E. Gay, Center for Experimental Rheumatology, Department of Rheumatology, University Hospital, CH-8091 Zürich, Switzerland

Steffen Gay, Center for Experimental Rheumatology, Department of Rheumatology, University Hospital, CH-8091 Zürich, Switzerland

Steven C. Ghivizzani, Center for Molecular Orthopaedics, Harvard Medical School, 221 Longwood Avenue, Room BL 152, Boston, MA 02115, USA

Nick Giannoukakis, Department of Molecular Genetics and Biochemistry, W1246 Biomedical Science Tower, University of Pittsburgh School of Medicine, Pittsburgh, PA 15261, USA

Alexis Paul Godillot, Division of Rheumatology, University of Pennsylvania School of Medicine, Philadelphia, PA 19104, USA

James H. Herndon, Partners Department of Orthopaedic Surgery, Massachusetts General Hospital, Gray 624-55 Fruit Street, Boston, MA 02114-2617, USA; e-mail: jherndon@partners.org

Simon P. Hogan, Division of Biochemistry and Molecular Biology, The John Curtin School of Medical Research, Australian National University, Canberra ACT 0200, Australia

Hui-Chen Hsu, University of Alabama at Birmingham, Department of Medicine, 701 South 19th Street, LHRB 473, Birmingham, AL 35294, USA; e-mail: hui-chen.hsu@ccc.uab.edu

Klaus M. Hummel, Department of Internal Medicine, University of Göttingen, D-37075 Göttingen

Daniel Jaffurs, Departments of Molecular Genetics and Biochemistry and Orthopaedic Surgery, University of Pittsburgh School of Medicine, Pittsburgh, PA 15261, USA

Richard Kang, Department of Orthopaedic Surgery, University of Pittsburgh School of Medicine, Pittsburgh, PA 15261 USA

Reiji Kasukawa, Department of Internal Medicine II, Fukushima University School of Medicine, Fukushima 960-1295, Japan

Eric R. Lechman, Departments of Molecular Genetics and Biochemistry and Orthopaedic Surgery, University of Pittsburgh School of Medicine, Pittsburgh, PA 15261, USA

Michael Madaio, Division of Nephrology, University of Pennsylvania School of Medicine, Philadelphia, PA 19104, USA

Sergei S. Makarov, Thurston Arthritis Research Center, University of North Carolina at Chapel Hill, 4109 Thurston, CB 7280, Chapel Hill, NC 27599-7280, USA; e-mail: smak@med.unc.edu

Zhibao Mi, Departments of Molecular Genetics and Biochemistry and Orthopaedic Surgery, University of Pittsburgh School of Medicine, Pittsburgh, PA 15261, USA

Masayuki Miyata, Department of Internal Medicine II, Fukushima University School of Medicine, Fukushima 960-1295, Japan; e-mail: metm@msg.biglobe.ne.jp

John D. Mountz, University of Alabama at Birmingham, 701 South 19th Street, LHRB 473, Birmingham, AL 35294-0007, USA; e-mail: John.Mountz@ccc.uab.edu

Ulf Müller-Ladner, Department of Internal Medicine, Division of Clinical Rheumatology and Immunulogy, University of Regensburg, 93042 Regensburg, Germany

Thomas Muzzonigro, Department of Orthopaedic Surgery, University of Pittsburgh School of Medicine, Pittsburgh, PA 15261, USA

Brian C. O'Connell, Department of Restorative Dentistry, School of Dental Science, Trinity College, Dublin, Ireland; e-mail: boconne@dental.tcd.ie

Thomas Pap, Center of Experimental Rheumatology, Department of Rheumatology, University Hospital, 8091 Zürich, Switzerland

Lihui Qin, Departments of Surgery and Pathology, Mt. Sinai School of Medicine, One Gustave L. Levy Place, Box 1104, New York, NY 10029-6574, USA

Alistair J. Ramsay, Discipline of Immunology and Microbiology, Faculty of Medicine, University of Newcastle, Newcastle NSW 2300, Australia; e-mail: aramsay@mail.newcastle.edu.au

Julio Reinecke, Orthogen GmbH, Düsseldorf, Germany

Paul D. Robbins, Department of Molecular Genetics and Biochemistry, W1246 Biomedical Science Tower, University of Pittsburgh School of Medicine, Pittsburgh, PA 15261, USA; e-mail: probb@pop.pitt.edu

Yukio Sato, Department of Internal Medicine II, Fukushima University School of Medicine, Fukushima 960-1295, Japan

Michael K. Shaw, Wayne State University School of Medicine, 540 E. Canfield, Detroit, MI 48201, USA; e-mail: mshaw@mediaone.net

Randall S. Sung, Departments of Surgery and Microbiology and Immunology, University of Michigan, Medical Center, Ann Arbor, MI 48109-0331, USA

Massimo Trucco, Division of Immunogenetics, Children's Hospital of Pittsburgh, University of Pittsburgh School of Medicine, W1246 Biomedical Science Tower, Pittsburgh, PA 15261, USA

Mary C. Wasko, Department of Medicine, Division of Rheumatology, University of Pittsburgh School of Medicine, Pittsburgh, PA 15261, USA

Peter Wehling, Praxis und Klinik für Orthopädie und Neurochirurgie, Steinstraße 2, 4000 Düsseldorf 1, Germany

David B. Weiner, Department of Pathology and Laboratory Medicine, University of Pennsylvania School of Medicine, Philadelphia, PA 19104, USA

William V. Williams, Department of Medicine, Rheumatology Division, University of Pennsylvania, 913 Stellar-Chance Laboratories, 422 Curie Drive, Philadelphia, PA 19104-6100, USA; e-mail: WWilliam@mail.med.upenn.edu

Yelin Xiong, Division of Immunology and Cell Biology, The John Curtin School of Medical Research, Australian National University, Canberra ACT 0200, Australia

Huang-Ge Zhang, University of Alabama at Birmingham, Department of Medicine, 701 South 19th Street, LHRB 473, Birmingham, AL 35294, USA;
e-mail: huang-ge.zhang@ccc.uab.edu

Tong Zhou, University of Alabama at Birmingham, Department of Medicine, 701 South 19th Street, LHRB 473, Birmingham, AL 35294, USA;
e-mail: tong.zhou@ccc.uab.edu

Preface

Inflammatory diseases cast a persistent shadow over the wellbeing of mankind. Their effects range from the acute and reversible symptoms that accompany, for example, transient microbial infection to the progressive misery resulting from chronic conditions such as rheumatoid arthritis. Despite a sustained, huge effort by the pharmaceutical industry for much of the present century, these diseases remain difficult to treat and almost impossible to cure.

Inflammation is a biological process; it seems axiomatic that any logical attempt to improve its medical management requires a thorough understanding of this biology. Modern molecular approaches to the study of inflammatory diseases have provided an appropriate conceptual framework, and we are beginning to see the first fruits of this in the clinical application of biological agents as anti-inflammatories. Gene therapy is the latest modality to emerge from this trend.

The genetic components of most inflammatory diseases are complex, polygenic and quantitatively less important than environmental influences. Why, then, use gene therapy to treat them? The answer is that genes are not, at this stage, being used to compensate for genetic alterations or polymorphisms in the patient. They are, instead, being used to deliver therapeutic gene products or to alter levels of gene expression in the host. In this sense, genes are being used as biological delivery systems for the RNA and protein molecules they encode, or as molecular regulators of gene expression.

Gene transfer systems are necessary because traditional methods of drug delivery fail to deliver proteins and nucleic acids in a clinically useful fashion, especially in chronic inflammatory diseases where therapeutic concentrations of these molecules need to be maintained for extended periods of time. Moreover, parenteral delivery of such agents exposes unaffected organs to concentrations of the drugs that are no less than those seen by the affected organs. This leads to undesirable side-effects, a problem for which anti-inflammatory drugs are notorious. Gene transfer technology, in contrast, can achieve the sustained, targeted, local production of therapeutic gene products. In theory, the level of production can be regulated as required by the level of disease activity.

Although recent, these concepts have found wide acceptance and a growing number of investigators are now involved in research in this area. Completion of the first human clinical trial of gene therapy for an inflammatory disease provides a timely juncture for the publication of this volume, the first to be dedicated to inflammation gene therapy. The focus of this book is on chronic inflammatory diseases, as this is the area where gene therapy is likely to have its greatest impact – biological treatment of acute inflammatory conditions such as septic shock is more likely to involve the direct infusion of gene products than the genes themselves.

Rather than ask every investigator in the field to contribute a short chapter and thereby risk producing a series of disjointed, redundant mini-reviews of each author's own research, we have selected a senior figure from each of the major disease areas to write an authoritative review. Most major inflammatory disorders including arthritis, diabetes, asthma, salivary duct conditions such as Sjögren's syndrome, lupus erythematosus, multiple sclerosis, and organ transplantation, are covered in detail. Additional disorders, such as colitis and keratitis, are mentioned. The chapter on organ transplantation provides an interesting example of how an iatrogenic problem illuminates areas of naturally occurring disease. Physicians involved in the first clinical trials of gene therapy in inflammation have contributed a chapter describing these landmark studies.

We have deliberately avoided chapters on vectors and other technological issues, as these have been extensively described in many other books on gene therapy. Instead, such issues are discussed within the introductory chapter that reviews briefly the basic concepts of gene therapy in inflammatory diseases. Nevertheless, we thought it appropriate to include two chapters on the use of naked DNA, as this may have a special niche in certain anti-inflammatory settings. One of these is in DNA vaccination to eliminate autoreactive T lymphocytes and the other to achieve immune deviation.

Finally, there is a chapter describing the use of gene transfer to establish models of inflammatory diseases which are more informative and authentic than those resulting from standard genetic or non-genetic manipulations. These models should improve both the understanding and treatment of inflammatory conditions, and they serve to remind us that the preclinical development of gene transfer and gene therapy is not merely an exercise in technology but also a novel scientific means of investigating wide areas of disease pathophysiology.

There is every expectation that genetic treatments will enhance the anti-inflammatory armamentarium early in the next millennium. The present volume describes the state-of-the-art as we stand on the threshold of this quantum leap.

Pittsburgh, Pennsylvania, July 1999

Christopher H. Evans
Paul D. Robbins

Gene therapy for inflammatory diseases – basic concepts

Christopher H. Evans[1] *and Paul D. Robbins*[2]

[1]Center for Molecular Orthopaedics, Harvard Medical School, 221 Longwood Avenue, Room BL 152, Boston, MA 02115, USA; [2]Department of Molecular Genetics and Biochemistry, University of Pittsburgh School of Medicine, W1246 Biomedical Science Tower, Pittsburgh, PA 15261, USA

Introduction

Although inflammatory diseases vary widely in the organs they affect and the symptoms they produce, as well as in their chronicity, morbidity and mortality, they share common pathophysiological pathways [1]. These pathways are illustrated in Figure 1.

The earliest changes occur in the vasculature where, in response to injury, infection or other initiating stimuli, the capillaries become leaky and the expression of adhesion molecules on their endothelial lining is increased. The latter leads to the capture of leukocytes which leave the circulation and enter the affected tissues by a process of diapadesis. The early infiltrate contains predominantly polymorphonuclear leukocytes which are replaced by mononuclear cells as inflammation progresses.

Within the inflamed tissue, both the infiltrating leukocytes and cells that are normally resident there secrete mediators, particularly cytokines and prostanoids, which perpetuate and magnify the inflammatory process in complex autocrine and paracrine fashions. These also provoke the production of proteinases, free radicals and other agents which destroy the integrity of the affected tissues.

This chain of events can be interrupted in a variety of ways. Traditional anti-inflammatory drugs include steroids, which suppress inflammation at multiple sites in the sequence shown in Figure 1, and cyclooxygenase inhibitors, which reduce the formation of prostanoids. Newer approaches target the adhesion molecules responsible for leukocyte recruitment and the cytokines that drive the disease locally. If the inflammation has an immune basis, there are various strategies for suppressing the immune response, particularly those which interfere with stimulation and co-stimulation of T lymphocytes by antigen-presenting cells (discussed in [2]).

Based upon the scheme shown in Figure 1, a number of gene products come to mind as potential anti-inflammatory agents (Tab. 1), including antibodies, soluble

Gene Therapy in Inflammatory Diseases, edited by C. H. Evans and P. D. Robbins

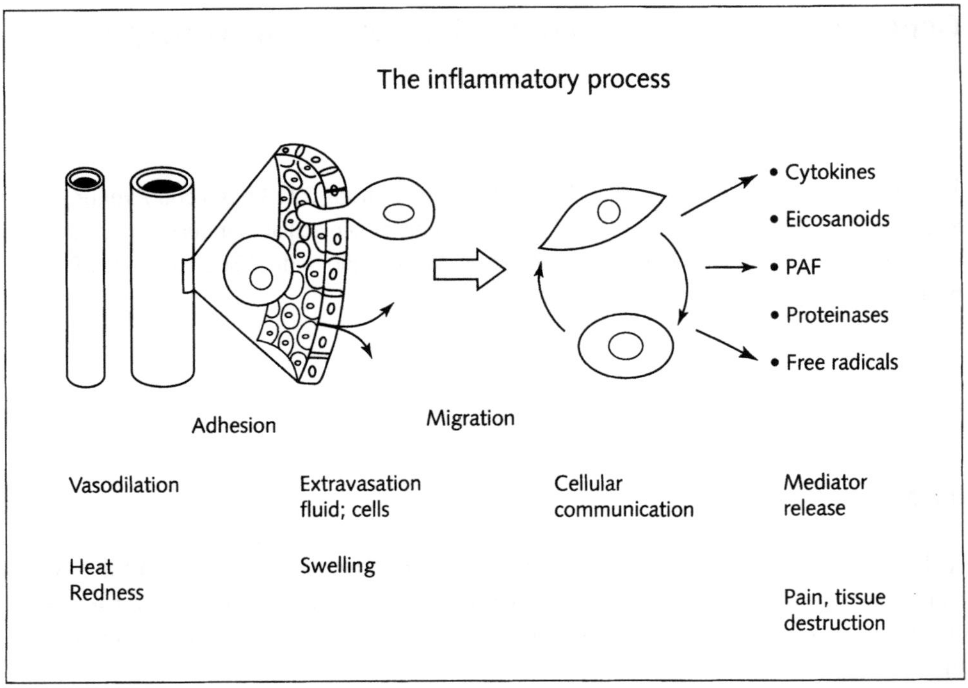

Figure 1
The inflammatory process. Taken from [1] with permission.

receptors or counterligands, type 2 cytokines or naturally occurring inhibitors such as the interleukin-1 receptor antagonist. These molecules have obvious potential application to the biological therapy of inflammatory diseases [3], but they are all proteins and proteins are poor drugs, especially in chronic conditions. The major problem is that of delivery.

Proteins are rarely effective when taken orally, as they are acidified and digested in the GI. They can be administered by various routes of injection, but this is unpleasant and impractical in chronic conditions. Moreover, because it is rarely possible to introduce the proteins in question directly and selectively into the site of disease, there is exposure of non-target organs and the prospect of deleterious side-effects. A particular concern with anti-inflammatory agents in this regard is the potential for increasing the incidence of infection and malignancy.

Gene therapy was proposed as a biological delivery system with which to circumvent these problems [2]. The original concept was to transfer genes encoding the therapeutic proteins of interest into sites of disease [4]. The affected tissues would then express the genes locally, thus producing the therapeutic gene products endoge-

Table 1 - Possible anti-inflammatory biological agents

Type of molecule	Examples
Anti-adhesion	Antibodies to, for example, ICAM-1 etc.; soluble forms of, for example, VLA4, CD44, etc.
Cytokine antagonist	Soluble receptors; IL-1 receptor antagonist
Anti-inflammatory cytokine	IL-4, IL-10, IL-13 and other Th-2 cytokines
Immunosuppressive	Soluble forms of T cell co-stimulatory molecules, e.g. sCTLA4; anti-TCR vaccines; antibodies to lymphocyte surface antigens; Th-1, Th-2 cytokines
Regulator of T cell differentiation	Type 1 cytokines (e.g. IL-12) in Th-2 driven disease Type 2 cytokines (e.g. IL-10) in Th-1 driven disease
Antioxidant	Superoxide dismutase, catalase, etc.
Anti-erosive	TIMPs, PAIs and other proteinase inhibitors
Regulators of gene expression	Antisense RNA, ribozymes, decoy nucleic acids, transcription factors, etc.

TIMP, tissue inhibitor of metalloproteinases; PAI, plasminogen activator inhibitor; ICAM, intercellular adhesion molecule; VLA, very late antigen

nously. In this way, systemic side-effects could be avoided and frequently repeated application would not be necessary. Moreover, there is the potential for regulating the level of gene expression to reflect disease activity.

Building upon these concepts, it is possible to envisage the delivery of not only proteins but also therapeutic species of RNA, such as ribozymes and anti-sense RNA [2]. Furthermore, the range of molecular targets has been expanded to include, for example, transcription factors (see Makarov, this volume) and certain death ligands (see Zhang et al., this volume) which induce apoptosis of inflammatory cells. DNA may also be used for the purpose of vaccinating against selected cell populations (see Godillot et al., this volume), and decoy oligonucleotides can act as regulators of gene expression (see Makarov, this volume).

Gene transfer vectors

Central to the success of any gene therapy protocol is an efficient means of transferring genes to the target cells in a way that gives appropriate levels of gene expression. Gene delivery vectors are employed to facilitate this process [5].

The simplest vector comprises a plasmid which contains the gene of interest under the control of a suitable promoter. Plasmids are inefficient gene delivery vehicles, but they hold much promise for DNA vaccination (see Godillot et al., this volume). For reasons that are not completely understood the introduction of plasmids into muscle and skin provokes strong, cell mediated immunity to the protein expressed from the plasmid. This property may be of use in vaccinating against autoreactive lymphocytes in autoimmune inflammatory diseases. There are also conditions where the low levels of gene expression that follow delivery of plasmid DNA are sufficient for an anti-inflammatory effect. As noted by Miyata et al., this volume, such effects have been reported for animal models of colitis, lupus, keratitis and arthritis.

The uptake and expression of plasmid DNA can be enhanced by associating it with a carrier. Liposomes, various proteins and certain polymers may be used for this purpose. Although these are usually more effective than naked DNA, the highest levels of gene transfer are achieved using viral vectors. These vectors exploit the natural ability of viruses to deliver their genomes to the cells they infect with great efficiency. For use as vectors, the wild-type viruses are genetically manipulated with the aim of eliminating their ability to replicate and cause disease, while retaining their infectivity. So far, four different classes of virus have been modified in this fashion with a success that permits their use in human clinical trials: retrovirus, adenovirus, adeno-associated virus and herpes simplex virus (Tab. 2).

Retroviruses have been used in the majority of human gene therapy trials, largely because of the ease with which they can be manipulated and manufactured, and because the cells they transduce express no viral proteins. Most of these vectors are derived from the Moloney murine leukemia virus and have as a major drawback their inability to transduce non-dividing cells. This has limited their use to *ex vivo* gene therapy where cells are removed from the body, infected with the retrovirus *in vitro*, and then re-implanted. The possibility of administering retroviruses *in vivo* by direct delivery has resulted from the development of recombinant retroviruses with titers as high as 10^{10} particles/ml. When the target cells are triggered to divide in situ, the *in vivo* delivery of high titer retroviruses can lead to efficient transduction [6]. Newer retroviral vectors derived from lentiviruses, which infect non-dividing cells, offer an alternative approach to the use of retroviruses for *in vivo* gene delivery [7].

Because retroviruses integrate their genomes into the chromosomal DNA of the cells they infect, they offer particular advantages in settings requiring long-term persistence of transgenes. Integration is, however, random and there is thus a finite, albeit small, possibility of insertional mutagenesis. There is thus much interest in utilizing adenoassociated virus (AAV) which, in its wild-type state, integrates into the host cell at a specific site at the tip of chromosome 19. Recent advances in the production of high titer, recombinant AAV have led to increasing experi-

Table 2 - Properties of present vectors

Vector	Advantages	Disadvantages
Integrating viral		
Retrovirus		
MoMLV-based	Straightforward production No viral proteins made Extensive use in human trials	Require target cell division Possible insertional mutagenesis
Lentivirus-based	Transduce non-dividing cells	More development required
AAV	Site-specific integration[1] Non-pathogenic Transduce non-dividing cells No viral proteins made	Difficult to produce Small packaging capacity (4 kb)
Viral non-integrating		
Adenovirus	Straightforward production High titers Transduce non-dividing cells	Inflammatory Immunogenicity of transduced cells
HSV	Large packaging capacity High titers Transduce non-dividing cells	Difficult to produce Cytotoxic
Non-viral		
Naked DNA	Simple Non-immunogenic Inexpensive Safe	Few cells transfect well
Liposomes	As above	Gene expression usually transient and low
Particle bombardment (gene gun)	Used in conjunction with plasmid DNA	Cumbersome; requires specialized equipment
DNA-ligand complexes	May be targetable Receptor-mediated uptake often efficient	Possible antigenicity Low expression

[1] *Wild-type AAV integrates in a site-specific fashion. Recombinant virus appears as if it does not. Note that all types of vectors are the subject of considerable research. This table summarizes the present state of development.*

MoMLV, moloney murine leukemia virus; AAV, Adeno-associated virus; HSV, Herpes simplex virus.

Reproduced from [2] with permission.

mental use of this vector. In several instances impressive persistence of transgene expression has been reported [8]. It is unclear, however, whether recombinant AAV retains the ability to integrate into mammalian genomic DNA and, if so, whether this occurs in a site-specific manner. Disadvantages of AAV include its small packaging capacity of 4 kb, and its high antigenicity which serves as a barrier to repeated dosing.

Probably the most powerful vectors are derived from adenovirus which can be grown to very high titers, is highly infectious towards a wide range of dividing and non-dividing cells and accommodates up to 14 kb of packaging. Extremely high levels of gene expression can be attained using viral promoters such as the cytomegalovirus early promoter. Expression, however, tends to be temporary. This is partly explained by the non-integrating nature of adenoviral DNA. Additional reasons for transient expression are not fully understood but appear to have an immunological basis. The earliest adenoviral vectors had deletions engineered into the E1 and E3 regions of the viral genome. Cells transduced with these viruses continue to express viral proteins. Because these proteins are antigenic they trigger powerful immune responses, a problem exacerbated by the fact that the E3 region encodes an immunosuppressive protein. In response to this, second generation viruses deleted in the E1 and E4 regions have been made, but it is not clear whether the duration of transgene expression is increased by this means. Recombinant adenoviruses, known as "gutted" viruses, lacking all coding sequences have been generated and their performance remains under evaluation [9]. In addition to triggering immune responses [10], infection with the first generation adenoviral vector, alters the metabolism of the host cell by, for instance, activating MAP kinases [11] and NFκB [12].

Herpes simplex virus (HSV) forms the basis of an alternative non-integrating high titer, highly infectious vector [13]. HSV has a large genome which may accept 30 kb or more of packaging. Early generations of HSV vectors were cytotoxic but considerable engineering of the viral genome is beginning to produce vectors with improved properties. Because HSV establishes a natural latency in neurons, vectors derived from HSV have the potential to achieve prolonged transgene expression after infection of nervous tissue [14].

Because gene delivery remains the single most important obstacle to human gene therapy, considerable effort is being devoted to the improvement of these and other vectors. As well as addressing issues of the level and duration of transgene expression, vectors are being engineered to improve targeting, safety, stability and ease of production.

Gene therapy strategies

Genes may be introduced into the patient by direct, *in vivo* delivery or indirect *ex vivo* delivery (Fig. 2). The choice of strategy is determined *inter alia*, by the anato-

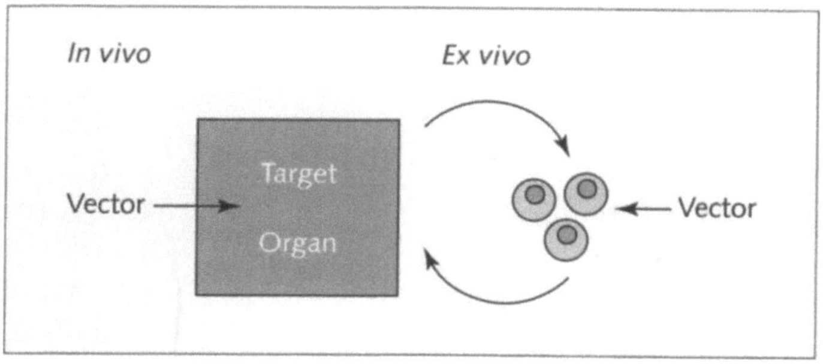

Figure 2
Models of gene delivery
In vivo *gene delivery involves the direct injection of genes into the body with the expectation that they will reach the target site and become incorporated into the target cell.* Ex vivo *gene delivery is a process whereby cells are removed from the body, are genetically altered* in vitro, *and are reimplanted in such a way as to reach the target organ. Taken from [20] with permission.*

my and physiology of the target organ and the vector that is used. For example, as discussed in the previous section, because Moloney-based retroviruses require division of the host cell for successful transduction, they are nearly always used in *ex vivo* protocols. Adenoviral vectors, in contrast, are most frequently used for *in vivo* gene delivery because they transduce non-dividing cells very effectively. Nevertheless, if it is difficult to gain access to the cells of choice *in situ* it may still be necessary to adopt *ex vivo* strategies regardless of the vector used. Examples of such cells include chondrocytes, stem cells and blood cells.

It is possible to draw a distinction between local and systemic gene delivery (Fig. 3). Local delivery implies that the genes are delivered to anatomically restricted sites where the gene product will accumulate, with minimal exposure of other organs. This has the advantage of minimizing side-effects while maximizing the local therapeutic effect. Local gene therapy is, however, poorly equipped to deal with disseminated disease. For this it may be necessary to utilize so-called systemic delivery where the secreted gene products gain access to the systemic circulation. This may be achieved by transferring genes to sites such as the liver, muscle and skin as well as by utilizing artificial organoids implanted into the host. Intravenous or intraperitoneal injection of adenovirus is one way to obtain high circulating levels of secreted transgene products.

It has recently become apparent that local gene delivery in models of inflammatory joint disease can bring impressive therapeutic effects at locations removed from the site of application (see Makarov, this volume). This appears to reflect the ability of inflammatory cells to traffick [15] and thereby blur the local/systemic distinc-

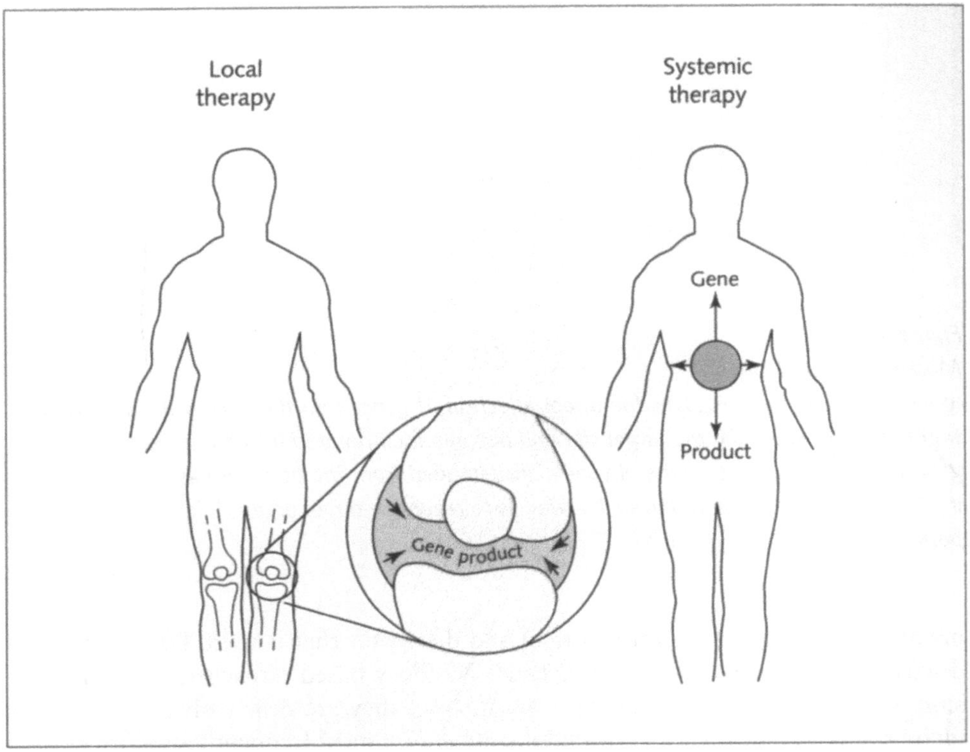

Figure 3
Local and systemic gene delivery
In local gene delivery, genes are delivered to individual sites of disease, such as the knee joint shown in this example. In systemic gene delivery, genes are delivered to sites where a secreted gene product has access to the systemic circulation. Taken from [20] with permission.

tion. Cells with the ability to home selectively to sites of inflammatory disease offer many advantages as vehicles for therapeutic gene delivery.

Regulation of gene expression

Although the expression of genes is regulated at several levels, in the context of gene therapy, attention has focused mainly on transcriptional regulation. Most investigators continue to use viral promoters that are either, as with the retroviral long terminal repeat, part of the original virus from which the vector was derived or, as with the SV40 and CMV early promoters, appropriated from other sources. Viral promoters drive high levels of gene expression in a largely unregulated fashion, but they show little tissue specificity and are considered vulnerable to promoter extinction in certain types of cells.

Use of eukaryotic promoters permits tissue-specific gene expression under conditions where targeting of the vector is imprecise. Moreover, inducible or constitutive endogenous promoters may be selected, as appropriate. Levels of gene expression obtained with eukaryotic promoters, however, are typically far lower than those obtained with viral promoters.

Because many chronic inflammatory diseases follow an uncertain course punctuated with flares and remissions, there is considerable interest in the use of inducible promoters. These may be selected or designed to regulate gene expression in response to endogenous stimuli such as inflammation, or to do so in response to an exogenous stimulus, such as a drug.

Nature provides a wide selection of inducible promoters of possible utility in the present context. Examples include the promoters responsible for the increase in production of inflammatory cytokines such as IL-1, IL-6, TNF etc. Inflammatory stimuli should rapidly enhance the expression of genes driven by such promoters. To increase the level of expression obtained by this means, Varley et al. [16] coupled an inducible mammalian promoter to the TAT transactivator gene of HIV. When this construct was used to regulate expression of a gene downstream from the TAT response element, there was an impressive combination of inducibility by inflammatory stimuli and high expression (see Makarov, this volume).

Although the use of an autoregulatory construct of this type is elegant, there are concerns. In the case of inflammation resulting from an infection, for example, it will be necessary to switch off the anti-inflammatory gene to enable host defense mechanisms to function. For this reason it may be better to regulate gene expression via inducible elements that respond to orally active drugs which can be taken by the patient as necessary. Examples already exist where genes can be switched on in response to tetracycline [17], non-abortive concentrations of RU486 [18] and rapamycin [19]. Systems which use human proteins as the regulatory elements stand a better chance of avoiding immune reactivity.

Conclusions

Gene therapy provides biological solutions to the problem of delivering anti-inflammatory gene products to sites of inflammatory disease. A variety of genes hold promise as therapeutic agents in this regard. Viral and non-viral vectors are available for the transfer of anti-inflammatory genes either locally or systemically by *ex vivo* or *in vivo* means. It remains difficult to achieve long-term gene expression but this should yield to further research. A variety of approaches are being taken to regulate the level of expression of the therapeutic genes to maximize their effectiveness.

References

1 Evans CH (1995) Nitric oxide – what role does it play in inflammation and tissue destruction? In: NS Doherty, BM Weichman, DW Morgan, L Marshall (eds): *Inflammation: mechanisms and therapeutics*. Birkhäuser Verlag, Basel, 107–116

2 Evans CH, Ghivizzani SC, Kang R, Muzzonigro T, Wasko MC, Herndon JH, Robbins PD (1999) Gene therapy for rheumatic diseases. *Arthritis Rheum* 42: 1–16

3 Moreland LW, Heck LW, Koopman WJ (1997) Biologic agents for treating rheumatoid arthritis: concepts and progress. *Arthritis Rheum* 40: 397–409

4 Bandara G, Robbins PD, Georgescu HI, Mueller GM, Glorioso JC, Evans CH (1992) Gene transfer to synoviocytes: prospects for gene treatment for arthritis. *DNA Cell Biol* 11: 227–231

5 Robbins PD, Ghivizzani SC (1998) Viral vectors for gene therapy. *Pharmacol Ther* 80: 35–47

6 Ghivizzani SC, Lechman ER, Tio C, Mulé KM, Chada S, McCormack JE, Evans CH, Robbins PD (1997) Direct retroviral mediated gene transfer to the synovium of the rabbit knee: implications for arthritis gene therapy. *Gene Therapy* 4: 977–982

7 Naldini L, Blomer U, Gallay P, Ory D, Mulligan R, Gage FH, Verma IM, Trono D (1996) *In vivo* delivery and stable transduction of non-dividing cells by lentiviral vector. *Science* 272: 263–267

8 Monahan PE, Samulski RJ, Tazelaar J, Xiao X, Nichols TC, Belliner DAA, Read MS, Walsh CE (1998) Direct intramuscular injection with recombinant AAV vectors results in sustained expression in a dog model of hemophilia. *Gene Ther* 5: 40–49

9 Chen HH, Mack LM, Kelly R, Ontell M, Kochanek S, Clemens PR (1997) Persistence in muscle of an adenoviral vector that lacks all viral genes. *Proc Natl Acad Sci USA* 94: 1645–1650

10 Yang Y, Nunes FA, Berenesi K, Furth EE, Gonczol E, Wilson JML (1994) Cellular immunity to viral antigens limits E1-deleted adenoviruses of gene therapy. *Proc Natl Acad Sci USA* 914401–4411

11 Bruder JT, Kovesdi I (1997) Adenovirus infection stimulates the Raf/MAPK signaling pathway and induces interleukin-8 expression. *J Virol* 71: 398–404

12 Clesham GJ, Adam PJ, Proudfoot D, Flynn PD, Efstathiou S, Weissberg PL (1998) High adenoviral loads stimulate NFκB-dependent gene expression in human vascular smooth muscle cells. *Gene Ther* 5: 174–180

13 Glorioso JC, Krisky D, Marconi P, Oligino T, Ghivizzani SC, Robbins PD, Schmidt MC,

Goins WF, Evans CH (1997) Progress in development of herpes simplex virus gene vectors for treatment of rheumatoid arthritis. *Adv Drug Del Rev* 27: 41–57
14 Fink DJ, Glorioso JC (1997) Engineering herpes simplex virus vectors for gene transfer to neurons. *Nature Med* 3: 357–359
15 Ghivizzani SC, Lechman ER, Kang R, Tio C, Kolls J, Evans CH, Robbins PD (1998) Direct adenoviral-mediated gene transfer of IL-1 and TNF-α soluble receptors to rabbit knees with experimental arthritis has local and distal antiarthritic effects. *Proc Natl Acad Sci USA* 95: 4613–4618
16 Varley AW, Geiszler SM, Gaynor RB, Munford RS (1997) A two-component expression that responds to inflammatory stimuli *in vivo*. *Nature Biotech* 15: 1002–1006
17 Gossen M, Freundlieb S, Bender G, Müller G, Hillen W, Bujard H (1995) Transcriptional activation of tetracyclines in mammalian cells. *Science* 268: 1766–1769
18 Wang Y, O'Malley BW Jr, Tsai SY, O'Malley BW (1994) A regulatory system for use in gene transfer. *Proc Natl Acad Sci USA* 91: 8180–8184
19 Magari SR, Rivera VM, Iuliucci JD, Gilman M, Cerasoli F (1997) Pharmacological control of a humanized gene therapy system implanted in to nude mice. *J Clin Invest* 100: 2865–2872
20 Evans CH, Robbins PD (1995) Possible orthopaedic applications of gene therapy. *J Bone Joint Surg* 77A: 1103–1114

Gene therapy for rheumatoid arthritis: preclinical studies

Sergei S. Makarov

Thurston Arthritis Research Center, University of North Carolina at Chapel Hill, 4109 Thurston, CB 7280, Chapel Hill, NC 27599-7280, USA

"Animals are such agreeable friends:
they ask no questions, they make no criticism."
Anonymous

Introduction

Originally intended as a tool for the correction of inborn errors of metabolism, gene transfer technology has revolutionized the development of novel treatments to acquired diseases, such as cancer, autoimmune, and chronic inflammatory conditions. The concept of gene therapy for rheumatoid arthritis (RA) was proposed as an alternative to inefficient conventional drug delivery to the affected joints [1]. In this approach, introduction of exogeneous genes into the synovium should afford expression of therapeutic proteins directly at the site of the disease, thereby obviating the problems of inefficient systemic protein delivery and sparing the host from the side-effects associated with the systemic exposure to recombinant proteins [2]. However, despite its conceptual simplicity, many principal problems of gene therapy for RA remain to be solved before it becomes a routine clinical procedure. Here, I will summarize what we have learned from the preclinical studies using animal models, and discuss some unresolved issues of gene therapy for RA.

Gene delivery to the synovium

Intraarticular (i.a.) injection of naked DNA results in a low frequency transduction and very transient transgene expression [3, 4], which necessitates the use of gene delivery vehicles. There are two possible approaches for local gene transfer to the synovium: *in vivo* and *ex vivo*. In a direct *in vivo* approach the transgene is expressed in the joint by using i.a. injection of a gene delivery construct. In the *ex*

Gene Therapy in Inflammatory Diseases, edited by C. H. Evans and P. D. Robbins

vivo approach, explanted synovial cells are transduced *in vitro* and re-implanted into the joint. Although different viral and non-viral constructs have been tested for *in vivo* and *ex vivo* gene delivery to the synovium [4, 5], so far, preclinical studies using therapeutic gene transfer in RA animal models have almost exclusively employed recombinant retroviral and adenoviral vectors.

Retrovirus-mediated gene delivery

Murine leukemia (MoMuLV)-based recombinant retroviral vectors (RV) are the best studied constructs for gene delivery, and most approved gene therapy trials in humans rely on such retroviral vectors. Lack of immunogenecity, and the stable incorporation of the transgene into the host chromosomal DNA, make RV ideal for many gene therapy applications. The feasibility of using RV for *in vivo* and *ex vivo* gene transfer to the synovium has been extensively explored in animal studies.

In vivo retroviral gene transfer to the synovium

Direct *in vivo* gene delivery to synovium has a distinct advantage with respect to clinical use. However, the applicability of RV is limited as transduction requires cell division, and early attempts to transduce normal rabbit synovium using i.a. injection of a low-titer RV (10^5–10^6 c.f.u./injection) failed [1]. The inflamed synovium contains significantly higher proportion of proliferating cells, and, as determined by our experiments in streptococcal cell wall (SCW)-induced arthritis in rats, arthritic joint was susceptible to RV transduction [6]. Inoculation of the inflamed rat joints with RV-producing packaging cells resulted in the transduction of approximately 1% of fibroblast-like synoviocytes. However, i.a. injection of RV itself (6×10^5 c.f.u./injection) failed to transduce the inflamed synovium [6]. More recent reports indicate the feasibility of using high-titer RVs for *in vivo* transduction of the synovium. In a study by Ghivizzani et al., i.a. injection of a reporter LacZ RV ($> 10^8$ c.f.u./injection) afforded transduction in both naïve and inflamed rabbit joints, although a significantly higher number of $LacZ^+$ cells were found in the inflamed synovium [7]. Remarkably, the transgene expression following *in vivo* gene transfer was at least equivalent to that of the *ex vivo* method in inflamed knees, and was detectable for at least 4 weeks following the transduction. In a similar study by Nguyen and co-workers, it was found that in adjuvant arthritis (AA) in rats, i.a. injection of a high titer (5×10^7 c.f.u./injection) reporter RV resulted in transient transgene expression which peaked between day 3 to 7 and then gradually declined [8]. The efficacy of the transduction was maximal while accelerating to chronic AA (days 15 and 25). An exponential dose response in the reporter β-gal activity was observed using RV titers in the range of 10^6–5×10^7 c.f.u./injection, suggesting that appropriate timing and high titers of RV were key determinants of *in vivo* RV gene transfer. These studies suggest the potential of a high-titer RV for *in vivo* gene transfer in human patients with active RA.

Ex vivo retroviral gene transfer to the synovium

Though more laborious compared to the *in vivo* approach, *ex vivo* RV gene delivery is more permissive. Even modest titers of RV allow for a high efficacy (20 to 50%) transduction of primary synoviocytes *in vitro*. Upon engraftment into normal rabbit joint, autologous lapine synoviocytes continued to express the transgene for a period of over 5 weeks, though the level of expression fell exponentially over time [9]. Similarly, we found that engraftment of syngeneic rat synoviocytes into the SCW rat arthritic joints allowed expression of the transgene for a period of approximately 2 weeks, with a gradual decline in the transgene expression [10].

Adenovirus-mediated gene transfer to synovium

Recombinant human adenoviruses (Ad) have been used extensively in animal models of gene therapy. These vectors are derived from human Ad serotypes 2 and 5, whose double-stranded DNA genomes span 36 kb and contain both early and late genes. The first generation of recombinant Ad vectors have been rendered replication defective by deleting the immediate early genes E1a and E1b [11]. In most models of adenoviral *in vivo* gene transfer, recombinant gene expression has been transient and associated with inflammation characterized by lymphocytic infiltrate [12]. Cells transduced with E1-deleted Ad express not only the transgene, but also viral proteins which cause activation of both cellular and humoral immune responses to Ad vectors. In tissues with a slow turnover, a T cell-driven response is believed to be the major factor limiting persistence of Ad transgene, whereas development of neutralizing antibodies to the Ad proteins and the transgene precludes repeated Ad transduction. I.v. administration of Ad vector permits transgene expression for a period of 1 to 2 weeks [11]. The liver is the primary target for i.v. injected Ad; in case of a soluble transgene, systemic Ad transduction affords appreciable plasma concentrations of the product (usually, in the range of several ng/ml) [11, 12]. As demonstrated by Roessler et al., local, i.a. injection of Ad vectors results in efficient transduction of the normal rabbit synovium, affording expression of the transgene in both type A (macrophages) and type B (fibroblasts) synoviocytes [13]. In this study, i.a. Ad administration did not provoke an inflammatory reaction, although circulating antibodies to Ad proteins gradually developed. Expression of the transgene declined after the first week, but transduced cells were detected in the synovium for as long as 8 weeks after transduction. A study by Nita and co-workers confirmed the high efficacy of Ad gene transfer to rabbit synovium, but titer-dependent synovitis was noted [4]. Similarly, i.a. Ad reporter gene transfer in normal mice resulted in a high frequency transduction of the synovium, but this was accompanied with lymphocytic infiltration, synovial inflammation, and a rapid decline in the transgene expression after the first week [14]. Consistent with these observations, our own studies with SCW arthritis in rats have demonstrated high efficacy of adenoviral transduction of the synovium *in vivo*, but i.a. injection of Ad into naïve animals resulted in a titer-dependent inflammation, and administration of the Ad vector into the SCW arthritic joint provoked the recurrence of the disease (A. Miagkov and S.Makarov, unpublished observations).

Ad vectors are uniquely capable of achieving high *in vivo* synovial transfer efficiency; however, immunogenecity of the current generation of Ad vectors is associated with aggravated inflammation in the synovium, limited transgene persistence, and impossibility of repeated administration. Rapid progress in the development of non- immunogenic Ad vectors has promise for RA human gene therapy.

Candidate therapeutic transgenes

Rheumatoid arthritis (RA) is a chronic systemic inflammatory disease of the connective tissue preferentially involving joints. The normal synovium is a delicate tissue lining the joint capsule. However, in RA, the synovium transforms into an aggressive, tumor-like structure called the pannus which invades and erodes both the articular cartilage and the subchondral bone [15]. Inflammation and hyperplasia of the synovium, and degradation of articular cartilage and bone are the hallmarks of RA [16]. The etiology of RA is still unknown, and thus it is not clear which therapeutic gene or combination of genes should be delivered in order to provide adequate suppression of the disease. Ideally, the transgene would restore the impaired homeostasis of the RA joint, but in lieu of a clear understanding of the basic mechanisms underlying the disease, therapeutic approaches to RA are by necessity designed as treatment rather than cure.

Although the etiological agent in RA remains elusive, the current paradigm is that initiation of the disease is associated with arthritogenic T cells which activate the resident synoviocytes to release numerous inflammatory molecules, chemoattractants, and growth factors into the synovium [17]. Established inflammation is believed to further enhance and perpetuate itself through recruiting of inflammatory cells and establishing multiple autocrine and paracrine loops of cytokines and growth factors [18]. There is also growing evidence that autonomous, T cell-independent mechanisms can contribute to RA pathology [16, 19, 20]. One striking feature of the RA synovium is the phenotype of synovial fibroblasts, usually associated with transformed tumor cells [15, 16, 21]. The RA synovial fibroblasts have high levels of expression of proto-oncogenes such as *ras*, *myc*, *c-fos*, and, in contrast to their normal counterparts, RA synoviocytes are capable of anchorage-independent growth *in vitro* [22, 23]. When co-engrafted with cartilage into immunodeficient SCID mice, RA fibroblasts invade and degrade the cartilage [19, 24, 25]. Recent observations demonstrated that RA synovial cells have frequent mutations in the p53 tumor-suppresser gene, similar to those observed in a variety of tumors [26]. This indicates that autonomous, T cell-independent mechanisms may contribute to the invasiveness and hyperplasia of the RA synovium. Therefore, the potential targets for gene therapy include both T cell-dependent and independent autonomous mechanisms as well as numerous inflammatory pathways.

Immunomodulatory gene therapy

Since T cell activation is an initial event in development of RA pathology, it represents a logical and attractive target for therapeutic intervention. The balance of Th1 and Th2 subsets of $CD4^+$ T helper cells is thought to play a crucial role in autoimmunity. Th1 cells, which secrete IL-2 and IFNγ, are considered pro-inflammatory and predominantly support macrophage activation. Th2 cells, which secrete IL-4, IL-5, IL-10, and IL-13, primarily provide help to B cells and are considered anti-inflammatory. Reciprocal regulation occurs between the Th cell subsets. Th1 cytokines favor the differentiation of naïve Th cells into Th1 subset and inhibit the development of Th2 subset, and *vice versa*. In RA, the Th1/Th2 balance is skewed toward the pro-inflammatory Th1 cell subset [27]. Experiments in animal models of RA demonstrated that systemic administration of recombinant Th2 cytokines, IL-4 and IL-10, shifted the Th1/Th2 balance toward the latter and alleviated the disease, whereas treatment with anti-IL-10 and anti-IL-4 Ab aggravated the severity of arthritis [28-30].

Gene transfer of IL-10 in animal arthritis

Intravenous administration of an Ad encoding viral IL-10 (AdvIL-10) in mice afforded detectable levels of vIL-10 in the circulation (with concentrations in the range of nanograms per ml) for approximately 1 week [31]. Intravenous administration of AdvIL-10 into mice with established CIA reduced the incidence of arthritis and joint swelling, bone and cartilage resorption, pannus formation, and synovitis. Thus, systemic gene transfer of vIL-10 exerted both anti-inflammatory and chondroprotective effects. The Th1/Th2 balance in AdvIL-10-treated animals was shifted toward the latter, as accounted by the increase of the ratio of IgG1:IgG2a anti-collagen antibodies. However, as demonstrated by studies in IL-10 transgenic animals, systemic expression of IL-10 can be detrimental to the normal functioning of the immune system, particularly with respect to anti-tumor immunity [32]. Data of Whalen and co-workers demonstrated that local, i.a. gene transfer of vIL-10 also significantly reduced the incidence of CIA in mice. Intriguingly, although vIL-10 could be detected only in AdvIL-10- injected joints, but not in the plasma, or uninjected, distal joints, the incidence of CIA was also significantly reduced in distal, untreated joints [33]. As described in the following sections, our own studies in SCW arthritis in rat demonstrated that "inflammation-regulated" i.a. expression of IL-10 gene effectively inhibited the recurrence of arthritis. Importantly, in addition to its immunomodulatory effects, IL-10 elicits numerous anti-inflammatory properties, such as inhibition of production of cytokines tumour necrosis factor α (TNFα), interleukin-1 (IL-1), IL-6, and IL-8 [34]. Taken together, the experimental data in animal models have established IL-10 as an excellent candidacy for gene therapy for human RA. The beneficial systemic effects of local treatment suggest that local, rather than systemic delivery of the IL-10 gene may represent safe and more appropriate strategy for treating human disease.

Antiinflammatory gene therapy

The cytokines IL-1 and TNFα are considered principal mediators of inflammation in the RA synovium [35]. IL-1 and TNFα share many pro-inflammatory properties and are implicated in many pathological processes in RA, including leukocytosis, synovial hyperplasia, cartilage breakdown, and inhibition of cartilage synthesis. Stimulation of macrophages and synovial fibroblasts with IL-1 and TNFα activates transcription of IL-1 and TNFα, which indicates autocrine/paracrine regulation of these cytokines in the RA synovium [35]. Beneficial effects of systemic administration of neutralizing molecules to IL-1 and TNFα in animal models and in clinical trials in human RA have validated these cytokines as attractive targets for therapeutic intervention.

Gene transfer of neutralizing molecules to IL-1

Initial studies on gene therapy for RA in our laboratory and by others focused on gene delivery of neutralizing molecules to IL-1. One naturally occurring inhibitor of IL-1 is the secreted IL-1 receptor antagonist protein (IRAP, or IL-1ra), which competitively binds the IL-1 receptor without eliciting cell activation, and inhibits numerous pro-inflammatory effects of IL-1 [36]. Therapeutic efficacy of IL-1ra gene transfer has been tested in several animal models of RA. The feasibility of expressing biologically active IL-1ra in the normal rabbit synovium using gene transfer technology was first demonstrated by Bandara et al. [9]. In this work, immortalized lapine synovial fibroblasts were transduced in culture with an IL-1ra RV, and engrafted into rabbit knee joints. The i.a. expressed IL-1ra was functionally active, as evidenced by the protection of IL-1ra producing joints against leukocytosis induced by an i.a. challenge with recombinant IL-1. It is noteworthy that the IL-1ra expressed in the synovium by gene transfer was found to be more efficient in antagonizing biological responses to i.a. administered recombinant IL-1 compared to i.a. injected recombinant IL-1ra. The *ex vivo* RV -mediated gene transfer of IL-1ra in antigen-induced arthritis (AIA) in rabbits produced a marked chondroprotective effect but a milder anti-inflammatory one [37]. Both the increased cartilage matrix catabolism and the inhibition of matrix synthesis that occur in antigen-induced arthritis were abrogated in the presence of the IL-1ra gene; the latter effect was particularly strong. Gene transfer of IL-1ra had no effect on joint swelling, although leukocyte influx into the joint space was significantly inhibited. Concentrations of endogenous rabbit IL-1 in joint lavages were reduced by the IL-1ra gene transfer, suggesting inhibition of an autocrine induction loop of IL-1 by exogenous IL-1ra.

In our study, we examined the therapeutic efficacy of *ex vivo* gene transfer of human IL-1ra in SCW arthritis in rats [10]. We found that the engraftment of syngeneic rat synoviocytes transduced in culture with a IL-1ra RV efficiently prevented the recurrence of SCW arthritis, as assessed by measuring joint swelling and the gross-observation score. However, morphological changes (pannus formation, and erosion of articular cartilage and subchondral bone) were attenuated but not abolished by IL-1ra expression. While the i.a. expression of IL-1ra did not significantly inhibit the severity of arthritis in the untreated contralateral joints, the flare-up of arthritis was resolved more rapidly in the contralateral ankle joints of animals with engrafted IL-1ra$^+$ cells as compared to the contralateral joints in a control (LacZ$^+$) group. Remarkably, IL-1ra expressed as a consequence of gene transfer was much more potent in suppressing arthritis than i.v. administered recombinant IL-1ra protein. Based on the data on the efficacy of systemically administered recombinant IL-1ra in SCW arthritis, we estimated that i.a. expressed IL-1ra was four orders of magnitude more therapeutically efficient than systemically administered recombinant IL-1ra [10].

Studies by Bakker and coworkers in collagen induced arthritis (CIA) in mice demonstrated that expression of human IL-1ra exerted both anti-inflammatory and chondroprotective effects [38]. In this work, histocompatible immortalized NIH3T3 fibroblasts were transduced in culture with an IL-1ra RV and engrafted into the knee cavities prior to the onset of CIA. It was found that development of CIA (arthritis incidence, joint swelling, leukocytosis, impairment of chondrocyte proteoglycan synthesis, and joint erosion) was almost completely prevented in knee joints containing IL-1ra-producing cells. Interestingly, engraftment of IL-1ra$^+$ cells precluded development of arthritis not only in the engrafted knees, but also in the draining ipsilateral paws, indicating distal effects of local suppression of the IL-1 pathway.

In human/SCID mouse model, Müller-Ladner and co-workers demonstrated the chondroprotective effects of IL-1ra gene transfer [39]. In this model, co-implantation of human RA synovial fibroblasts with human cartilage into the renal cavity of SCID mice resulted in T cell-independent destruction of cartilage by invasive fibroblasts and chondrocyte-mediated degradation [25]. Expression of IL-1ra in RA fibroblasts inhibited progressive, chondrocyte-mediated cartilage degradation, although fibroblast invasion into the cartilage was not abolished.

Gene transfer of neutralizing molecules to TNFα

Le and co-workers examined the therapeutic efficacy of gene transfer of neutralizing molecules to TNFα in CIA in rats [40]. The gene for a soluble TNFα receptor (TNFR)-Ig fusion protein was expressed systemically using an i.v. injection of an AdTNFR vector, or locally, through i.a. injection. Intravenous injection of Ad vector afforded transient expression of soluble TNFR in serum (up to 5 ng/ml) which was detectable for 8 days following gene transfer. Intravenous administration of AdTNFR inhibited the severity of arthritis both in preventive (when Ad was given prior to arthritis onset) and therapeutic (after arthritis onset) protocols. However, i.a. injection of control AdLacZ, or AdTNFR vector into CIA joints elicited strong inflammatory reaction, without any beneficial net effects.

Combinatorial gene transfer of IL-1 and TNFα soluble receptors

Direct comparison of the efficacy of the gene transfer of neutralizing molecules to IL-1 and TNFα in AIA in rabbits was done by Ghivizzani and co-workers [41]. In their study, Ad vectors were used for the *in vivo* delivery of genes encoding a soluble IL-1-type I receptor (IL-1R)-IgG fusion protein and/or a soluble type I TNFR-IgG fusion protein into the knees of rabbits with AIA. Ad gene delivery of soluble receptor molecules for IL-1 and TNFα substantially blocked an acute inflammatory and erosive response. The soluble IL-1R gene was found to be considerably more effective at inhibiting synovial fluid leukocytosis and cartilage matrix degradation than the soluble TNFR gene. Remarkably, although neither inhibitor had a significant effect on synovitis, simultaneous gene transfer of soluble TNFR and IL-1R resulted in a strong synergy in inhibiting leukocytosis and cartilage breakdown, and considerably reduced synovitis. Anti-arthritic effects of the gene transfer of the soluble IL-1R alone or the combination of soluble TNFR and IL-1R were also seen in the contralateral control knees receiving only a marker gene. This suggests that sustained local inhibition of disease activity in one joint might exert an anti-arthritic effect on other joints (see the following sections).

Experimentation with gene delivery of neutralizing molecules to IL-1 and TNFα in animal models of RA yielded several important conclusions:

- Although the therapeutic effects varied depending on the model of arthritis, beneficial anti-inflammatory and chondroprotective properties of IL-1ra gene transfer were noted in all examined models.
- IL-1ra delivered by local, i.a. gene transfer, was found to be much more effective in antagonizing exogenous IL-1 and in suppression of SCW arthritis, as compared to recombinant IL-1ra protein. It is possible that the high efficacy of the transgene expression can be attributed to the combination of various factors, such as glycosylation of the expressed protein, different tissue localization of expressed IL-1ra compared to that of injected recombinant protein, and to a short half-life of systemically administrated recombinant IL-1ra. In any event, these results indicate superiority of approaches based on gene delivery compared to systemic or i.a. administration of recombinant proteins.
- The high efficacy of locally expressed IL-1ra suggests a predominant role of local rather than systemic effects of IL-1 in the pathogenesis of RA. Consistent with this hypothesis, mice engineered to express high (micrograms/ml) concentrations of plasma IL-1ra [42] were found to be more resistant to endotoxemia [43], but as prone to developing arthritis as their normal counterparts (C.H. Evans and P.D. Robbins, personal communication). In contrast, while moderate (ng/ml) plasma concentrations of soluble TNFR effectively inhibited CIA arthritis, local expression of soluble TNFR was found either ineffective [40], or exerted only marginal effects [41]. This suggests that circulating TNFα has more impact on arthritis than i.a. produced TNFα.

The remarkable therapeutic efficacy of the combinatorial gene transfer of soluble IL-1R and TNFR indicates that simultaneous suppression of multiple autocrine/paracrine loops of cytokines produces strong synergistic effects. At present, it is not clear which combination of therapeutic genes will afford adequate treatment. An attractive alternative to combinatorial gene transfer may be provided by suppression of transcription factors which control numerous pathological pathways in the synovium.

Transcription factors as targets of gene therapy for RA

Cells in the RA synovium are both the targets and the sources of extracellular inflammatory mediators, and thus cell activation appears to be the point where the action of multiple pathways converge. Transcription of inflammatory genes is controlled by intracellular messengers, inducible transcription factors. There is growing evidence that two transcription factors, NF-κB and AP-1, are of particular importance in RA pathology.

The transcription factor NFκB in RA

The transcription factor NFκB [44–46] is particularly important in the regulation of inflammatory responses. Five members of the mammalian NFκB family exist: NFκB1 (p50), RelA (p65), c-Rel, RelB, and NFκB2 (p52). Although NFκB is considered to be any dimer of these proteins, classic NFκB is the p50-RelA dimer. In unstimulated cells, NFκB is retained in the cytoplasm through an interaction with inhibitory proteins known as IκB. Cell stimulation causes rapid phosphorylation and degradation of IκB, leading to the concomitant appearance of NFκB in the nucleus. Phosphorylation of IκB is controlled by inducible IκB kinases (IKK) [47–49]. In the nucleus, NFκB binds to κB sites in promoters and enhancers of targeted genes and activates transcription. An alternative mechanism of regulation of NFκB transactivation function involves phosphorylation of the NFκB RelA subunit [50]. Inducers of NFκB include IL-1, TNFα, PDGF, LPS, oxidative stress, viruses and viral products. In turn, NFκB can activate transcription of IL-1, TNFα, IL-6, IL-8, the adhesion molecules ICAM-1, VCAM-1, E-selectin, the growth factor GM-CSF, and inducible nitric oxide synthase (iNOS) [44,46]. Data from our laboratory and by others demonstrated that gene transfer of IκBα inhibited expression of IL-1, IL-6, IL-8 messages in endothelial cells [51], and suppressed IL-1- and LPS-stimulated inflammatory responses (IL-1, IL-8 and Groγ messages induction and IL-6 and IL-8 secretion) in fibroblasts and monocytic cells [52].

Several lines of evidence suggest an important role of NFκB in the pathogenesis of RA: (i) NFκB is activated in human RA synovium [53–55]; (ii) HTLV-1 *tax*, a potent activator of NFκB, causes synovial hyperplasia in humans and in transgenic animals [56, 57]; (iii) the therapeutic efficacy of many antiarthritic compounds such as glucocorticoids, gold, and acetylsalicylates correlates with their ability to inhibit NFκB activation [58]; and (iv) the list of known inducers and targets of NFκB almost perfectly matches the profile of the pivotal mediators of inflammation in RA synovium. Recent reports demonstrated that the activation of NFκB by TNFα served as a protective mechanism against the cytotoxicity of this cytokine [59], which suggested the potential involvement of NFκB in regulating apoptosis in the inflamed synovium.

In our studies, we examined the role of NFκB in the expression of inflammatory cytokines, control of apoptosis, and proliferation of synovial cells in animal models of RA [60]. We found that multiple inflammatory stimuli, such as IL-1, TNFα, LPS, PDGF, and serum, induced NFκB activity in rat synovial fibroblasts *in vitro*, and in turn, activation of NFκB was required for inducible expression of IL-1β and TNFα, and cell adhesion receptor VCAM-1. Specific suppression of NFκB by the adenoviral gene transfer of a undegradable "super-repressor" IκBα (srIκBα) greatly potentiated cytotoxicity of TNFα and FasL in synovial fibroblasts *in vitro*, indicating that activation of NFκB served as a protective mechanism against the cytotoxicity of these molecules. Similar to that observed in human RA, we found that the onset of SCW arthritis in rats coincided with persistent activation of NFκB in the synovium. In SCW- and pristane-induced arthritis in rats, suppression of NFκB in the synovium by proteasomal inhibitors and by Ad gene transfer of srIκBα profoundly enhanced apoptosis. This indicated that the persistent activation of NFκB by inflammatory mediators inhibited apoptosis in the arthritic synovium *in vivo* [60]. Our studies also revealed an important role of NFκB in mitogenic responses to growth factors in synovial fibroblasts ([62] and J. Romashkova and S. Makarov, unpublished observations). Activation of NFκB DNA-binding activity was found essential for platelet-derived growth factor (PDGF) and basic fibroblast growth factor (bFGF)-induced DNA synthesis. Since PDGF and bFGF are among the most potent mitogens found in the RA synovium [61], our data indicate the importance of NFκB in proliferation of RA synovial cells. Therefore, NFκB emerges as a pivotal regulator of both inflammation and hyperplasia in the RA synovium.

In animal models of RA, specific inhibitors of NFκB had strong therapeutic effects. In our studies, we found that i.a. administration of liposomal complexes of NFκB decoys (short double-stranded (ds) oligodeoxynucleotides (ODNs) containing NFκB- binding sites) prior to reactivation of SCW arthritis in rats efficiently suppressed the severity of recurrence. Unexpectedly, administration of NFκB decoys in a single joint inhibited the severity of arthritis not only in the ipsilateral, treated joint, but also in the contralateral, untreated joint [60]. Consistent with these observations, Tomita et al., found that hemagglutinating virus of Japan (HVJ) liposome-mediated delivery of NFκB DNA decoys to the joint significantly reduced the severity of CIA arthritis in rats, as assessed by clinical, histological, and radiological examination [63].

The transcription factor AP-1 in RA

AP-1 (activating protein-1) is a collective term referring to dimeric transcription factors composed of Jun, Fos or ATF (activating transcription factor) subunits that bind to a common DNA site, the AP-1-binding site [64]. Different AP-1 factors may regulate different target genes and thus execute distinct biological functions. In addition to regulation by heterodimerization between Jun, Fos and ATF proteins, AP-1 activity is regulated on transcriptional and post-translational levels, by specific mitogen-activated protein (MAP) kinases and a variety of transcriptional coactivators [65, 66]. AP-1 is thought to be critically involved in the abnormal growth regulation and joint destruction observed in the RA joint. This is based on increasing evidence that (i) expression of the *c-fos* gene and AP-1 DNA-binding activity in the RA synovium correlate with disease severity [54, 67]; (ii) IL-1, TNFα, and collagenase genes have AP-1 binding sites in their promoters [64, 66]; (iii) overexpression of the *c-fos* gene in synovial cells potentiated cell growth, indicating the importance of AP-1 in synovial proliferation [68]; (iv) overexpression of the *c-fos* gene in osteoblasts stimulated release of soluble factors enhancing the osteoclastic bone resorption [69], and (v) immunization of H2-*c-fos* transgenic mice with a type II collagen reproduced the major features of RA joint pathology, such as extensive joint destruction by the invasive pannus; most interestingly, this occurred in the absence of lymphocyte infiltration, suggesting an important role of AP-1 in T cell-independent mechanisms of joint destruction [70].

Recent studies by Shiozawa et al., directly demonstrated the therapeutic efficacy of specifically suppressing AP-1 in CIA in mice [71]. Systemic administration of AP-1 ds DNA decoys reduced the arthritis score, inhibited inflammatory cell infiltration and attenuated joint destruction. It is noteworthy that the AP-1 decoys were found to be more effective in preventing joint destruction than inflammatory cell infiltration.

A large body of experimental evidence strongly implicates the transcription factors NFκB and AP-1 in maintaining RA joint pathology. NFκB appears to be important in the regulation of inflammation, synovial proliferation, and apoptosis, whereas AP-1 seems to be important in the control of the synovial stroma proliferation, production of matrix metalloproteinases, and bone resorption. The local suppression of these transcription factors in the RA synovium should afford simultaneous inhibition of numerous pathological mechanisms, and thus NFκB and AP-1 appear to be extremely attractive targets for therapeutic intervention in RA. One challenging issue for gene therapy for RA based on targeting intracellular transcription factors is inefficient delivery of intracellular inhibitors. Therapeutic gene delivery of transcription factors inhibitors (such as srIκBα, and dominant negative mutants of NFκB and AP-1) requires vectors allowing for a high-frequency transduction of the majority of cells in the RA synovium, while using DNA decoys requires an efficient and reproducible liposomal delivery system. One way to circumvent this problem can be provided by delivery of genes encoding the extracellular antagonists of NFκB pathway, such as IL-10 [34]; it is conceivable that at least a part of antiarthritic effects of IL-10 gene transfer described in the previous sections can be attributed to suppression of NFκB in the synovium.

Suppression of hyperplasic growth of the RA synovium

Cell mass is determined by the balance between cell production (cell proliferation and recruitment) and cell death. Experimental evidence exists that both abnormal proliferation and impaired apoptosis contribute to the RA synovial tissue hyperplasia [16, 18, 72]. This suggests that regression of proliferative RA synovium may be achieved by delivery of molecules that inhibit proliferation and/or accelerate apoptosis. Fas/FasL interactions are believed to be particularly important in the regulation of apoptosis in the RA synovium [72]. High levels of Fas are expressed on activated RA synovial cells and infiltrating leukocytes in the inflamed joints; however, the levels of FasL expressed in the arthritic joints are low [73–75]. I.a. administration of a functional monoclonal anti-Fas antibody in transgenic HTLV-1 arthritic mice inhibited paw swelling and histopathological features of arthritis by inducing apoptosis in synovial fibroblasts and macrophages, indicating the feasibility of a strategy based on accelerating apoptosis [76]. However, leakage of recombinant FasL or anti-Fas antibody into circulation may have devastating effects, such as lethal hepatic injury. Gene delivery can provide a high concentration of pro-apoptotic molecules in the synovium, while drastically reducing systemic host exposure. As demonstrated by Zhang and co-workers, i.a. injection of an Ad vector carrying FasL gene induced apoptosis of synovial cells, and ameliorated collagen-induced arthritis in DBA/1 mice [77]. Additionally, in a study in SCID-RA model, Okamoto et al. found that local injection of T cells transduced with FasL gene accelerated apoptosis and eliminated synoviocytes in engrafted human RA synovium [78]. These data indicate that gene transfer of pro-apoptotic molecules may induce regression of the hyperplastic synovium. However, the long-term benefits of the "molecular synovectomy" are not clear. One potential issue is the safety of this approach due to induction of apoptosis in the bystander cells, such as articular chondrocytes, which also express Fas. Another concern is that self-elimination of FasL transduced cells through Fas/FasL-interaction may preclude a long-term transgene expression.

An alternative approach to suppression of hyperplastic growth was proposed by Kohsaka et al. [79]. In this approach, the proliferation of synovial cells is suppressed by gene delivery of intracellular cell cycle inhibitors, such as inhibitors of cyclin-dependent kinases (CDKI). The CDKI arrest cell cycle progression by inhibiting the cyclin-dependent kinases which are responsible for the phosphorylation of the Rb protein and subsequent E2F-dependent DNA replication. The p16 gene, a naturally occurring CDK inhibitor of CyclinD-CDK4/6 complexes, was expressed in knee joints of rats with adjuvant arthritis using adenovirus gene transfer. Expression of p16 in the synovium significantly inhibited inflammation in established adjuvant arthritis [79]. Similar to the delivery of inhibitors of transcription factors, an unresolved problem of this approach is inefficient gene delivery of intracellular inhibitors.

Regulated transgene expression

In the most common scenario of RA, the disease progresses through the episodes of acute recurrence alternating with periods of remission. To make the production of therapeutic proteins correspond to the severity of the disease, transgene expression should be appropriately regulated. Unphysiologic, constitutive production of exogenous proteins could lead to deleterious consequences, including inappropriate downregulation of effector systems, cellular toxicity, and aberrant joint physiology. One possible way to regulate the production of a therapeutic product can be provided by using vectors with molecular gene switches that are regulated by systemic administration of small molecule drugs, such as tetracycline or rapamycine [80, 81]. Vectors with drug-inducible promoters permit tightly regulated dose-dependent transgene expression and afford precise regulation of the transgene production *in vivo*. However, using these kind of constructs require the physician or patient to control production of a therapeutic protein within a defined therapeutic window.

An alternative approach is based on autonomous regulation of the transgene expression by using vectors with inflammation-sensitive promoters. In this approach, production of therapeutic proteins is regulated by inflammation, thereby providing a negative feedback to the severity of the disease. Varley et al. demonstrated that by using cytokine-inducible promoters, it was possible to produce exogenous proteins in a direct relationship to the intensity of inflammation [82]. In this study, promoters of the acute-phase proteins (APP) complement factor 3 (C3) and serum amyloid A3 (SAA3), were introduced into a recombinant Ad vector containing a reporter luciferase gene. Adenovirus-mediated expression of APP-luciferase in mouse liver increased in response to inflammatory stimuli, such as systemic challenge with LPS and turpentine. The construction of the inflammation-inducible promoter was further improved by designing a two-component C3-*tat*/HIV construct in which the C3 promoter controlled the production of the human immunodeficiency virus (HIV) transactivator of transcription (Tat), and the Tat protein then bound the HIV promoter controlling a transgene expression [83]. An Ad reporter vector with this construct (Ad.C3-*tat*/HIV-luc) resulted in a high level, inflammation-inducible expression of the transgene *in vivo*. After systemic challenge with turpentine and LPS, luciferase production in the liver increased by more than 400-fold and reached levels similar to those observed in mice infected with an Ad with a strong constitutive CMV promoter [83].

In our own studies, we have examined the utility of inflammation-regulated C3-*tat*/HIV promoter for therapeutic treatment of recurrent SCW arthritis in rats (A. Miagkov, A. Varley, R. Munford and S. Makarov, unpublished observations). We found that stimulation of primary rat synovial fibroblasts *in vitro* with TNFα and LPS increased expression of Ad.C3-*tat*/HIV-luc by four to five orders of magnitude. To assess the feasibility of therapeutic treatment using the inducible system, we constructed an adenoviral vector Ad.C3-*tat*/HIV-hIL-10 which carried the human IL-10 gene controlled by the C3-*tat*/HIV promoter. I.a. injection of Ad.C3-*tat*/HIV-hIL-10 vector prior to reactivation of SCW arthritis afforded efficacious protection of joints against the recurrence of arthritis, as assessed by inhibited joint swelling and leukocytosis. Most interestingly, expression of adenoviral hIL-10 was virtually undetectable in unreactivated joints, but increased more than 300-fold during the first 2 days after reactivation of SCW arthritis, and fell to very low levels thereafter. These results establish the feasibility of inflammation-regulated gene therapy in chronic inflammatory diseases.

Systemic vs local gene delivery

RA is a multisystemic disease. In most cases, the disease develops symmetrically and involves multiple joints, and extraarticular manifestations are common. Therefore, efficacious therapeutic approaches must suppress the disease at multiple sites. This is one of the most challenging issues of RA gene therapy. There are several possible approaches to this problem.

Therapeutic genes can be delivered systemically by using *ex vivo* or *in vivo* delivery. The primary targets of systemically administrated Ad vectors are extraarticular tissues, such as liver and lung. Beneficial therapeutic effects of systemic *in vivo* Ad gene transfer of soluble TNFR [40] and vIL-10 [31] in animal arthritis have been described in the previous sections. Apparent disadvantages of extraarticular gene expression are rapid protein degradation in the circulation, poor protein delivery to the RA joint, and systemic host exposure to the potentially harmful proteins. Extraarticular expression of a transgene lacks many attractive features of local gene transfer, such as a high therapeutic efficacy of locally expressed proteins. In fact, this approach can be considered as a mere improvement of already existing technologies for sustained delivery of proteins into circulation, e. g. osmotic pumps and continuous s.c. infusion. Another principal limitation of extraarticular transgene expression is that this approach is restricted to using secreted therapeutic genes and rules out delivery of intracellular inhibitors (such as inhibitors of transcription factors or cell-cycle inhibitors). Systemic *in vivo* gene transfer can be potentially improved by designing vectors with selective tropism and/or tissue-specific promoters affording a selective, local transgene expression in the RA joints [84].

Systemic *ex vivo* gene delivery can be achieved by transducing circulating cells *in vitro* and re-injecting them into the circulation. Chernajovsky et al. demonstrated that expression of TGFβ in splenocytes and T cells precluded adoptive transfer of CIA in SCID mice and alleviated established CIA arthritis [85]. A distinct advantage of systemic *ex vivo* gene delivery is that by using circulating cells with a long life span (e.g. mature T cells), it may be possible to achieve a long-term expression of therapeutic genes; additionally, transduced cells can be engineered to home the RA joints. However, existing vectors do not permit efficient transduction of primary lymphoid cells.

As described in the previous sections, we and others have found that the local suppression of joint pathology may have beneficial systemic effects. In our studies, suppression of NFκB in SCW arthritic joints by i.a. injection of NFκB decoys inhibited the recurrence of arthritis not only in treated, but also in the contralateral, untreated joints [62]. I.a. administration of Ad vectors encoding soluble IL-1 and TNFα receptors in AIA in rabbits also inhibited the disease in both treated and untreated, contralateral joints [41]. Similar effects were noted in CIA in mice treated by i.a. injection of Ad vIL-10 [33]. Taken together, these findings suggest that the local inhibition of disease activity in one joint may confer an anti-arthritic effect on other joints, and that local i. a. gene transfer could be used to treat systemic arthritides. Although the mechanisms underlying this effect are largely unknown, these findings have wide ramifications for clinical approaches to human RA.

Concluding comments

Gene therapy for human RA has stirred great expectations. The progress has been impressive: the idea of turning the arthritic joint into the factory producing therapeutic molecules was proposed in 1992 [1], and only 4 years later, the first clinical trials in human RA patients started in two clinical centers (see Muzzonigro et al., this volume). There is little doubt that beneficial therapeutic effects of gene therapy in human disease will be demonstrated in the near future; however, routine clinical applications will demand developing the constructs affording a long-term, convenient, and cost-effective treatment. This will require tedious work in animal models for testing the novel approaches. In all likelihood, clinical protocols designed for routine use in RA patients will have no more resemblance to the first animal experiments than the Boeing 747 airplane resembles the flying machines of the Wright brothers.

Another important aspect of gene transfer technology is that it provides an invaluable tool for understanding the basic mechanisms of the disease. Since the previous *in vivo* data in human RA and animal models have been almost exclusively derived from the experiments with systemic administration of inhibitory molecules, the role of systemic vs local mechanisms in the pathogenesis of the disease is poorly understood. The extent to which activation of synovial T cells occurs prior to or following entry into the synovium is not yet known. Also largely unknown are the mechanisms regulating proliferation and apoptosis in the synovium and the role of cell-cell interaction between the major participants in the arthritic joint: macrophages, fibroblasts, chondrocytes, T and B lymphocytes, and dendritic cells. Gene transfer is uniquely capable of achieving local expression of exogenous molecules in the synovium, and thus affords addressing these questions. As discussed in this chapter, gene transfer experimentation in animal models has already brought unexpected findings, such as demonstration of beneficial systemic effects of intraarticular gene delivery. There is no doubt that new discoveries will follow.

Acknowledgements

My thanks are due to all my colleagues who collaborated on the experimental work described herein, to Alexei Miagkov and Julia Romashkova for their agreement to present unpublished data, to Joanna Watson for her patient editorial assistance, and to Darcy Berger for even greater patience in editing the manuscript and for an everlasting sense of humor. The work was supported by the NIH grants AR/AI 44564 and 5-P60-AR30701-14, and a grant from the Arthritis Foundation.

References

1 Bandara G, Robbins PD, Georgescu HI, Mueller GM, Glorioso JC, Evans CH (1992) Gene transfer to synoviocytes: prospects for gene treatment of arthritis. *DNA Cell Biol* 11: 227–231

2 Evans CH, Robbins PD (1996) Pathways to gene therapy in rheumatoid arthritis. *Curr Opin Rheumatol* 8: 230–234

3 Yovandich J, O'Malley B, Jr., Sikes M, Ledley FD (1995) Gene transfer to synovial cells by intra-articular administration of plasmid DNA. *Hum Gene Ther* 6: 603–610

4 Nita I, Ghivizzani SC, Galea-Lauri J, Bandara G, Georgescu HI, Robbins PD, Evans CH (1996) Direct gene delivery to synovium. An evaluation of potential vectors *in vitro* and *in vivo*. *Arthritis Rheum* 39: 820–828

5 Tomita T, Hashimoto H, Tomita N, Morishita R, Lee SB, Hayashida K, Nakamura N, Yonenobu K, Kaneda Y, Ochi T (1997) *In vivo* direct gene transfer into articular cartilage by intraarticular injection mediated by HVJ (Sendai virus) and liposomes. *Arthritis Rheum* 40: 901–906

6 Makarov SS, Olsen JC, Johnston WN, Schwab JH, Anderle SK, Brown RR, Haskill JS (1995) Retrovirus mediated *in vivo* gene transfer to synovium in bacterial cell wall-induced arthritis in rats. *Gene Ther* 2: 424–428

7 Ghivizzani SC, Lechman ER, Tio C, Mule KM, Chada S, McCormack JE, Evans CH, Robbins PD (1997) Direct retrovirus-mediated gene transfer to the synovium of the rabbit knee: implications for arthritis gene therapy. *Gene Ther* 4: 977–982

8 Nguyen KH, Boyle DL, McCormack JE, Chada S, Jolly DJ, Firestein GS (1998) Direct synovial gene transfer with retroviral vectors in rat adjuvant arthritis. *J Rheumatol* 25: 1118–1125

9 Bandara G, Mueller GM, Galea-Lauri J, Tindal MH, Georgescu HI, Suchanek MK, Hung GL, Glorioso JC, Robbins PD, Evans CH (1993) Intraarticular expression of biologically active interleukin 1-receptor-antagonist protein by *ex vivo* gene transfer. *Proc Natl Acad Sci USA* 90: 10764–10768

10 Makarov SS, Olsen JC, Johnston WN, Anderle SK, Brown RR, Baldwin AS, Jr., Haskill JS, Schwab JH (1996) Suppression of experimental arthritis by gene transfer of interleukin 1 receptor antagonist cDNA. *Proc Natl Acad Sci USA* 93: 402–406

11 Kozarsky KF, Wilson JM (1993) *Gene Therapy*: adenovirus vectors. *Curr Opin Genet Dev* 3: 499–503

12 Wilson JM (1996) Adenoviruses as gene-delivery vehicles. *N Engl J Med* 334: 1185–1187

13 Roessler BJ, Allen ED, Wilson JM, Hartman JW, Davidson BL (1993) Adenoviral-mediated gene transfer to rabbit synovium *in vivo*. *J Clin Invest* 92: 1085–1092

14 Sawchuk SJ, Boivin GP, Duwel LE, Ball W, Bove K, Trapnell B, Hirsch R (1996) Anti-T cell receptor monoclonal antibody prolongs transgene expression following adenovirus-mediated *in vivo* gene transfer to mouse synovium. *Hum Gene Ther* 7: 499–506

15 Zvaifler NJ, Firestein GS (1994) Pannus and pannocytes. Alternative models of joint destruction in rheumatoid arthritis. *Arthritis Rheum* 37: 783–789
16 Firestein GS (1996) Invasive fibroblast-like synoviocytes in rheumatoid arthritis. Passive responders or transformed aggressors? *Arthritis Rheum* 39: 1781–1790
17 Fox DA (1997) The role of T cells in the immunopathogenesis of rheumatoid arthritis: new perspectives. *Arthritis Rheum* 40: 598–609
18 Wilder RL, Remmers EF, Sano H, Case JP, Lafyatis R (1991) The cytokine network in rheumatoid arthritis. Br *J Rheumatol* 30 (2): 44–47
19 Müller-Ladner U (1996) Molecular and cellular interactions in rheumatoid synovium. *Curr Opin Rheumatol* 8: 210–220
20 Gay S, Gay RE, Koopman WJ (1993) Molecular and cellular mechanisms of joint destruction in rheumatoid arthritis: two cellular mechanisms explain joint destruction? *Ann Rheum Dis* 52 (1): S39–47
21 Wilder RL, Case JP, Crofford LJ, Kumkumian GK, Lafyatis R, Remmers EF, Sano H, Sternberg EM, Yocum DE (1991) Endothelial cells and the pathogenesis of rheumatoid arthritis in humans and streptococcal cell wall arthritis in Lewis rats. *J Cell Biochem* 45: 162–166
22 Lafyatis R, Remmers EF, Roberts AB, Yocum DE, Sporn MB, Wilder RL (1989) Anchorage-independent growth of synoviocytes from arthritic and normal joints. Stimulation by exogenous platelet-derived growth factor and inhibition by transforming growth factor-beta and retinoids. *J Clin Invest* 83: 1267–1276
23 Yocum DE, Lafyatis R, Remmers EF, Schumacher HR, Wilder RL (1988) Hyperplastic synoviocytes from rats with streptococcal cell wall-induced arthritis exhibit a transformed phenotype that is thymic-dependent and retinoid inhibitable. *Am J Pathol* 132: 38–48
24 Müller-Ladner U, Gay RE, Gay S (1997) Cellular pathways of joint destruction. *Curr Opin Rheumatol* 9: 213–220
25 Müller-Ladner U, Kriegsmann J, Franklin BN, Matsumoto S, Geiler T, Gay RE, Gay S (1996) Synovial fibroblasts of patients with rheumatoid arthritis attach to and invade normal human cartilage when engrafted into SCID mice. *Am J Pathol* 149: 1607–1615
26 Firestein GS, Echeverri F, Yeo M, Zvaifler NJ, Green DR (1997) Somatic mutations in the p53 tumor suppressor gene in rheumatoid arthritis synovium. *Proc Natl Acad Sci USA* 94: 10895–10900
27 Miossec P, van den Berg W (1997) Th1/Th2 cytokine balance in arthritis. *Arthritis Rheum* 40: 2105–2115
28 Joosten LA, Lubberts E, Durez P, Helsen MM, Jacobs MJ, Goldman M, van den Berg WB (1997) Role of interleukin-4 and interleukin-10 in murine collagen-induced arthritis. Protective effect of interleukin-4 and interleukin-10 treatment on cartilage destruction. *Arthritis Rheum* 40: 249–260
29 Persson S, Mikulowska A, Narula S, O'Garra A, Holmdahl R (1996) Interleukin-10 suppresses the development of collagen type II-induced arthritis and ameliorates sustained arthritis in rats. *Scand J Immunol* 44: 607–614

30 Horsfall AC, Butler DM, Marinova L, Warden PJ, Williams RO, Maini RN, Feldmann M (1997) Suppression of collagen-induced arthritis by continuous administration of IL-4. *J Immunol* 159: 5687–5696

31 Apparailly F, Verwaerde C, Jacquet C, Auriault C, Sany J, Jorgensen C (1998) Adenovirus-mediated transfer of viral IL-10 gene inhibits murine collagen-induced arthritis. *J Immunol* 160: 5213–5220

32 Hagenbaugh A, Sharma S, Dubinett SM, Wei SHY, Aranda R, Cheroutre H, Fowell DJ, Binder S, Tsao B, Locksley RM et al (1997) Altered immune responses in interleukin 10 transgenic mice. *J Exp Med* 185: 2101–2110

33 Whalen JD, Carlos CA, Robbins PD, Evans CH (1997) Periarticular *Gene Therapy* with viral IL-10 can prevent collagen-induced arthritis in mice. *Arthritis Rheum* 40: S158 (Abstract)

34 Wang P, Wu P, Siegel MI, Egan RW, Billah MM (1995) Interleukin (IL)-10 inhibits nuclear factor kappa B (NF kappa B) activation in human monocytes. IL-10 and IL-4 suppress cytokine synthesis by different mechanisms. *J Biol Chem* 270: 9558–9563

35 Arend WP, Dayer JM (1995) Inhibition of the production and effects of interleukin-1 and tumor necrosis factor alpha in rheumatoid arthritis. *Arthritis Rheum* 38: 151–160

36 Arend WP, Malyak M, Guthridge CJ, Gabay C (1998) Interleukin-1 receptor antagonist: role in biology. *Annu Rev Immunol* 16: 27–55

37 Otani K, Nita I, Macaulay W, Georgescu HI, Robbins PD, Evans CH (1996) Suppression of antigen-induced arthritis in rabbits by *ex vivo Gene Therapy*. *J Immunol* 156: 3558–3562

38 Bakker AC, Joosten LA, Arntz OJ, Helsen MM, Bendele AM, van de Loo FA, van den Berg WB (1997) Prevention of murine collagen-induced arthritis in the knee and ipsilateral paw by local expression of human interleukin-1 receptor antagonist protein in the knee. *Arthritis Rheum* 40: 893–900

39 Müller-Ladner U, Roberts CR, Franklin BN, Gay RE, Robbins PD, Evans CH, Gay S (1997) Human IL-1Ra gene transfer into human synovial fibroblasts is chondroprotective. *J Immunol* 158: 3492–3498

40 Le CH, Nicolson AG, Morales A, Sewell KL (1997) Suppression of collagen-induced arthritis through adenovirus-mediated transfer of a modified tumor necrosis factor alpha receptor gene. *Arthritis Rheum* 40: 1662–1669

41 Ghivizzani SC, Lechman ER, Kang R, Tio C, Kolls J, Evans CH, Robbins PD (1998) Direct adenovirus-mediated gene transfer of interleukin 1 and tumor necrosis factor alpha soluble receptors to rabbit knees with experimental arthritis has local and distal anti-arthritic effects. *Proc Natl Acad Sci USA* 95: 4613–4618

42 Boggs SS, Patrene KD, Mueller GM, Evans CH, Doughty LA, Robbins PD (1995) Prolonged systemic expression of human IL-1 receptor antagonist (hIL-1ra) in mice reconstituted with hematopoietic cells transduced with a retrovirus carrying the hIL-1Ra cDNA. *Gene Ther* 2: 632–638

43 Doughty LA, Patrene KD, Evans CH, Boggs SS, Robbins PD (1997) Constitutive sys-

temic expression of IL-1Ra or soluble TNF receptor by genetically modified hematopoietic cells suppresses LPS induction of IL-6 and IL-10. *Gene Ther* 4: 252–257

44 Baeuerle PA, Henkel T (1994) Function and activation of NF-kappa B in the immune system. *Annu Rev Immunol* 12: 141–179

45 Verma IM, Stevenson JK, Schwarz EM, Van Antwerp D, Miyamoto S (1995) Rel/NF-kappa B/I kappa B family: intimate tales of association and dissociation. *Genes Dev* 9: 2723–2735

46 Baldwin AS Jr (1996) The NF-kappa B and I kappa B proteins: new discoveries and insights. *Annu Rev Immunol* 14: 649–83: 649–683

47 Woronicz JD, Gao X, Cao Z, Rothe M, Goeddel DV (1997) IkappaB kinase-beta: NF-kappaB activation and complex formation with IkappaB kinase-alpha and NIK. Science 278: 866–869

48 Mercurio F, Zhu H, Murray BW, Shevchenko A, Bennett BL, Li J, Young DB, Barbosa M, Mann M, Manning A, et al (1997) IKK-1 and IKK-2: cytokine-activated IkappaB kinases essential for NF- kappaB activation. *Science* 278: 860–866

49 DiDonato JA, Hayakawa M, Rothwarf DM, Zandi E, Karin M (1997) A cytokine-responsive IkappaB kinase that activates the transcription factor NF-kappaB. *Nature* 388: 548–554

50 Zhong H, SuYang H, Erdjument-Bromage H, Tempst P, Ghosh S (1997) The transcriptional activity of NF-kappaB is regulated by the IkappaB-associated PKAc subunit through a cyclic AMP-independent mechanism. *Cell* 89: 413–424

51 Wrighton CJ, Hofer-Warbinek R, Moll T, Eytner R, Bach FH, de Martin R (1996) Inhibition of endothelial cell activation by adenovirus-mediated expression of I kappa B alpha, an inhibitor of the transcription factor NF-kappa B. *J Exp Med* 183: 1013–1022

52 Makarov SS, Johnston WN, Olsen JC, Watson JM, Mondal K, Rinehart C, Haskill JS (1997) NF-kappa B as a target for anti-inflammatory *Gene Ther*apy: suppression of inflammatory responses in monocytic and stromal cells by stable gene transfer of I kappa B alpha cDNA. *Gene Ther* 4: 846–852

53 Marok R, Winyard PG, Coumbe A, Kus ML, Gaffney K, Blades S, Mapp PI, Morris CJ, Blake DR, Kaltschmidt C et al (1996) Activation of the transcription factor nuclear factor-kappaB in human inflamed synovial tissue. *Arthritis Rheum* 39: 583–591

54 Handel ML, McMorrow LB, Gravallese EM (1995) Nuclear factor-kappa B in rheumatoid synovium. Localization of p50 and p65. *Arthritis Rheum* 38: 1762–1770

55 Asahara H, Asanuma M, Ogawa N, Nishibayashi S, Inoue H (1995) High DNA-binding activity of transcription factor NF-kappa B in synovial membranes of patients with rheumatoid arthritis. *Biochem Mol Biol Int* 37: 827–832

56 Iwakura Y, Tosu M, Yoshida E, Takiguchi M, Sato K, Kitajima I, Nishioka K, Yamamoto K, Takeda T, Hatanaka M (1991) Induction of inflammatory arthropathy resembling rheumatoid arthritis in mice transgenic for HTLV-I. *Science* 253: 1026–1028

57 Nishioka K, Sumida T, Hasunuma T (1996) Human T lymphotropic virus type I in arthropathy and autoimmune disorders. *Arthritis Rheum* 39: 1410–1418

58 Baeuerle PA, Baichwal VR (1997) NF-kappa B as a frequent target for immunosuppressive and anti-inflammatory molecules. *Adv Immunol* 65: 111–137

59 Baichwal VR, Baeuerle PA (1997) Activate NF-kappa B or die? *Curr Biol* 7: R94–6

60 Miagkov AV, Kovalenko DV, Brown CE, Didsbury JR, Cogswell JP, Stimpson SA, Baldwin AS, Makarov SS (1998) NF-κB activation provides the potential link between inflammation and hyperplasia in the arthritic joint. *Proc Natl Acad Sci USA* 95: 13859–13864

61 Remmers EF, Lafyatis R, Kumkumian GK, Case JP, Roberts AB, Sporn MB, Wilder RL (1990) Cytokines and growth regulation of synoviocytes from patients with rheumatoid arthritis and rats with streptococcal cell wall arthritis. *Growth Factors* 2: 179–188

62 Romashkova JA, Makarov SS (1999) NF-κB is a target of AKT in anti-apoptotic PDGF signaling. *Nature (London)* 401: 86–90

63 Tomita T, Takeuchi E, Tomita N, Morishita R, Hashimoto H, Kaneko M, Yamamoto K, Kaneda Y, Ochi T (1997) *In vivo* transfection of NF-kB decoy reduced severity of rat collagen-induced arthritis as a *Gene Therapy*. *Arthritis Rheum* 40: S220 (Abstract)

64 Karin M, Liu Zg, Zandi E (1997) AP-1 function and regulation. *Curr Opin Cell Biol* 9: 240–246

65 Minden A, Karin M (1997) Regulation and function of the JNK subgroup of MAP kinases. *Biochim Biophys Acta* 1333: F85–104

66 Karin M (1996) The regulation of AP-1 activity by mitogen-activated protein kinases. *Philos Trans R Soc Lond B Biol Sci* 351: 127–134

67 Asahara H, Fujisawa K, Kobata T, Hasunuma T, Maeda T, Asanuma M, Ogawa N, Inoue H, Sumida T, Nishioka K (1997) Direct evidence of high DNA binding activity of transcription factor AP-1 in rheumatoid arthritis synovium. *Arthritis Rheum* 40: 912–918

68 Kuroki Y, Shiozawa S, Yoshihara R, Hotta H (1993) The contribution of human c-fos DNA to cultured synovial cells: a transfection study. *J Rheumatol* 20: 422–428

69 Kuroki Y, Shiozawa S, Sugimoto T, Kanatani M, Kaji H, Miyachi A, Chihara K (1994) Constitutive c-fos expression in osteoblastic MC3T3-E1 cells stimulates osteoclast maturation and osteoclastic bone resorption. *Clin Exp Immunol* 95: 536–539

70 Shiozawa S, Tanaka Y, Fujita T, Tokuhisa T (1992) Destructive arthritis without lymphocyte infiltration in H2-c-fos transgenic mice. *J Immunol* 148: 3100-3104

71 Shiozawa S, Shimizu K, Tanaka K, Hino K (1997) Studies on the contribution of c-fos/AP-1 to arthritic joint destruction. *J Clin Invest* 99: 1210–1216

72 Nishioka K, Hasunuma T, Kato T, Sumida T, Kobata T (1998) Apoptosis in rheumatoid arthritis: a novel pathway in the regulation of synovial tissue. *Arthritis Rheum* 41: 1–9

73 Asahara H, Hasumuna T, Kobata T, Yagita H, Okumura K, Inoue H, Gay S, Sumida T, Nishioka K (1996) Expression of Fas antigen and Fas ligand in the rheumatoid synovial tissue. *Clin Immunol Immunopathol* 81: 27–34

74 Cantwell MJ, Hua T, Zvaifler NJ, Kipps TJ (1997) Deficient Fas ligand expression by synovial lymphocytes from patients with rheumatoid arthritis. *Arthritis Rheum* 40: 1644–1652

75 Matsumoto S, Muller-Ladner U, Gay RE, Nishioka K, Gay S (1996) Ultrastructural demonstration of apoptosis, Fas and Bcl-2 expression of rheumatoid synovial fibroblasts. *J Rheumatol* 23: 1345–1352
76 Fujisawa K, Asahara H, Okamoto K, Aono H, Hasunuma T, Kobata T, Iwakura Y, Yonehara S, Sumida T, Nishioka K (1996) Therapeutic effect of the anti-Fas antibody on arthritis in HTLV-1 tax transgenic mice. *J Clin Invest* 98: 271–278
77 Zhang H, Yang Y, Horton JL, Samoilova EB, Judge TA, Turka LA, Wilson JM, Chen Y (1997) Amelioration of collagen-induced arthritis by CD95 (Apo-1/Fas)-ligand gene transfer. *J Clin Invest* 100: 1951–1957
78 Okamoto K, Asahara H, Kobayashi T, Matsuno H, Hasunuma T, Kobata T, Sumida T, Nishioka K (1998) Induction of apoptosis in the rheumatoid synovium by Fas ligand gene transfer. *Gene Ther* 5: 331–338
79 Kohsaka H, Inoue N, Taniguchi K, Miyasaka N (1998) *In vivo* gene therapy of arthritis with exogenous cell cycle regulator. In: *Abstracts of the Keystone symposia "Pathogenesis of Rheumatoid Arthritis: Implications for Future Therapy"*, Tamarron, CO: 39 (Abstract)
80 Allgood VE, Eastman EM (1997) Chimeric receptors as gene switches. *Curr Opin Biotechnol* 8: 474–479
81 Miller N, Whelan J (1997) Progress in transcriptionally targeted and regulatable vectors for genetic therapy. *Hum Gene Ther* 8: 803–815
82 Varley AW, Coulthard MG, Meidell RS, Gerard RD, Munford RS (1995) Inflammation-induced recombinant protein expression *in vivo* using promoters from acute-phase protein genes. *Proc Natl Acad Sci USA* 92: 5346–5350
83 Varley AW, Geiszler SM, Gaynor RB, Munford RS (1997) A two-component expression system that responds to inflammatory stimuli *in vivo*. *Nat Biotechnol* 15: 1002–1006
84 Chernajovsky Y, Annenkov A, Herman C, Triantaphyllopoulos K, Gould D, Dreja H, Moyes SP, Croxford JL, Mageed RA, Podhajcer OL et al (1998) *Gene Therapy* for rheumatoid arthritis. Theoretical considerations. *Drugs Aging* 12: 29–41
85 Chernajovsky Y, Adams G, Triantaphyllopoulos K, Ledda MF, Podhajcer OL (1997) Pathogenic lymphoid cells engineered to express TGF beta 1 ameliorate disease in a collagen-induced arthritis model. *Gene Ther* 4: 553–559

Cartilage erosion in rheumatoid arthritis: studies in SCID mouse model

Thomas Pap[1], Ulf Müller-Ladner[2], Klaus M. Hummel[3], Renate E. Gay[1] and Steffen Gay[1]

[1]Center for Experimental Rheumatology, Department of Rheumatology, University Hospital, 8091 Zürich, Switzerland; [2]Department of Internal Medicine I, Division of Clinical Rheumatology and Immunology, University of Regensburg, 93042 Regensburg, Germany; [3]Department of Internal Medicine, University of Göttingen, 37075 Göttingen, Germany

Introduction

In the past few years there has been a growing interest in gene therapy to be used not only for the treatment of inherited, but also acquired, diseases. Although genetic factors have been frequently implicated in the pathogenesis of rheumatoid arthritis (RA) [1], and recent reports suggest mutations of tumor suppressor genes to play a role [2], RA is not caused by a specific genetic mutation. Much more likely it is an acquired disorder with a complex pathogenesis and yet unknown etiology. Gene therapy approaches in diseases such as RA differ from those in defined genetic disorders. Apart from the problem of how to correct a specific genetic abnormality, in RA another question appears to be crucial: that of which pathogenic pathway to modulate. Therefore, a suitable animal model for gene therapy approaches in RA should not only reflect relevant features of human disease but also permit one to analyze alterations in key disease processes as closely as possible to the conditions found in people.

Pathogenesis of RA and animal models

It is well recognized that RA is characterized by the triad of synovial hyperplasia, chronic inflammation and numerous immunological phenomena which, by mutual interaction, lead to progressive destruction of affected joints [3]. Although the last decade has brought considerable progress in elucidating the molecular and cellular basis of rheumatoid joint destruction, and growing evidence suggests T cell independent mechanisms to contribute significantly to this disease [3, 4], the debate on which factors initiate and perpetuate RA still continues. In the context of the present work we will focus on established mechanisms that are pivotal in joint destruction and represent potential targets for gene transfer studies.

Gene Therapy in Inflammatory Diseases, edited by C. H. Evans and P. D. Robbins

It has been demonstrated that destruction of joints is mediated by synovial cells attached to articular cartilage [3]. Apart from numerous macrophages, the synovial lining consists mainly of fibroblast-like cells that differ from normal synovial fibroblasts [5]. These transformed-appearing fibroblasts are found at the very site of invasion into cartilage and bone and possess an aggressive invasive phenotype [4,6,7].

Several studies have shown that these cells produce matrix-degrading enzymes such as matrix-metalloproteinases (MMPs) and cathepsins, and thereby contribute significantly to cartilage and bone degradation [8-20]. Undoubtedly, overproduction of these enzymes has to be regarded as the key mechanism of joint destruction that determines the outcome of disease in the vast majority of patients.

Finally, there is an inflammatory cytokine milieu present in RA joints which is characterized by abundant expression of macrophage- and fibroblast-derived cytokines such as interleukin (IL)-1, tumor necrosis factor α (TNFα), and IL-6. Although the question of to which extent this cytokine milieu is responsible for driving the disease has not been conclusively answered, it has been widely accepted that cytokines such as IL-1 and TNFα contribute considerably to an enhanced production of matrix-degrading enzymes [21–25]. In addition, some cytokines have also been demonstrated to increase proliferation of synovial cells [26, 27].

Although many of these insights into the pathogenesis of RA have been obtained from animal models, there exists no animal model that reflects human RA *in toto*. It was mostly the adjuvants arthritis model and later that of collagen induced arthritis (CIA) in rodents by which important features of inflammation could be studied. Utilizing the MRL-lpr/lpr mouse strain led to important insights into early events in the pathogenesis of RA [28]. The latter model has been of particular interest because MRL-lpr/lpr mice develop an RA-like destructive arthritis, and the sequence of events may resemble certain aspects of human RA. However, all these animal models are lacking the ability to study specific human features of RA.

Development of the SCID mouse model for use in studies of rheumatoid arthritis

It was Bosma et al. who were the first to describe an autosomal recessive mutation in mice of the C.B-17 strain that resulted in animals showing severe combined immunodeficiency (SCID) [29]. Due to this mutation, SCID mice have significantly smaller lymphoid organs with only few lymphocytes. A defective DNA repair enzyme and a VDJ recombinase-associated defect affects somatic rearrangement of antigen receptor genes in T lymphocytes and immunoglobulin genes in B lymphocytes, as a consequence of which these mice are lacking both functional T and B cells [30].

The intriguing potential of this model began to emerge when Mosier et al. demonstrated that a functionally intact human immune system can survive in SCID mice recipients [31]. Numerous experiments followed in which SCID mice were used to study autoimmune phenomena by engraftment of human immune cells. First studies addressing RA pathophysiology showed rheumatoid factor IgM production by SCID mice which were reconstituted with RA synovial lymphocytes [32]. Based on these experiments, and on an earlier observation by Brinckerhoff and Harris, who showed that synovial cells are able to form nodular structures when implanted into nude mice [33], Adams et al. [34] and Rendt et al. [35] implanted rheumatoid synovial tissue under the renal capsule of SCID mice. Most interestingly, these experiments demonstrated that rheumatoid fibroblast-like synoviocytes not only survive in SCID mice but also maintain their characteristic biological features [34, 35]. Based on these results our laboratory developed a novel model for studying molecular mechanisms of rheumatoid joint destruction *in vivo* – the SCID mouse co-implantation model for RA.

Description of the SCID mouse co-implantation model

In the primary SCID mouse studies, human RA synovial tissue implanted into the SCID mice was termed "target tissue", because human peripheral blood lymphocytes of the same patients when injected into the SCID mouse, homed to the RA synovium [36]. However, the term "target tissue" is somewhat misleading as, with respect to human rheumatoid joint destruction, the actual targets are human cartilage and bone. To imitate the situation in a rheumatoid joint we, therefore, established a novel SCID mouse model in which human RA synovium was co-implanted with normal human cartilage under the renal capsule of SCID mice [37].

This experimental approach provided us with important insights into the molecular and cellular events leading to destruction of human cartilage by RA synovium. Both RA synovial tissue and normal human cartilage could be successfully implanted into SCID mice for more than 300 days without alteration of their characteristic biological features. Moreover, implanted RA synovium showed the same invasive growth as it does in human rheumatoid joints [37].

Most interestingly, the vast majority of synovial cells found at sites of cartilage invasion resembled transformed-appearing synovial fibroblasts. To specifically study the molecular properties of these fibroblasts in the absence of other human cells and especially their contribution to cartilage degradation, we used subsequently normal human cartilage together with isolated synovial fibroblasts from RA patients to analyze the matrix-degrading properties of these cells in the absence of both lymphocytes and macrophages. Utilizing this model we have been able to show that RA synovial fibroblasts maintain their phenotypic appearance and invasive behavior by degrading the cartilage progressively [7].

Characteristics of the SCID mouse model

For experimental studies, SCID mice are commercially available and can be obtained from several companies and laboratories both in Europe and in the United States. However, there are some pitfalls in handling these mice.

In about 15% of young mice functional antigen receptor rearrangement occurs through "illegitimate" recombination . Thus, a few T and B cell clones survive and expand *in vivo* after antigen exposure. This phenomenon is called "leakiness" and increases in frequency with age especially in mice that are not kept under strict germ free conditions. At the age of 12 to 14 months, the majority of SCID mice becomes leaky [29, 30, 38]. Therefore, the use of young animals at an age of 6 to 8 weeks that are tested for leakiness by the provider is recommended. In addition, it is essential to ensure strictly aseptic conditions at the breeding colonies, the animal housing facilities and during the complete surgical procedure. This is not only required because of the mentioned leakiness but also due to the susceptibility of these animals to infections.

Finally, any animal should be examined for macroscopic abnormalities before and during surgery, as well as for macro- and histopathological abnormalities after sacrifice.

Preparation of cultured synovial fibroblasts and cartilage

While implantation of complete synovial tissue causes no major problems, using synovial fibroblasts requires a special procedure for preparing and cultivating these cells prior to implantation. First, synovial tissue specimens need to be obtained from patients with active RA at synovectomy, joint replacement surgery or through biopsies. Synovial tissue specimens from OA patients and fresh *post mortem* samples or amputations from individuals without any history of joint disease are used as controls. Tissue samples are digested enzymatically and attached synovial cells are transfered into culture flasks, in which they are grown for 3–6 passages. Eventually cells are harvested, tested for mycoplasma infections and characterized as synovial fibroblasts ($CD68^-$, anti-fibroblast antibody$^+$ [7]). Immediately before implantation cells are trypsinized, spun down and resuspended [39]. Normal human cartilage is obtained from non-arthritic amputation of the lower limb (knee cartilage).

Implantation technique

For co-implantation of cultured RA synovial fibroblasts and normal human cartilage into the SCID mice we use a newly developed sponge technique, which is illustrated in Figure 1.

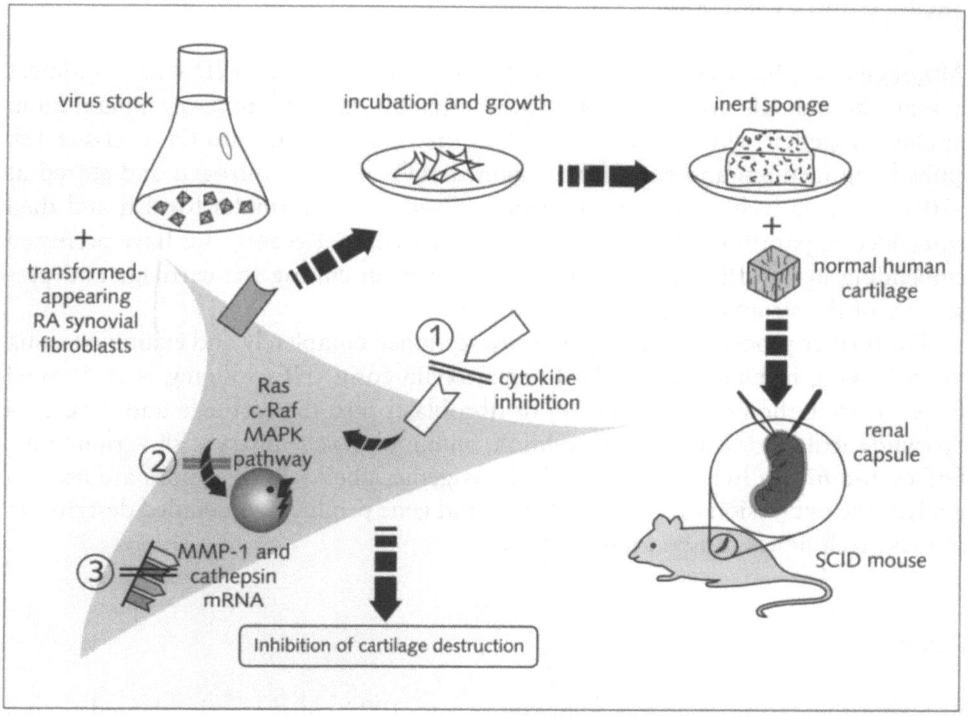

Figure 1
The system of delivering the different genes into human RA synovial fibroblasts, their possible modulating mechanisms and the SCID mouse co-implantation model. The MFG-retrovirus containing the gene of choice is co-cultured with passaged human RA synovial fibroblasts to facilitate the transduction of the gene into the fibroblast genome. Depending on the gene delivered, it becomes possible to inhibit cytokine action (①), block signal transduction (②) or cleave the mRNA of matrix-degrading enzymes (③). After incubation and growth of the cells, they are co-implanted with normal human cartilage under the renal capsule of SCID mice using an inert sponge as a carrier for the fibroblasts.

First, fibroblasts and cartilage are inserted microscopically into a cavity within an inert sterile gel sponge in a total volume of 2 mm^3. This step guarantees close contact between fibroblasts and cartilage. Following careful disinfection of the skin, an incision of approximately 1 cm length is made in the left flank of the intraperitoneally anesthetized SCID mice. After exterioration of the left kidney a small incision of the renal capsule is made, and the gel sponge is placed directly under the capsule using a small forceps. Finally, the peritoneum and the skin wound are sutured and the skin is disinfected again [39].

Sacrifice and evaluation

Although it has been shown that such implants can survive in SCID mice for almost a year, the animals are usually sacrificed after 60 days. At time of explantation, implants together with the adjacent kidney are removed, put into OCT Tissue Tek embedding medium and snap frozen immediately in liquid nitrogen and stored at –70°C. Alternatively, implants can also be fixed in 4% formalin for 4 h and then embedded in paraffin according to standard procedure. Recently, we have preferred embedding in paraffin due to certain advantages in cutting the cartilage and preserving of the structural integrity of the sections.

For further procedures all implants are sectioned completely and examined using the following techniques: Standard hematoxylin-eosin (HE) staining is performed for evaluating the grade of invasion of fibroblasts into the cartilage and perichondrocytic cartilage destruction. In addition, immunohistochemistry with various antibodies and *in situ* hybridization with digoxigenin labeled RNA probes are used to analyze the expression of specific mRNAs and gene products. A detailed description of these techniques can be found in [40].

Results

Applying the above described technique, up to 100% of the co-implanted tissues and cells can be retrieved. There is only minimal scarring around the implants and no necrosis occurs.

Microscopic evaluation of HE-stained sections reveals intense and directed invasive growth of RA synovial fibroblasts into the co-implanted cartilage (Fig. 2A). Most interestingly, the RA synovial fibroblasts maintain their transformed-appearing phenotype, especially at sites of invasion. The area between these fibroblasts and the adjacent cartilage appears loosely fibrillar, which implies direct degradation of matrix components by enzymes released from the fibroblasts. In contrast, OA synovial fibroblasts do not exhibit this invasive growth when co-implanted with normal human cartilage (Fig. 2B). In some implants of OA synovial fibroblasts only isolated, superficial erosions can be seen, which do not significantly differ from those produced by normal skin fibroblasts [7].

Using *in situ* hybridization techniques to examine the presence of mRNA for matrix degrading enzymes a number of cartilage degrading enzymes can be demonstrated. These include mostly cathepsins (B, L and K) as well as matrix-metalloproteinases (e.g. MMP1, MMP2, MMP13 and also MT1-MMP). The expression pattern of these enzymes varies depending on whether or not the RA synovial fibroblasts are directly attached to the cartilage and on the extent of invasion. In contrast, none of these matrix-degrading enzymes can be found, when normal skin or OA synovial fibroblasts are examined in this model [7].

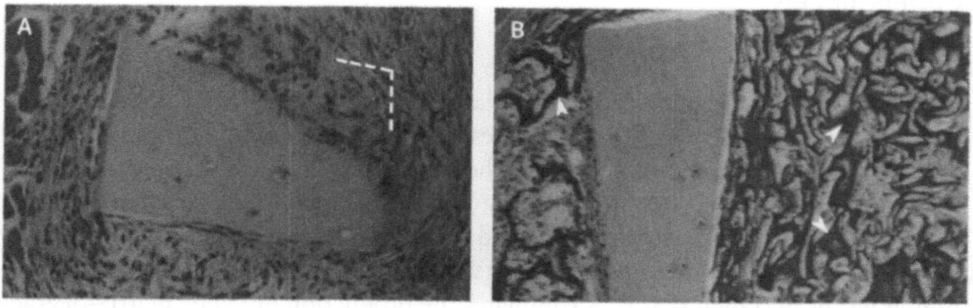

Figure 2
RA and OA synovial fibroblasts engrafted together with normal human cartilage under the renal capsule of SCID mice. RA synovial fibroblasts produce destruction of the cartilage (--- delineates original shape) after 60 days of implantation with diffuse margins at the sites of invasion (A). In contrast, OA synovial fibroblasts exhibit only isolated, shallow erosions at the surface of the cartilage (B). In addition, this figure also demonstrates the implantation technique with the fibroblasts and the cartilage located in a pocket of an inert sponge (➤) (Reproduced from [7] with permission by the publisher).

In addition, RA synovial fibroblasts maintain their ability to express vascular adhesion molecule 1 (VCAM-1), which has been found abundantly expressed in the lining layer of RA synovium, most likely mediating the attachment of RA synovial fibroblasts to cartilage [41].

In summary, RA synovial fibroblasts maintain their aggressive phenotype towards cartilage even after several passages in cell culture and at least 60 days implanted into SCID mice. They express adhesion molecules and invade normal human cartilage through the production of matrix-degrading enzymes in the absence of human macrophages and T cells. As cartilage and bone destruction determines the outcome of RA, gene therapy approaches that target the invasive and destructive properties of RA synovial fibroblasts appear to be a most promising therapeutic approach for treatment.

Gene transfer studies

As described above, gene therapy in RA is aimed at inhibiting destruction of cartilage and bone. In theory, this goal can be achieved by several approaches which target the production and/or activation of matrix-degrading enzymes.

Current targets

When searching for the factors that are involved in the upregulation of matrix-degrading enzymes a number of proinflammatory cytokines were found to contribute to enhanced levels of these enzymes [24, 42]. Among those molecules, which may be targets for gene therapy approaches to treating RA, are IL-1 and TNFα.

IL-1, which is mainly produced by fibroblasts, macrophages and vascular endothelial cells, has been demonstrated to be one of the key proinflammatory cytokines in rheumatoid synovium [43]. With respect to rheumatoid joint destruction, it has been shown that IL-1 stimulates the production of major matrix-degrading enzymes such as collagenase and stromelysin in synovial fibroblasts [22]. It also induces the release of these enzymes by chondrocytes [12] and contributes significantly to the upregulation of other proinflammatory pathways [44]. Therefore, inhibition of IL-1 is an interesting approach to reduce cartilage degradation and inflammation. Fortunately, there exists a naturally occurring inhibitor of IL-1, the IL-1 receptor antagonist (IL-1Ra) [45]. In normal synovium, IL-1Ra is mainly produced by fibroblasts and macrophages. By competitively binding to the IL-1 receptor without intrinsic activity, IL-1Ra counteracts the effects of IL-1 and contributes to cytokine homeostasis in synovium [46, 47]. As IL-1 is overexpressed in RA synovium, increasing IL-1Ra might be a feasible approach to reduce the proinflammatory effects of IL-1 [48]. However, to achieve this goal, a large molar excess of IL-1Ra is required, as the affinity of IL-1Ra does not exceed that of IL-1, and IL-1 has a pronounced spare receptor effect.

The properties of TNFα, the second proinflammatory cytokine which might be targetable for gene therapy in RA, are similar to those of IL-1 with respect to its induction of inflammation and matrix degradation [49]. TNFα has been shown to increase the levels of several matrix-degrading enzymes, especially those of MMPs [25, 50, 51]. Furthermore, it enhances the proinflammatory effects of IL-1 in inflammatory pathways [44, 52]. Similar to IL-1, there exists a natural inhibitor for TNFα, which is its shed, soluble receptor. There also appears to be an imbalance between the expression of this naturally occurring inhibitor of TNFα and TNFα itself in rheumatoid synovium. This imbalance has been proposed to be the major cause of TNFα mediated upregulation of inflammation pathways and matrix degradation [53]. Thus, increasing the amount of TNFα receptor proteins, e.g. its p55 form (TNFRp55), is a promising way to reduce inflammation and possibly joint destruction. This conclusion has been supported by numerous clinical studies, that have proven TNFα blockade to be a safe and effective approach to the treatment of RA. Among these there are some recent trials, which used fusion proteins of the soluble TNFRp55 and TNFRp75 receptors fused, in each case, to the Fc domain of IgG [54, 55].

IL-10 is an anti-inflammatory cytokine, which by downregulation of IL-1, TNFα as well as of IL-2 , IL-6 and interferon gamma, exerts an inhibitory effect on inflammation and matrix degradation. In rheumatoid synovium, IL-10 is largely produced by macrophages and T cells and, despite the fact that it has anti-inflammatory effects, IL-10 has been found to be elevated in RA synovial fluids and sera. Therefore, it has been speculated that this increase reflects an insufficient inhibitory response of the activated immune system in the synovium. As IL-10 has also been shown to inhibit tyrosine kinase activity and the Ras signaling pathway [56] which upregulates cathepsin L [20], IL-10 is a promising candidate to be locally delivered into RA joints [57].

Transduction of cells

The transfer of genes into target cells can be achieved by various methods. Generally, viral gene transfer in *ex vivo* models has been shown to be very efficient [58, 59]. Recently, the group of Evans and Robbins developed an approach, in which the Moloney murine mouse leukemia virus is engineered into a replication-defective retrovirus and used as a vector to transduce synovial fibroblast cells [60]. In this vector, designated "MFG," the env gene, which is needed by the virus to synthesize proteins for its envelope, is replaced by the gene of choice, e.g. IL-1Ra, sTNFRp55 or IL-10. Incubation of human RA synovial fibroblasts with the MFG-vector containing the target gene leads to the incorporation of this gene into the fibroblast genome. In addition to implanting untransduced cells, fibroblasts, transduced with the lacZ gene can be used as an additional negative control (Fig. 1).

In general, the transduction procedure is performed as follows: synovial fibroblasts are suspended in appropriate medium (DMEM + 10% FCS) and plated on culture dishes. 24 h later, when cells are 20–25% confluent, they are washed and then incubated with the viral vector preparation for a total of 12 h. Immediately before implantation, cells are trypsinized and then treated as described before (for details of this procedure see [39]). The efficacy of transduction usually reaches 70% of the fibroblasts being marked by the expression of the lacZ marker gene product, β-galactosidase, 48 h after transduction [39]. Efficacy of transduction can also be determined by measuring the concentration of the gene product (e.g. IL-1Ra, sTNFRp55 or IL-10) by ELISA in the cell supernatants. When transduced RA fibroblasts are cultivated in parallel during the entire implantation period, it is also possible to monitor gene expression *in vitro* until explantation. For example, in our experiments with IL-1Ra gene transduced RA synovial fibroblasts, increased production of IL-1Ra by these cells could be observed for at least 60 days in culture.

Study results

Several studies have been performed to determine whether inhibition of the destructive properties of RA synovial fibroblasts occurs after transduction with the above-mentioned genes: IL-1Ra, TNFRp55 and IL-10. Comparison of cartilage degradation by these cells with that by genetically unmodified RA fibroblasts revealed considerable differences (Figs. 3 and 4).

The incorporation of the IL-1Ra gene into the genome of RA synovial fibroblasts did not alter the invasive behavior of these cells. No significant differences could be observed in the grade of invasion between IL-1Ra-transduced, lacZ-transduced and mock-transduced RA fibroblasts [39]. However, significant differences could be observed in perichondrocytic cartilage degradation. While mock- and lacZ-transduced RA fibroblasts showed considerable perichondrocytic cartilage destruction, this pericellular degradation was markedly reduced in IL-1Ra transfected RA fibroblasts (Fig. 3). This maintenance of the chondrocyte-matrix integrity, therefore, was the main result of IL-1Ra gene transfer into human RA synovial fibroblasts, indicating that chondrocytic chondrolysis appears to be, at least in part, an IL-1 driven process. In addition, it can be concluded that IL-1 independent pathways contribute most significantly to the adhesion of RA fibroblasts to cartilage and to its subsequent fibroblast-mediated destruction.

In contrast, the results obtained following IL-10 gene transfer, demonstrated a significant reduction of invasion with the grade of invasiveness being the lowest among all experiments performed so far. However, IL-10 transduction did not reduce perichondrocytic cartilage degradation [61].

Most interestingly, transduction of RA synovial fibroblasts with bivalent, sTNFRp55 resulted in neither a substantial reduction of invasiveness nor in a decrease of perichondrocytic cartilage degradation. Only few implants showed a slight reduction of invasiveness by synovial fibroblasts, which failed to reach statistical significance [62].

Lessons and perspectives

As long as the exact etiology of rheumatoid arthritis remains unsolved, it is difficult to envision a cure for this disease which, by affecting about 1% of Western population, is of outstanding medical and social importance. However, each piece of new information on the molecular and cellular basis of RA is also a potential piece of hope for the patients suffering from RA and for those physicians who are involved in treating these patients. The present model of human RA, in which genetically unmodified vs genetically altered RA synovial fibroblasts are co-implanted with normal human cartilage under the renal capsule of SCID mice has a dual advantage. Reducing the cellular complexity of rheumatoid synovial tissue, it permits one to investigate the molecular basis of rheumatoid joint destruction by studying selectively the behavior of those cells which most likely drive this process. Yet, at the same time, this model offers unique opportunities to study modulation of pathways of cartilage destruction in RA by transfer of protective genes. In sum-

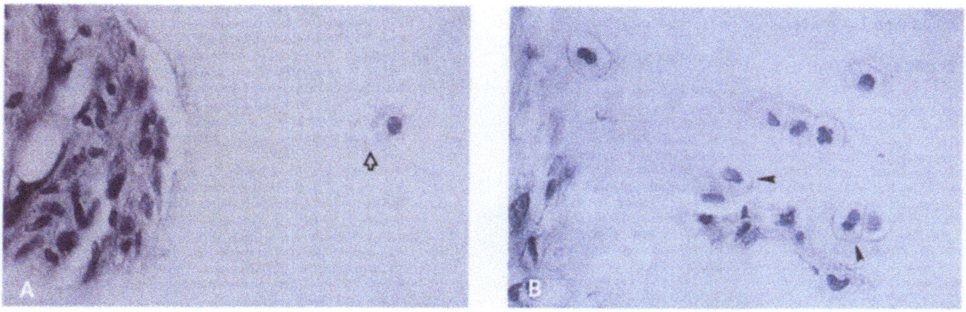

Figure 3
Intensive pericellular chondrocyte-mediated cartilage degradation (⇨) in a specimen with mock-transfected RA fibroblasts (A). Considerable reduction of this pericellular chondrocyte-mediated cartilage degradation can be detected in the implants utilizing IL-1Ra transduced RA fibroblasts. Intact pericellular regions (➤) are detectable (B).
(Reproduced from [39] with permission by the publisher).

marizing the data of the experiments outlined above, the following conclusions can be drawn:

Synovial tissue as well as cultured RA synovial fibroblasts and normal human cartilage can be maintained in SCID mice for several months without losing their pathologic properties. The utilization of an inert sponge is a most useful method to ensure close contact between synovial fibroblasts and cartilage. Employing this experimental setting, RA synovial fibroblasts retain their "transformed" appearance and attach to human cartilage, followed by intensive degradation of the cartilage. The experiments revealed also that the MFG retroviral vector is a most suitable tool to transduce human synovial fibroblasts with cartilage protective genes. These were incorporated into the genome of these cells and overexpressed for the entire implantation period of at least 60 days. However, our results also demonstrate that although proinflammatory cytokines enhance significantly the release of matrix degrading enzymes, blocking the effect of one single cytokine does not appear sufficient to stop both invasion and perichondrocytic cartilage degradation. Therefore, we are currently investigating gene transfer approaches in our laboratory, which extend the above described experimental setting.

The data from the IL-1Ra and the IL-10 experiments together suggest that transduction of RA synovial fibroblasts with both IL-1Ra and IL-10 should reduce perichondrocytic degradation as well as synovial cell invasion. Although the level on which such a double gene transfer approach interferes with the secretion of matrix degrading enzymes is basically the same as in the single gene transfer experiments, it takes into account the complexity of the cytokine network and thereby appears to

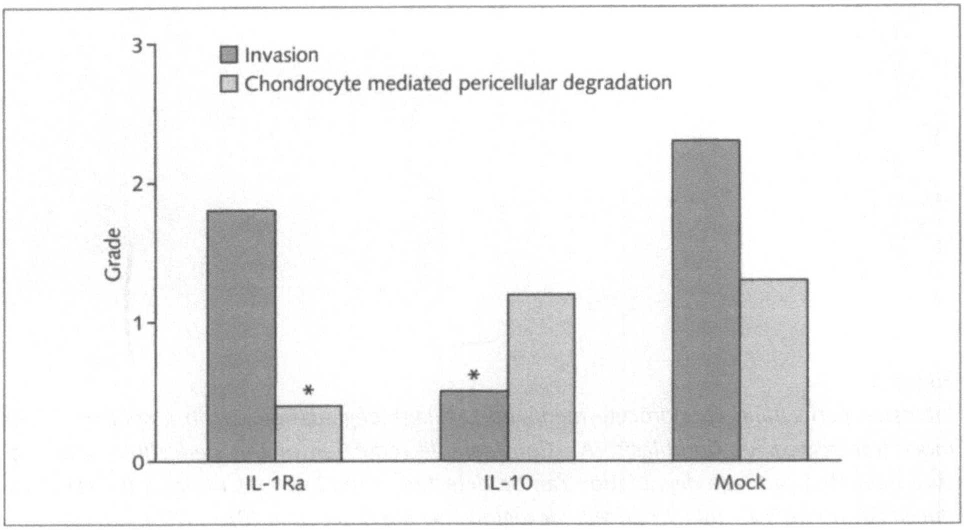

Figure 4
Scores for invasion and chondrocyte mediated pericellular degradation by IL-1Ra-, IL-10- and mock-transduced RA synovial fibroblasts. Invasiveness is significantly reduced in IL-10 transduced cells, while transduction with IL-1Ra leads to a significant decrease of perichondrocytic degradation ($p < 0.05$ vs. mock).*

be more promising than transfection of RA synovial fibroblasts with genes encoding only one cytokine or soluble cytokine receptor (Fig. 1).

The complexity of the cytokine milieu also points to another potential way of modulating the invasive behavior of RA synovial fibroblasts: that of blocking signaling pathways and cellular activation within these cells. It has been suggested that the expression of several matrix degrading enzymes such as collagenase, cathepsin B, D, and L is regulated by proto-oncogenes, and reports from our laboratory demonstrated that the early response genes egr-1 and c-fos contribute to the production of collagenase in RA synovial fibroblasts [63]. Although the exact pathways and cascades, by which these proto-oncogenes are stimulated are just beginning to emerge, some pathways are already well documented. It has been shown that extracellular signals are forwarded by the Ras-Raf-MAPK cascade to the nucleus and certain proto-oncogenes therein (Fig. 1). Thus, one interesting approach to reduce the production of MMPs and cathepsins is to transfect RA synovial fibroblasts with dominant negative mutants of signaling molecules like c-Raf in order to block specific activation pathways and study the effects on the invasive behavior of RA synovial fibroblasts (Fig. 1). However, the complexity of these pathways has been demonstrated by most recent data, revealing that the activation of synovial fibroblasts in RA depends on Raf-independent signaling pathways [64].

Lastly, an additional promising approach that is aimed at modulating the terminal phase of MMP and cathepsin upregulation, involves cleaving the mRNAs for these enzymes. This can be achieved by the delivery and expression of so called hammerhead ribozymes to RA synovial fibroblasts. Hammerhead ribozymes are RNA molecules, which share a special structural motive known as the "hammerhead" and are able to site-specifically cleave RNA. Such ribozymes can be used to destroy specific messages inside cells. RA synovial fibroblasts in which ribozymes capable of cleaving collagenase are expressed will, therefore, produce reduced amounts of this enzyme. The usefulness of this method in reducing the invasiveness of RA synovial fibroblasts is currently evaluated together with Wolfgang Zacharias from the University of Alabama at Birmingham (Fig. 1).

In conclusion the SCID mouse model represents a valuable tool for genetically targeting pivotal pathways in rheumatoid joint destruction and thereby offering new avenues for treatment.

References

1 Weyand CM, Goronzy JJ (1997) Pathogenesis of rheumatoid arthritis. *Med Clin N Am* 81: 29–55

2 Firestein GS, Echeverri F, Yeo M, Zvaifler NJ, Green DR (1997) Somatic mutations in the p53 suppressor gene in rheumatoid arthritis synovium. *Proc Natl Acad Sci USA* 94: 10895–10900

3 Gay S, Gay RE, Koopman WJ (1993) Molecular and cellular mechanisms of joint destruction in rheumatoid arthritis. *Ann Rheum Dis* 52: S39–S47

4 Firestein GS (1996) Invasive fibroblast-like synoviocytes in rheumatoid arthritis – passive responders or transformed aggressors. *Ann Rheum Dis* 39: 1781–1790

5 Fassbender HG (1983) Histomorphologic basis of articular cartilage destruction in rheumatoid arthritis. *Coll Relat Res* 3: 141–155

6 Lafyatis R, Remmers EF, Roberts AB, Yocum DE, Sporn MB, Wilder RL (1989) Anchorage-independent growth of synoviocytes from arthritic and normal joints. Stimulation by exogenous platelet-derived growth factor and inhibition by transforming growth factor-beta and retinoids. *J Clin Invest* 83: 1267–1276

7 Müller-Ladner U, Kriegsmann J, Franklin BN, Matsumoto S, Geiler T, Gay RE, Gay S (1996) Synovial fibroblasts of patients with rheumatoid arthritis attach to and invade normal human cartilage when engrafted into SCID mice. *Am J Pathol* 149: 1607–1615

8 Trabandt A, Gay RE, Fassbender HG, Gay S (1991) Cathepsin B in synovial cells at the site of joint destruction in rheumatoid arthritis. *Arthritis Rheum* 34: 1444–1451

9 Firestein GS, Paine MM (1992) Expression of stromelysin and TIMP in rheumatoid arthritis synovium. *Am J Pathol* 140: 1309–1314

10 Hummel KM, Petrow PK, Jeisy E, Franz J, Gay RE, Brömme D, Gay S (1997) Cathepsin K mRNA is expressed in synovium of patients with rheumatoid arthritis (RA) at sites of bone destruction. *Arthritis Rheum* 40: S250(Abstract)

11 Petrow PK, Hummel KM, Franz J, Kriegsmann J, Müller-Ladner U, Gay RE, Gay S (1997) In situ-detection of MMP13 messenger RNA in the synovial membrane and cartilage-pannus junction in rheumatoid arthritis. *Arthritis Rheum* 40: S336(Abstract)

12 Mort JS, Dodge GR, Roughley PJ, Liu J, Finch SJ, DiPasquale G, Poole AR (1993) Direct evidence for active metalloproteinase mediating matrix degradation in interleukin-1 stimulated human articular cartilage. *Matrix* 13: 95–102

13 Okada Y, Konomi H, Yada T, Kimata K, Nagase H (1989) Degradation of type IX collagen by matrix metalloproteinase 3 (stromelysin) from human rheumatoid synovial cells. *FEBS Lett* 244: 473–476

14 Ahrens D, Koch AE, Pope RM, Stein-Picarella M, Niedbala MJ (1996) Expression of matrix metalloproteinase 9 (96-kd gelatinase B) in human rheumatoid arthritis. *Arthritis Rheum* 39: 1576–1587

15 Okada Y, Morodomi T, Enghild JJ, Suzuki K, Yasui A, Nakanishi I, Salvesen G, Nagase H (1990) Matrix metalloproteinase 2 from human rheumatoid synovial fibroblasts. Purification and activation of the precursor and enzymic properties. *Eur J Biochem* 194: 721–730

16 Okada Y, Nagase H, Harris ED Jr (1987) Matrix metalloproteinases 1, 2, and 3 from rheumatoid synovial cells are sufficient to destroy joints. *J Rheumatol* 14: 41–42

17 Hiraoka K, Sasaguri Y, Komiya S, Inoue A, Morimatsu M (1992) Cell proliferation-related production of matrix metalloproteinases 1 (tissue collagenase) and 3 (stromelysin) by cultured human rheumatoid synovial fibroblasts. *Biochem Int* 27: 1083–1091

18 Sorsa T, Konttinen YT, Lindy O, Ritchlin C, Saari H, Suomalainen K, Eklund KK, Santavirta S (1992) Collagenase in synovitis of rheumatoid arthritis. *Semin Arthritis Rheum* 22: 44–53

19 Xue C, Takahashi M, Hasunuma T, Aono H, Yamamoto K, Yoshino S, Sumida T, Nishioka K (1997) Characterisation of fibroblast-like cells in pannus lesions of patients with rheumatoid arthritis sharing properties of fibroblasts and chondrocytes. *Ann Rheum Dis* 56: 262–267

20 Keyszer GM, Heer AH, Kriegsmann J, Geiler T, Trabandt A, Keysser M, Gay RE, Gay S (1995) Comparative analysis of cathepsin L, cathepsin D, and collagenase messenger RNA expression in synovial tissues of patients with rheumatoid arthritis and osteoarthritis by *in situ* hybridization. *Arthritis Rheum* 38: 976–984

21 Dayer JM, Beutler B, Cerami A (1985) Cachectin/tumor necrosis factor stimulates collagenase and prostaglandin E2 production by human synovial cells and dermal fibroblasts. *J Exp Med* 162: 2163–2168

22 Dayer JM, de Rochemonteix B, Burrus B, Demczuk S, Dinarello A (1986) Human recombinant interleukin-1 stimulates collagenase and protaglandin E2 production by human synovial cells. *J Clin Invest* 77: 86

23 Lemaire R, Huet G, Zerimech F, Grard G, Fontaine C, Duquesnoy B, Flipo RM (1997) Selective induction of the secretion of cathepsins B and L by cytokines in synovial fibroblast-like cells. *Br J Rheumatol* 36: 735–743
24 Firestein GS, Zvaifler NJ (1997) Anticytokine therapy in rheumatoid arthritis. *N Engl J Med* 337: 195–197
25 Migita K, Eguchi K, Kawabe Y, Ichinose Y, Tsukada T, Aoyagi T, Nakamura H, Nagataki S (1996) TNF-alpha-mediated expression of membrane-type matrix metalloproteinase in rheumatoid synovial fibroblasts. *Immunology* 89: 553–557
26 Alvaro Gracia JM, Zvaifler NJ, Brown CB, Kaushansky K, Firestein GS (1991) Cytokines in chronic inflammatory arthritis. VI. Analysis of the synovial cells involved in granulocyte-macrophage colony-stimulating factor production and gene expression in rheumatoid arthritis and its regulation by IL-1 and tumor necrosis factor-alpha. *J Immunol* 146: 3365–3371
27 Remmers EF, Lafyatis R, Kumkumian GK, Case JP, Roberts AB, Sporn MB, Wilder RL (1990) Cytokines and growth regulation of synoviocytes from patients with rheumatoid arthritis and rats with streptococcal cell wall arthritis. *Growth Factors* 2: 179–188
28 O'Sullivan FX, Gay RE, Gay S (1995) Spontaneous arthritis models. In: B Henderson, JCW Edwards, ER Pettipher (eds): *Mechanisms and models in theumatoid arthritis.* Academic Press, London, 471–483
29 Bosma GC, Custer RP, Bosma MJ (1983) A severe combined immunodeficiency mutation in the mouse. *Nature* 301: 527–530
30 Vladutiu AO (1993) The severe combined immunodeficient (SCID) mouse as a model for the study of autoimmune diseases. *Clin Exp Immunol* 93: 1–8
31 Mosier DE, Gulizia RJ, Baird SM, Wilson DB (1988) Transfer of a functional human immune system to mice with severe combined immunodeficiency. *Nature* 335: 256–259
32 Tighe H, Silverman GJ, Kozin F, Tucker R, Gulizia R, Peebles C, Lotz M, Rhodes G, Machold K, Mosier DE et al (1990) Autoantibody production by severe combined immunodeficient mice reconstituted with synovial cell from rheumatoid arthritis patients. *Eur J Immunol* 20: 1843–1848
33 Brinckerhoff CE, Harris ED (1981) Survival of rheumatoid synovium implanted into nude mice. *Am J Pathol* 103: 411–419
34 Adams CD, Zhou T, Mountz JD (1990) Transplantation of human rheumatoid synovium into a SCID mouse as a model for disease activity. *Arthritis Rheum* 33: S120(Abstract)
35 Rendt KE, Barry TS, Jones DM, Richter CE, McCachren SS, Haynes BF (1991) An *in vivo* model of human rheumatoid arthritis (RA) using RA synovium engrafted into severe combined immune-deficient (SCID) mice. *FASEB J* 5: 1371(Abstract)
36 Rendt KE, Barry TS, Jones DM, Richter CE, McCachren SS, Haynes BF (1993) Engraftment of human synovium into severe combined deficient (SCID) mice: migration of human peripheral blood T-cells to engrafted human synovium and to mouse lymph nodes. *J Immunol* 151: 7324–7336
37 Geiler T, Kriegsmann J, Keyszer GM, Gay RE, Gay S (1994) A new model for rheuma-

toid arthritis generated by engraftment of rheumatoid synovial tissue and normal human cartilage into SCID mice. *Arthritis Rheum* 37: 1664–1671
38 Bosma GC, Fried M, Custer RP, Carroll A, Bosma MJ (1988) Evidence of functional lymphocytes in some (leaky) scid mice. *N Engl J Med* 167: 1016–1033
39 Müller-Ladner U, Roberts CR, Franklin BN, Gay RE, Robbins PD, Evans CH, Gay S (1997) Human IL-1Ra gene transfer into human synovial fibroblasts is chondroprotective. *J Immunol* 158: 3492–3498
40 Kriegsmann J, Müller-Ladner U, Gay RE, Gay S (1997) Molecular immunopathology. In: LA Herzenberg, C Blackwell, D Weir (eds): *The handbook of experimental immunology.* 133.1–133.16
41 Kriegsmann J, Keyszer GM, Geiler T, Bräuer R, Gay RE, Gay S (1993) Expression of vascular cell adhesion molecule-1 mRNA and protein in rheumatoid arthritis synovium demonstrated by in situ hybridization and immunohistochemistry. *Lab Invest* 68: 682–688
42 Firestein GS, Alvaro Gracia JM, Maki R (1990) Quantitative analysis of cytokine gene expression in rheumatoid arthritis. *J Immunol* 144: 3347–3353
43 Henderson B, Pettipher ER (1989) Arthritogenic actions of recombinant IL-1 and tumour necrosis factor alpha in the rabbit: evidence for synergistic interactions between cytokines *in vivo*. *Clin Exp Immunol* 75: 306–310
44 Harigai M, Hara M, Kitani A, Norioka K, Hirose T, Hirose W, Suzuki K, Kawakami M, Masuda K, Shinmei M et al (1991) Interleukin 1 and tumor necrosis factor-alpha synergistically increase the production of interleukin 6 in human synovial fibroblast. *J Clin Lab Immunol* 34: 107–113
45 Arend WP (1993) Interleukin-1 receptor antagonist. *Adv Immunol* 54: 167–227
46 Berger AE, Carter DB, Hankey SO, McEwan RN (1993) Cytokine regulation of the interleukin-1 receptor antagonist protein in U937 cells. *Eur J Immunol* 23: 39–45
47 Firestein GS, Boyle DL, Yu C, Paine MM, Whisenand TD, Zvaifler NJ, Arend WP (1994) Synovial interleukin-1 receptor antagonist and interleukin-1 balance in rheumatoid arthritis. *Arthritis Rheum* 37: 644–652
48 Chikanza IC, Roux-Lombard P, Dayer JM, Panayi GS (1995) Dysregulation of the *in vivo* production of interleukin-1 receptor antagonist in patients with rheumatoid arthritis: Pathogenetic implications. *Arthritis Rheum* 38: 642–648
49 Brennan FM, Maini RN, Feldmann M (1992) TNF alpha – a pivotal role in rheumatoid arthritis. *Br J Rheumatol* 31: 293–298
50 Borden P, Heller RA (1997) Transcriptional control of matrix metalloproteinases and the tissue inhibitor of matrix metalloproteinases. *Crit Rev Eukaryot Gene Expr* 7: 159–178
51 Dayer JM, Burger D (1994) Interleukin-1, tumor necrosis factor and their specific inhibitors. *Eur Cytokine Netw* 5: 563–571
52 Probert L, Plows D, Kontogeorgos G, Kollias G (1995) The type 1 interleukin-1 receptor acts in series with tumor necrosis factor (TNF) to induce arthritis in TNF transgenic mice. *Eur J Immunol* 25: 1794–1797

53 Weckmann AL, Alcocer Varela J (1996) Cytokine inhibitors in autoimmune disease. *Semin Arthritis Rheum* 26: 539–557

54 Williams RO, Ghrayeb J, Feldmann M, Maini RN (1995) Successful therapy of collagen-induced arthritis with TNF receptor-IgG fusion protein and combination with anti-CD4. *Immunology* 84: 433–439

55 Moreland LW, Baumgartner SW, Schiff MH, Tindall EA, Fleischmann RM, Weaver AL, Ettlinger RE, Cohen S, Koopman WJ, Mohler K et al (1997) treatment of rheumatoid arthritis with recombinant human tumor necrosis factor receptor (p75)-Fc-fusion protein. *N Engl J Med* 337: 141–147

56 Geng Y, Gulbins E, Altman A, Lotz M (1994) Monocyte deactivation by interleukin 10 via inhibition of tyrosine kinase activity and the Ras signaling pathway. *Proc Natl Acad Sci USA* 91: 8602–8606

57 Maini RN, Elliott M, Brennan FM, Williams RO, Feldmann M (1997) TNF blockade in rheumatoid arthritis: implications for therapy and pathogenesis. *APMIS* 105: 257–263

58 Evans CH, Robbins PD, Ghivizzani SC, Herndon JH, Kang R, Bahnson AB, Barranger JA, Elders EM, Gay S, Tomaino MM et al (1996) Clinical trial to assess the safety, feasibility, and efficacy of transferring a potentially anti-arthritic cytokine gene to human joints with rheumatoid arthritis. *Hum Gene Ther* 7: 1261–1280

59 Evans CH, Robbins PD (1996) Pathways to gene therapy in rheumatoid arthritis. *Curr Opin Rheumatol* 8: 230–234

60 Nita I, Ghivizzani SC, Galea Lauri J, Bandara G, Georgescu HI, Robbins PD, Evans CH (1996) Direct gene delivery to synovium. An evaluation of potential vectors *in vitro* and *in vivo*. *Arthritis Rheum* 39: 820–828

61 Müller-Ladner U, Franklin BN, Roberts CR, Gay RE, Robbins PD, Evans CH, Gay S (1996) Gene transfer of interleukin-10 into human synovial fibroblasts and implantation into the SCID mouse. *Arthritis Rheum* 39: S160 (Abstract)

62 Müller-Ladner U, Roberts CR, Franklin BN, Gay RE, Robbins PD, Evans, CH, Gay S (1996) Gene transfer of TNF-alpha receptor p55 into human synovial fibroblasts and implantation into the SCID mouse. *Arthritis Rheum* 39: S307 (Abstract)

63 Trabandt A, Aicher WK, Gay RE, Sukhatme VP, Fassbender HG, Gay S (1992) Spontaneous expression of immediately-early response genes c-fos and egr-1 in collagenase-producing rheumatoid synovial fibroblasts. *Rheumatol Int* 12: 53–59

64 Hummel KM, Petrow PK, Nawrath M, Müller-Ladner U, Neidhart M, Pavlovic J, Gay RE, Mölling K, Gay S (1997) Retroviral gene transfer of a c-Raf dominant negative mutant does not inhibit synovial fibroblasts (SF) from patients with rheumatoid arthritis (RA) to invade normal human cartilage in the SCID mouse model. *Arthritis Rheum* 40: S120 (Abstract)

Gene therapy for rheumatoid arthritis: clinical studies

Thomas S. Muzzonigro[1], Richard Kang[1], Julio Reinecke[3], Peter Wehling[3], Mary C. Wasko[2] and James H. Herndon[4]

Departments of [1]Orthopaedic Surgery and [2]Rheumatology, University of Pittsburgh School of Medicine, Pittsburgh, PA 15261, USA; [3]Orthogen Gmbh, Düsseldorf, Germany; [4]Partners Department of Orthopaedic Surgery, Massachusetts General Hospital, Gray 624-55 Fruit Street, Boston, MA 02114-2617, USA

Introduction

Collectively, over 35 million Americans suffer from the various arthritidies with an annual cost estimated to be greater than 18 billion dollars annually [1]. Rheumatoid arthritis (RA) is a progressive, autoimmune disease that primarily affects diarthrodial joints. It has a world-wide incidence of approximately four per 10 000 in the population aged greater than 15 years, and causes significant increases in morbidity and even mortality in affected patients [2–4]. 150 000 patients are diagnosed with RA each year in the United States at a cost of approximately $ 30 000 per case [5]. Women are twice as likely to be affected as men, and the prevalence increases with age. Although the prevalence of RA varies across the globe, no etiologic agents have been unequivocally identified [6–9].

Patients with RA have a remarkable reduction in life expectancy, although confounding variables relating to the toxicity of long-term anti-rheumatic medications obscure the reasons for this [10, 11]. Although some patients experience remission of disease, the vast majority progress in a chronic fashion. It has been reported that fewer than 50% of patients with a disease duration of 10 years or more can continue to work [2]. Most are forced to alter their activities of daily living, substantially impacting on social and economic aspects of their lives. In this sense, it is impossible to quantify the effects of this disease in the rheumatoid population.

Classical pharmacological approaches to treating RA have largely failed to control the progression of the disease. Newer, biological approaches, recently reviewed by Moreland et al. [12], promise to improve the management of RA. Thus far, antibodies to tumor necrosis factor (TNF), TNF soluble receptors, and the interleukin-1 receptor antagonist (IL-1Ra) have shown efficacy as anti-arthritic biologic agents in human trials [13–16]. However, the potential utility of these anti-arthritic pro-

Gene Therapy in Inflammatory Diseases, edited by C. H. Evans and P. D. Robbins

teins in RA may be limited by the clinicians' ability to safely deliver them to the joints in a sustained fashion. To overcome this difficulty, we have explored gene transfer to the synovial lining of joints as a means to achieve therapeutic, intra-articular levels of anti-arthritic proteins [17, 18]. To this end, gene therapy has evolved as a biologic drug delivery system , capable of transferring sustained levels of therapeutic proteins to the principal sites of disease.

For the current clinical trials we have focused on the *ex vivo* delivery of the cDNA encoding human IL-1Ra to the synovial lining of rheumatoid joints. The *ex vivo* approach permits use of Moloney-based retroviral vectors for delivery of the human IL-1Ra (hIL-1Ra) gene, allows for extensive safety testing of the genetically modified cells before reimplantation, and does not introduce infectious viral particles into the joint.

Pre-clinical studies

IL-1 is an important mediator of joint inflammation and cartilage degradation in the rheumatoid joint. IL-1Ra is a naturally occurring antagonist of IL-1 that has been shown to have anti-arthritic effects in experimental models of RA [19–21].

We have previously demonstrated in experimental animals that the gene encoding IL-Ra can be transferred to the synovial lining of joints, and express its product intra-articularly in a biologically active form [22]. Moreover, this procedure has been shown to suppress arthritis in four different animal models of RA [23–25]. Thus we have sought to develop transfer of IL-1Ra gene to treat RA in humans. After reporting efficacy and feasibility in animal models of RA, as well as safety, we proposed the first clinical trial of gene therapy for RA [26]. Permission was sought to initiate a phase I trial, first in the USA at the University of Pittsburgh, and then in Germany at the University of Düsseldorf.

Regulatory issues

USA

In the United States, the regulatory bodies governing clinical gene therapy trials are present at both the local and federal levels. Locally, the Institutional Review Board (IRB) and the Institutional Biohazard Safety Committee (IBSC) evaluate the research proposal and govern its advancement. The IRB operates in accordance with the regulations of the Department of Health and Human Services (DHHS) and the Food and Drug Administration (FDA), and has authority to review, approve or disapprove any and all research activities involving humans that fall within its jurisdiction. The Office for Protection from Research Risks (OPRR) is the unit within the

DHHS that oversees IRB compliance with federal mandates. This office provides instruction, support, and guidance on ethical issues related to research on human subjects.

Central to IRB approval is that appropriate measures to protect the rights and welfare of research subjects are taken. Further, participants must understand all risks and possible benefits. It is incumbent upon the researcher to ensure that proper informed consent is obtained and documented. The safety of participants is the highest concern, and provisions to monitor therapy are emphasized. The patients privacy must be guarded and respected.

After approval by the local IRB, the research proposal is evaluated at the federal level by the Recombinant DNA Advisory Committee (RAC) of The National Institutes of Health (NIH). At this level, the protocol is evaluated on ethical, medical and scientific merits. The meetings of the RAC are open to the public, and investigators must appear and defend their proposals. The records of these meeting are a matter of public knowledge and are openly published in the Federal Register. After the RAC has evaluated and approved a protocol, the director of the NIH must personally review and approve it.

The role of the RAC in reviewing human gene therapy protocols has recently been reduced such that most new protocols now proceed directly to the FDA after IRB and IBC approval. The human arthritis protocol however was subjected to the full RAC review.

Further oversight and approval from the FDA is then required. An application for an Investigational New Drug (IND) is lodged and then evaluated. The Office of Therapeutics Research and Review (OTRR) has a Division of Applications Review and Policy (DARAP) which reviews annual reports and is responsible for investigating any adverse effects in patients within clinical studies.

The US clinical trial described here is supported by an RO1 grant from the National Institute of Arthritis and Musculoskeletal and Skin Diseases (NIAMS). Funding was contingent upon the establishment of an External Monitoring Board composed of leaders in rheumatology, orthopaedic surgery, ethics and gene therapy. This board evaluates and monitors the clinical trial, and its members have no other formal connection with the University of Pittsburgh.

Only after approval at all levels was the clinical trial allowed to proceed.

Germany

In Germany, a clinical gene therapy study is regulated by the *Arzneimittelgesetz* (AMG) and prerequisites are equivalent to a conventional clinical drug trial. A valid patient insurance and the approval of the local ethics commission is required.

By the time of the application for this clinical trial several local regulatory bodies were to be involved. The steps were:

1. Application for the clinical study lodged with the local ethics committee of the University in 1994.
2. Patient insurance
3. Detailed report to the *Bezirksregierung* (district Governor) and the district pharmacist's office (*Amtsapotheker*).

On a voluntary basis the federal Paul Ehrlich Institute (FDA equivalent) and the federal *Zentrale Kommission für Biologische Sicherheit* (ZKBS) were informed about the trial. These bodies were each supplied with a copy of the clinical protocol structured according to the RAC "points to consider" and an FDA master drug file.

Involved in the establishment of a laboratory equipped and suited for gene technology work are the State Environment Office 9 (*Landesumweltamt*) and bodies of the local Düsseldorf administration. They are concerned with the usual labor and laboratory safety issues such as biohazard, toxic waste and fire regulations.

Recently, the *Bundesärztekammer* (federal bureau of physicians) ethics commission has also been established with responsibility for the permission process for gene therapy trials. This is the first federal body whose involvement in the evaluation of gene therapy trials is compulsory. Until the German federal government passes specific laws and guidelines for gene therapy the procedure of a normal clinical trial needs to be followed.

Clinical design

As this is the first protocol to apply gene transfer techniques to a non-lethal disease, safety is the principal design focus. We have addressed safety at multiple levels in the design of the current clinical trial of gene therapy for RA. The results of the pre-clinical studies demonstrated that *ex vivo* gene delivery of the hIL-1Ra gene to the synovial lining of the joint was feasible and safe in experimental models. Extensive studies in humans previously showed that the protein itself had an excellent safety profile.

The challenge was to design a clinical trial that ensured the safety and welfare of patients suffering from a non-lethal disease while obtaining scientifically valuable information. Further, the clinical trial should not alter in any way the care of the patient or expose the patient to any unnecessary procedures.

Based on our pre-clinical studies we decided to use local delivery of the gene therapy to minimize systemic exposure to the therapy. Further, it was decided to utilize the ex vivo system of gene delivery to maximize our control over the transduced, autologous cells. End-stage rheumatoid joints are often surgically removed and replaced by prosthetic joints. This provided an opportunity to insert the IL-1Ra genes into rheumatoid joints and then to remove them afterwards during joint replacement surgery. Not only does this provide a strong safety cushion, but it also makes available surgically retrieved tissue for analysis. Accordingly, it was decided to study rheumatoid patients with end-stage disease in the metacarpophalangeal (MCP) joints of their hands who required replacement of their MCP joints as part of the surgical management of the disease. The MCP joints are a common site of disease, and the associated deformities and dysfunction often require MCP joint replacement. Furthermore, human MCP joints are approximately equal in size to the rabbit knee joints used for much of the pre-clinical studies. Genes were transferred to MCP joints 2–5, 1 week before the joints were to be surgically removed. In this way few, if any, of the transduced cells remain in the patient to pose potential long-term risks. Further, the bulk of tissues exposed to the gene transfer are excised at the time of surgery and are available for detailed *ex vivo* analysis. In order to harvest autologous tissue for cell culture, eligible patients also need another clinically indicated joint surgery such as synovectomy, total joint replacement or fusion during which synovial tissue is excised and expanded in culture.

Eligible patients are evaluated by the chief orthopaedic surgeon as well as a rheumatologist to determine if they are candidates for the clinical trial. If they are indeed candidates, blood is drawn and analyzed to determine if the patient is a reasonable surgical candidate, and to provide baseline laboratory data.

To prevent the theoretical possibility of gene transfer to germ-line cells, only post-menopausal or post-ovariectomized women are eligible to participate.

To maximize control and safety, an ex vivo gene transfer is utilized. This enables investigators both to control which cells are transduced and to perform extensive safety testing on the cells prior to re-implantation. In addition, no infectious viral particles are introduced into the patients' joints. The MFG-IRAP retrovirus is used to transduce the cells.

After removal of the MCP joints during joint replacement surgery, the retrieved tissues are analyzed for evidence of successful gene transfer and gene expression. Further analysis looks for indications that the transgene product had been biologically active within the joint. The procedure is summarized in Figure 1.

As described below, the design of the German trial is very similar to the US trial. The major differences are that the genes remain in the joints for 1 month rather than 1 week, and that they may be removed by synovectomy as well as by joint replacement surgery.

Clinical trials

USA

Eligible patients are identified, and advised of the risks and benefits of the clinical trial. Informed consent is then given by an orthopaedic surgeon not actively involved in the care of the patient. After the first surgery, the patient recuperates while the cells recovered from the synovial biopsy are expanded in cell culture under sterile conditions. After expansion, the cells are split in half. One-half are retrovirally transduced with MFG-IRAP, and one-half are maintained as control cells. The transduced cells are tested to ensure that production of IL-1Ra is equal to, or greater than 30 ng/10^6 cells/48 h. At this point, the majority of the cells undergo rigorous safety testing for adventitious agents, endotoxin and replication-competent retrovirus at an independent laboratory. Once the samples have received favorable test results, the cells are thawed, recultured and re-tested for production of the IL-1Ra protein. Prior to gene transfer, the patients' MCP joints are lavaged to determine the baseline levels of endogenous IL-1Ra. Three groups of patients have received IL-1Ra gene transfer in a dose-escalation format. The first group received 10^6 cells per MCP joint, the second group received up to 5×10^6 cells per MCP joint, and the third group received up to 10^7 cells per MCP joint.

Genetically modified cells were transferred to two MCP joints and untransduced cells to the other two MCP joints, under sterile conditions in the orthopaedic office. This was performed in a double blinded fashion 1 week before scheduled replacement of these joints. Each day after gene transfer, we called the patients to check for adverse effects according to World Health Organization recommendations. One week later, at the time of MCP joint replacement, the joints were lavaged, and synovium, and cartilage if present, were harvested for analysis. After participation in this clinical trial, patients were evaluated by the orthopaedic surgeon and rheumatologist. Blood is drawn and analyzed at week 1, months 1, 3, 6, 12, and annually thereafter. At these appointments the patients undergo routine orthopaedic postoperative follow-up. The blood is evaluated for the presence of replication-competent retrovirus by a PCR-based assay for expression of the retroviral env gene as well as for deviations from baseline laboratory values.

Synovial tissue retrieved at the time of surgery is transported to the laboratory for analysis of success of gene transfer and transgene expression. Transgene expression is evaluated by reverse transcriptase polymerase chain reaction (RT-PCR), in situ hybridization (ISH) to detect IL-1Ra mRNA and by immunohistochemistry to detect the IL-1Ra protein. The concentration of IL-1Ra in the synovial lavage fluid is analyzed by enzyme linked immunosorbent assay (ELISA). Additional in situ analyses will be performed to determine whether local, synovial responses occurred in response to intraarticular expression of the transgene.

Germany

In the trial safety is of paramount importance. The trial protocol used the Pittsburgh design as a template. It was designed to examine carefully whether any side effects or risks occur in addition to those already known. In the following section mainly those features differing from the characteristics of the Pittsburgh trial described above will be stressed.

Permission has been granted to treat six women with no child-bearing capacity in an advanced stage of rheumatoid arthritis. Synovial tissue obtained during a joint replacement surgery or a therapeutic synovectomy is used to isolate autologous synovial cells. The cells are cultured and transduced *ex vivo* using the MFG-IRAP system. Transduced and non-transduced control cells are expanded to the desired numbers and checked for IL-1Ra expression (minimum *in vitro* expression: 30 ng/48 h/ 10^6 cells).

Sterility, adventitious agents and replication competent retrovirus (RCR) are tested under GMP conditions by a third party. Transduced and non-transduced cells (negative control) are injected into rheumatoid joints. In the trial, we prefer to treat adjacent MCP joints, but the protocol does not specifically restrict us to these joints.

The cells remain *in situ* for 4 weeks. Synovial fluid is obtained by lavage from these joints before injection of cells and twice (after 2 weeks and before second surgery) during the 4 weeks of treatment. Analysis of intraarticular inflammation parameters and IL-1Ra expression is performed on these specimens. Surgical joint replacement or therapeutic synovectomy is performed after the 4-week period.

The protocol is designed to inflict as little additional inconvenience on the patients as possible. The injection of engineered and control cells, and lavages, are the only procedures added to the therapeutic joint replacement or synovectomy surgeries that the patients would have had anyway.

In summary, the Düsseldorf protocol differs from the published Pittsburgh protocol as follows:

1. No restriction with respect to the joints to be treated.
2. Tissue may be obtained by a therapeutic synovectomy and not only for endoprosthesis surgery.
3. Transgenic and control cells remain *in situ* for 4 weeks.
4. Transgenic and control tissue may be removed by synovectomy and not only for endoprosthesis surgery.

By choosing an extended timespan during which transgenic cells remain in situ we hope to gain more information about the kinetics of transgene expression in the patients' joints. Blood analysis for the parameters published in the clinical protocol are performed before, during and after treatment period.

Preliminary results

USA

All nine patients have been recruited and treated (Tab. 1). One of these patients has been followed for more than 2 years. There have been no complications or adverse effects noted in any of these patients, although four of the women noted ecchymosis and tenderness after the injections. In all of the cases the procedure has been well tolerated. Transgene expression has been confirmed in all specimens yet analyzed by RT-PCR and by ISH. Other analyses are currently ongoing.

Germany

So far two patients have been treated at the University of Düsseldorf, Germany. The first patient is a 35-year-old female with an 8-year history of disease. The second patient is a 60-year-old female. Both patients suffered from recurrent joint inflammations with progressive cartilage destruction.

Patient 1 received transgenic cells into her thumb MCP and index finger MCP joint. Control cells were injected into the middle finger MCP joint.

Patient 2 received transgenic cells into her thumb MCP joint, and control cells into the adjacent MCP joint.

Reverse transcriptase PCR (RT-PCR) data show that the transgene is active after 4 weeks in tissue samples and cells regrown from specimens obtained from joints treated with transduced cells.

Patient 1 cells from control and transgenic joints secreted high levels of IL-1Ra in culture. Transgenic IL-1Ra mRNA represented the by far greater part of the IL-1Ra message in the cells obtained from transgenic joints. Analysis is underway to determine the effects on other genes. First results indicate that matrix metalloproteinase mRNA expression is more pronounced in cells from the control joint. IL-1Ra amounts produced by transgenic cells obtained from the first patients joints are in the range of 50–100 ng/10^6 cells/48 h *in vitro*.

From the second patient only small amounts of tissue could be harvested: all the tissue was frozen for later histologic analysis.

No side-effects or adverse reactions attributable to the gene therapy treatment have been observed.

Clinically, the first patient characterized by a more intact joint morphology did show some improvement as judged from reduction of swelling and pain. The second patient experienced only mild improvement in terms of swelling and pain.

Conclusion

To date, nine patients in the US and two patients in Germany have received arthritis gene therapy. The current clinical trials have demonstrated that genes can be safely and successfully transferred to human rheumatoid joints, with resulting intraarticular expression of the transgene. All patients have tolerated the procedure well, without any serious side-effects. Success in this clinical trial would pave *iTable 1 - Status of American arthritis gene therapy trial*

Patient	1st procedure	IL-1Ra[1]	Cells/MCPJ	RT-PCR	ISH
1	Thumb fusion	208	1×10^6	+	+
2	Wrist fusion	35	1×10^6	+	+
3	Thumb fusion	188	1×10^6	+	+
4	Thumb fusion	103	1.5×10^6	+	+
5	Thumb fusion	489	2.5×10^6	+	+
6	Wrist fusion	81	5×10^6	+	*
7	Thumb fusion	152	6.5×10^6	+	*
8	First toe fusion	74	1×10^7	+	*
9	Thumb fusion	64	1×10^7	+	*

[1], *production of IL-1Ra ng/10^6 cells/48 h by transduced cells prior to implantation. MCPJ, metacarpophalangeal joint; RT-PCR, reverse transcriptase-polymerase chain reaction; ISH,* in situ *hybridization; +, positive result; *, work in progress*

the way for additional human studies of gene transfer in arthritis and other inflammatory diseases, and disorders of the musculoskeletal system.

References

1 Smyth C, Clayton M (1992) Medical perspectives of surgery for rheumatoid arthritis. In: *Surgery for rheumatoid arthritis*. Churchill, Livingstone, New York, 3–8

2 Lindgren JU (1996) Arthritis review. In: *Orthopaedic knowledge update* 5. American Academy of Orthopaedic Surgeons, IL, 169–171

3 Kaipiainen S, Aho K, Isomaki H, Laakso M (1996) Incidence of rheumatoid arthritis in Finland during 1980–1990. *Ann Rheum Dis* 55: 608–611

4 Series V (1987) Rheumatology epidemiology. *National Center for Health Statistics* 10: 164

5 Harris E (1997) Clinical features of rheumatoid arthritis. In: *Textbook of rheumatology*, 5th ed. WB Saunders, Philadelphia, 898–933

6 Beasley R, Wilkens R, Bennett P (1973) High prevalence of rheumatoid arthritis in Yakima Indians. *Arthritis Rheum* 16: 743–748

7 Harvey J, Lotze M, Stevens M (1983) Rheumatoid arthritis in a Chippewa band. *Rheumatology* 10 (1): 28–32

8 Solomon L, Robin G, Valkenberg H (1975) Rheumatoid arthritis in an urban South African Negro population. *Ann Rheum Dis* 34 (2): 128–135

9 Lawrence J (1970) Rheumatoid arthritis: Nature or nurture? *Ann Rheum Dis* 29 (4): 235–241
10 Myllykangas R, Aho K, Isomaki H (1995) Mortality in rheumatoid arthritis. *Sem Arthritis Rheum* 25: 193–202
11 Pincus T, Callahan L (1992) Early mortality in rheumatoid arthritis predicted by poor clinical status. *Bull Rheum Dis* 41: 1–4
12 Moreland LW, Heck LW, Koopman WJ (1997) Biologic agents for treating rheumatoid arthritis. *Arthritis Rheum* 40: 397–409
13 Moreland LW, Baumgartner SW, Schiff MH, Tindall EA, Fleischmann RM, Weaver AL, Ettlinger RE, Cohen S, Koopman WJ, Mohler K, Widner KM, Blosch CM (1997) Treatment of rheumatoid arthritis with a recombinant human tumor necrosis factor receptor (p75)-Fc fusion protein. *N Engl J Med* 337: 141–147
14 Elliott MJ, Maini RN, Feldmann M, Kalden JR, Anoni C, Smoler JS, Leeb B, Breedveld FC, Macfarlane JD, Bijl H, Woody JN (994) Randomised, double blind comparison of a chimaeric: monoclonal antibody to tumor-necrosis factor alpha (cA2) versus placebo in rheumatoid arthritis. *Lancet* 344: 1105–1110
15 Drevlow BE, Louis R, Haag MA, Sinacore JM, Jacobs C, Blusche C, Landay A, Moreland LW, Pope RM (1996) Recombinant human interleukin-1 receptor antagonist in patients with rheumatoid arthritis. *Arthritis Rheum* 39: 257–265
16 Campion G, Lebsack M, Lookabough J, Gordon G, Catalano M (1996) Dose-range and dose-frequency study of recombinant human interleukin-1 receptor antagonist in patients with rheumatoid arthritis. *Arthritis Rheum* 39: 1092–1101
17 Evans CH, Ghivizzani SC, Kang R, Muzzonigro T, Wasko MC, Herndon JH, Robbins PD (1999) Gene therapy for rheumatic diseases. *Arthritis Rheum* 42: 1–16
18 Bandara G, Robbins PD, Georgescu HI, Mueller GM, Glorioso JC, Evans CH (1992) Gene transfer to synoviocytes: prospects for gene treatment of arthritis. *DNA Cell Biol* 11: 227–231
19 Arend WP, Dayer JM (1995) Inhibition of the production and effects of interleukin-1 and tumor necrosis factor alpha in rheumatoid arthritis. *Arthritis Rheum* 38: 151–160
20 Schwab JH, Anderle SK, Brown RR, Dalldorf FR, Thompson RC (1989) Pro- and anti-inflammatory effects of interleukin-1in recurrence of bacterial, cell wall-induced arthritis in rats. *Infect Immunol* 59: 4436–4442
21 Wooley PH, Whalen JD, Chapman DL, Berger AE, Richard KA, Aspar DG, Staite ND (1993) The effect of interleukin-1 receptor antagonist protein on type II collagen-induced arthritis and antigen-induced arthritis in mice. *Arthritis Rheum* 36: 1305–1312
22 Hung GL, Galea-lauri J, Mueller GM, Georgescu HI, Larkin LA, Tindal M., Robbins PD, Evans CH (1993) Suppression of intraarticular responses to interleukin-1 by transfer of the interleukin-1 receptor antagonist gene to synovium. *Gene Ther* 1: 64–69
23 Otani K, Nita I, Macaulay W, Georgescu HI, Robbins PD, Evans CH (1996) Suppression of antigen-induced arthritis in rabbits by *ex vivo* gene therapy. *J Immunol* 156: 3558–3562
24 Makarov SS, Olsen JC, Johnston WN, Anderle SK, Brown RR, Baldwin AS, Haskill JS,

Schwab JH (1996) Suppression of experimental arthritis by gene transfer of interleukin-1 receptor antagonist cDNA. *Proc Natl Acad Sci USA* 93: 402–406

25 Bakker AC, Joosten LAB, Arntz OJ, Helser MMA, Bendele AM, Van De Loo FAJ, Van den Berg WB (1997) Prevention of murine collagen-induced arthritis in the knee and ipsilateral paw by local expression of human interleukin-1 receptor antagonist protein in the knee. *Arthritis Rheum* 40: 893–900

26 Evans CH, Robbins PD, Ghivizzani SC, Herndon JH, Kang R, Bahnson AB, Barranger JA, Elders EM, Gay S, Tomaino MM et al (1996) Clinical trial to assess the safety, feasibility, and efficacy of transferring a potentially antiarthritic cytokine gene to human joints with rheumatoid arthritis. *Hum Gene Ther* 7: 1261–1280

Cytokine gene therapy of allergic airways inflammation

Alistair J. Ramsay[1], *Simon P. Hogan*[3], *Paul S. Foster*[3] *and Yelin Xiong*[2]

[1]Discipline of Immunology and Microbiology, Faculty of Medicine, University of Newcastle, Newcastle NSW 2300, Australia; Divisions of [2]Immunology and Cell Biology and [3]Biochemistry and Molecular Biology, The John Curtin School of Medical Research, Australian National University, Canberra ACT 0200, Australia

Introduction

Although the chain of events leading to asthma is highly complex, the dysregulated production of type 2 cytokines, notably IL-4 and IL-5, by allergen-specific T cells, has emerged as an important causative factor [1, 2]. The symptoms of allergic asthma, including reversible airways occlusion and airways hyperreactivity (AHR), correlate with a local infiltration of the airways mucosa by inflammatory cells, whose recruitment and activation is influenced by IL-3, IL-4, IL-5, granulocyte-macrophage colony stimulating factor and other chemotactic agents produced by activated Th2 cells [3–6]. Indeed, the severity of disease appears to correlate with the degree of airways inflammation and the level of local Th2 cell activity [7, 8]. The molecular and cellular mechanisms underlying the presence of large numbers of Th2 cells in allergic airways remain to be resolved, however their products appear to have profound and specific effects in promoting allergic disease. IL-5, for example, regulates all stages of the development of eosinophils, which are consistently the predominant leukocyte population in the inflammatory infiltrate of asthmatics [5]. IL-4 modulates mast cell activity [4] and, through its influence on Ig class switching, regulates the production of IgE [3] which may specifically sensitize inflammatory cells implicated in allergic airways disease, including mast cells, eosinophils, basophils and macrophages. This leads to the release of inflammatory substances including histamine, leukotrienes, platelet-activating factor, cationic proteins and chemokines which may, in turn, augment the inflammatory process. *In vivo* studies in murine models of allergic airways inflammation have also strongly implicated Th2 cells and/or their products in the pathogenesis of allergic asthma. Firstly, antibody-mediated depletion of $CD4^+$ T cells or IL-5 abrogates eosinophilia and AHR associated with disease [9, 10]. Secondly, IL-4-deficiency may result in marked attenuation of inflammation, either by its effects on Th2 cell-derived IL-5 production and eosinophil recruitment [11], or through modulation of IgE production and mast cell activity [12]. Thirdly, we have shown that allergen-induced eosinophilia, damage to airways epithelium and airways hyperreactivity are abol-

Gene Therapy in Inflammatory Diseases, edited by C. H. Evans and P. D. Robbins

ished in IL-5-deficient mice but are restored following reconstitution of IL-5 production [13].

Cytokines produced by Th1-type cells inhibit Th2 cell development and have been shown to suppress Th2-driven immune responses [14–16]. IL-12 is a recently-described heterodimeric cytokine which strongly promotes naive $CD4^+$ T cell differentiation to the Th1 phenotype and suppresses the expression of type 2 cytokines [17–19]. IL-12 is produced largely by APCs and is a critical regulator of Th1-driven immune responses, greatly enhancing T cell and NK cell production of interferon-γ (IFNγ) and IL-2 and inducing lytic functions of CTL and NK cells [20]. An increasing number of studies have reported that rIL-12 has adjuvant effects on both cell-mediated and humoral immune responses when used in vaccines against a variety of infectious diseases [21–24] and may also suppress potentially damaging Th2-driven responses against parasites and allergens [17, 25–30]. These effects were mediated largely through the activity of IFNγ, although there is evidence that IL-12 may also down regulate IL-4 expression and Th2-driven immune responses independently of IFNγ [26–28].

Gene therapy has been used, both experimentally and clinically, as a tool for modifying the progression of a number of diseases [31]. We have shown that localized, transient gene expression achieved following immunization with a single inoculum of poxviral vectors encoding immune modifiers, particularly cytokines, selectively modulated host immune responses in a profound manner [32–34]. Here, we have engineered recombinant vaccinia virus (VV) vectors and DNA vaccines designed to deliver genes encoding type 1 cytokines to respiratory tissues in order to establish their effectiveness in the treatment of allergic airways disease. In our disease model, exposure to aeroallergen induces airways inflammation and AHR which are strongly associated with eosinophilia and localized expression of type 2 cytokines [13]. Using this approach, we have shown that vector-directed gene transfer of type 1 cytokines into the lungs of sensitized mice resulted in the suppression of local type 2 cytokine production and prevented the development of allergic airways disease and AHR to cholinergic stimuli.

A murine model for allergic airways disease

For the purpose of these studies we have employed a mouse model of allergic airways disease which is based on many published studies and is illustrated in Figure 1. In the basic model, mice were sensitised by two intraperitoneal injections with the dietary protein ovalbumin (OVA) in adjuvant (50 μg OVA/1 mg alhydrogel) on days 0 and 12, whilst control mice were given saline in alhydrogel. On day 24 of the protocol, sensitized mice were exposed to aerosolized OVA (10 mg/ml in normal saline) for 3 × 30 min periods at hourly intervals and this procedure was repeated every second day for 7 days (i.e. 4 days of exposure over 7 days). Non-sensitized (control)

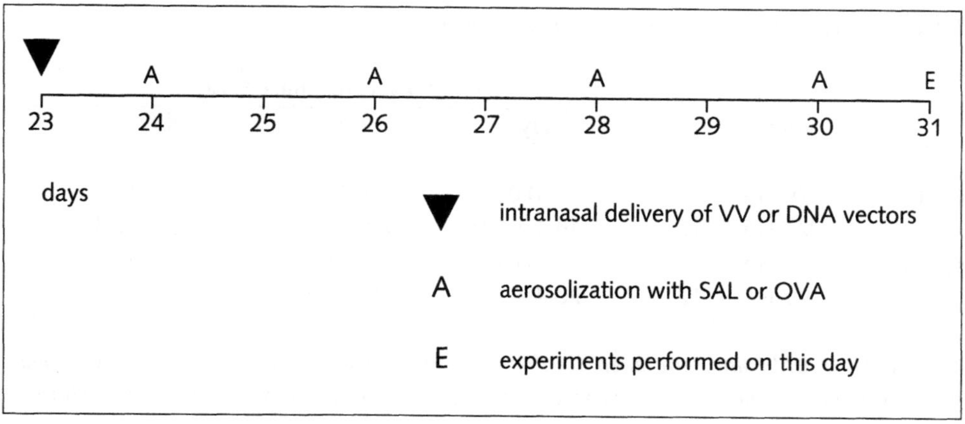

Figure 1
The vector delivery and aeroallergen challenge protocol used in these studies. Mice were sensitized with OVA by intraperitoneal injection on days 0 and 12.

mice were given aerosolized saline without OVA. Mice were sacrificed at different times for assessment of disease, although in most cases this was done 24 h after the last aeroallergen challenge. This treatment protocol resulted in eosinophilic lung inflammation which was widespread but mostly observed in the peribronchial and perivascular regions. Eosinophilia correlated with the development of gross alterations in the structural integrity of the airway walls and with microvascular leakage, mucosal edema and particulate exudation in the lumina of the airways. Inflammation following allergen challenge was also directly associated with AHR to the spasmogen, β-methacholine. The above-mentioned manifestations of disease resemble those occurring in late phase asthma and we have described them in more detail elsewhere [13].

Construction of vectors for mucosal cytokine gene therapy

We used both recombinant VV and DNA vaccines as vectors for delivering cytokine genes, particularly IL-12 and IFNγ, for the treatment of allergic airways inflammation in this model. Each of the vectors was constructed according to established protocols as detailed elsewhere [35, 36]. For example, the construction procedure for rVV involved removal of the coding sequence for the p40 subunit of murine IL-12 from the plasmid pED40 as an *Eco*RI fragment, subcloning into pBluescript KS, removal as a *Bam*HI/*Hind*III fragment and ligation into the VV plasmid pPS7.5A to create the plasmid, pPS7.5A-p40. We amplified the coding sequence for the p35 subunit from pED35 by PCR as a *Xho*I fragment, subcloned it into pBluescript KS and

Table 1 - Levels of IL-12 in BALF and sera of mice given rVV

	virus	IL-12 levels (ng/ml ± SEM) day 1	day 3	day 5
BALF	VV-HA-X	<0.01	<0.01	<0.01
	VV-HA-IL-12	15.4 ± 5.9	29.1 ± 9.5	22.2 ± 6.3
serum	VV-HA-X	<0.01	<0.01	<0.01
	VV-HA-IL-12	20.4 ± 4.3	38.1 ± 7.8	35.2 ± 5.6

IL-12 levels in BALF and sera taken at intervals from mice given rVV vectors i.n. were measured by bioassay. Data are expressed as mean levels ± SEM groups of 4 mice at each time point.

ligated it into the VV plasmid pSC65 as a *SalI/KpnI* fragment. A *Hind*III fragment, containing the PSE/L promoter and p35 was removed from this vector and subcloned into pPS7.5A-p40 in the reverse orientation distal to the p40 fragment. *In vitro* homologous recombination of the resultant plasmid with the recombinant virus VV-HA-TK$^-$ [37] gave rise to VVHA-IL-12, which contained the genes for p35 and p40 together with the herpes simplex virus thymidine kinase (TK) gene in the VV *Hind*III F region and the HA gene of influenza virus, strain A/PR/8, in the J region. VV-HA-X was used as the control virus [35]. Testing of VV-HA-IL-12 for IL-12 expression, using bioassay of 24 h supernatants taken from virus infected 143B cell monolayers, confirmed that biologically active IL-12 was secreted by this construct. Production of IL-12 in mice given this vector, but not in mice given the control vector, VV-HA-X, was confirmed by bioassay of serum samples and bronchoalveolar lavage fluid (BALF) taken up to 5 days after infection via the intranasal route (Tab. 1). This confirmed that VV-HA-IL-12 was able to sustain expression of IL-12 both locally in the lungs and systemically for a significant period following infection. In the case of DNA vaccines, bioassay of supernatants overlying transfected 143B cells confirmed their expression of IL-12 *in vitro*, whilst reverse transcriptase PCR analysis of pulmonary tissues indicated local expression of vector-directed IL-12 for up to 30 days after their delivery into the lungs.

The influence of vector-directed cytokine expression on allergic airways inflammation, AHR, cytokine production and antibody responses

To establish whether IL-12 gene transfer could ameliorate the airways inflammation and AHR which occurs following exposure to allergen, sensitized wild-type mice were given either a single intranasal inoculum of the vector VV-HA-IL-12, or an

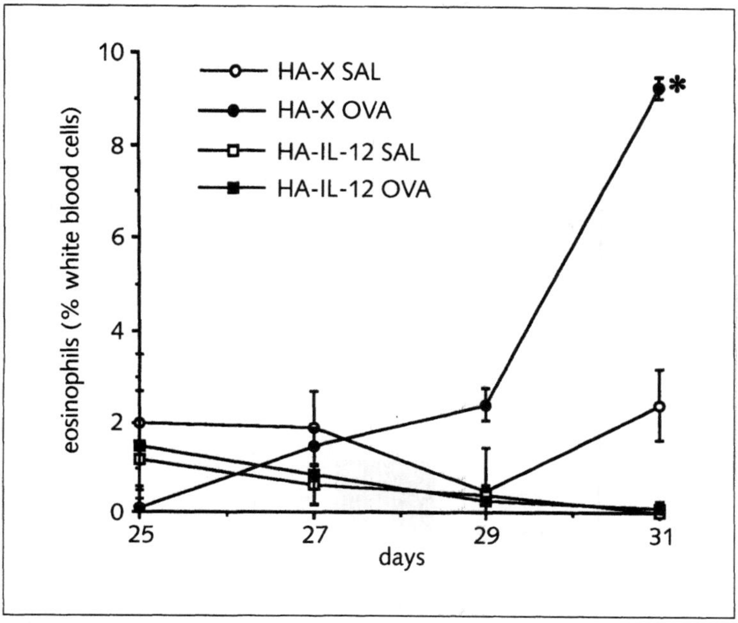

Figure 2
*Eosinophil numbers in peripheral blood in C57BL/6 mice given VV-HA-X or VV-HA-IL-12. Mice were sensitized and treated with virus and aeroallergen as described in Materials and Methods and according to the protocol outlined in Figure 1. Data represent the mean ± SEM for groups of five mice. *$p < 0.005$ compared with mice given VV-HA-IL-12 and aerosolized OVA.*

intratracheal dose of a cocktail of the DNA vaccines encoding p35 and p40 and mixed in lipofectamine, at 1 day prior to aeroallergen challenge (see Fig. 1). Aerosol challenge of mice sensitized with OVA and given the control vector, VV-HA-X resulted in a significant increase in numbers of eosinophils in the bloodstream (Fig. 2) and BALF (Fig. 3) in comparison to control mice given aerosolized saline. Pulmonary eosinophilic inflammation was widespread and was directly associated with AHR to β-methacholine (Fig. 4) occurring at similar levels to those observed in sensitized mice challenged with OVA but not given the control vector. In sharp contrast, aerosol challenge of sensitized animals given VV-HA-IL-12 did not induce eosinophilia in the blood (Fig. 2), whilst airways eosinophilia was markedly reduced (Fig. 3) and AHR was detected only at similar levels to those observed in controls (Fig. 4). Histological examination revealed only minimal morphological changes in the airways of the VV-HA-IL-12-treated animals, indeed their lungs resembled those from mice that had not been actively sensitized, except that highly localized pockets of non-eosinophilic, lymphocytic inflammation were seen and correlated with

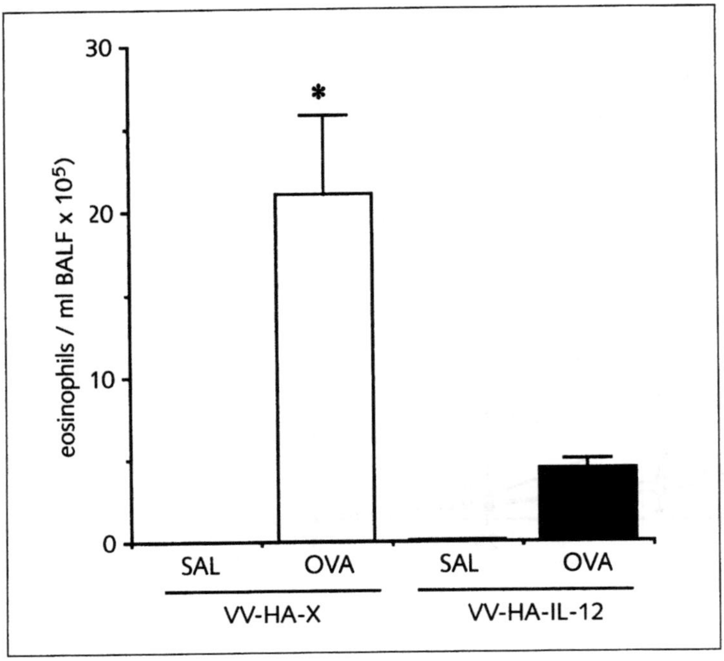

Figure 3
*Eosinophil numbers in BALF on day 31 in C57BL/6 mice given VV-HA-X or VV-HA-IL-12. Mice were sensitized and treated with virus and aeroallergen as described in Figure 2. Data represent the mean ± SEM for groups of five mice. Differences between experimental groups on day 31 were analyzed. *$p < 0.005$ compared with mice given VV-HA-IL-12 and aerosolized OVA.*

sites of vector virus infection. Both IL-12-encoding and control vectors displayed similar tissue tropism, with foci of infected cells localised near airways. Importantly, none of the symptoms of allergic airways disease were seen in sensitized mice infected with either of the viral vectors in the absence of aeroallergen.

The intratracheal instillation of DNA vaccines encoding IL-12 also resulted in many of the protective effects against allergic airways disease mediated by VV encoding this factor. When DNA-IL-12 was administered to sensitized mice at 1 day prior to aeroallergen exposure (see Fig. 1), eosinophil numbers in BALF were markedly reduced and the histological appearance of treated lung tissues following the full course of exposure to aerosolized OVA was similar to that seen in control mice.

Examination of cytokine expression by T cells isolated from the lungs of aeroallergen-treated mice given control VV or DNA vaccine and which exhibited allergic disease revealed marked expression of IL-4 and IL-5 but low expression of IFNγ

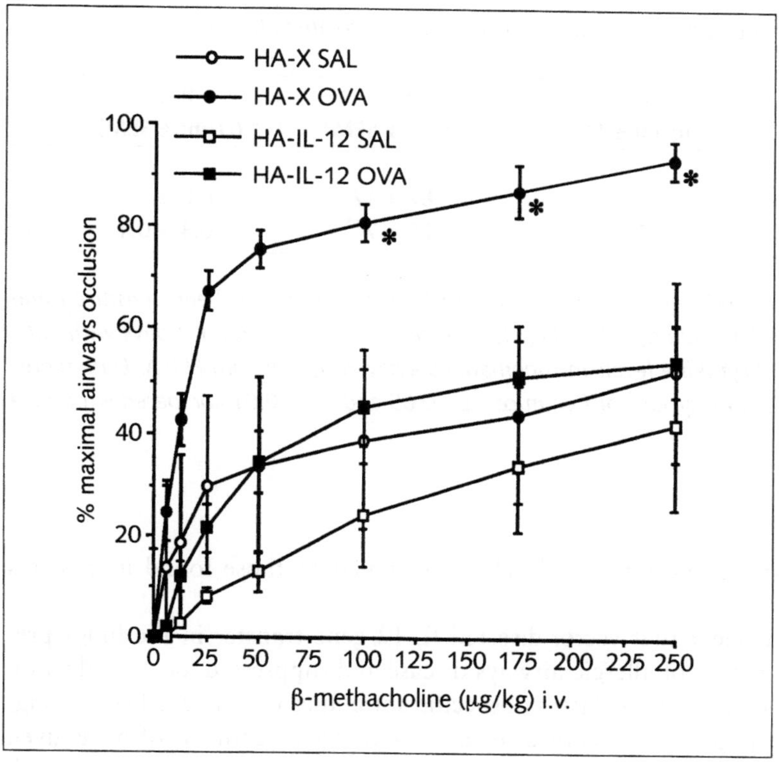

Figure 4
*Airways hyperreactivity on day 31 in C57BL/6 mice given VV-HA-X or VV-HA-IL-12. Mice were sensitized and treated with virus and aeroallergen as described in Figure 2. Airways constriction was measured with a bronchospasm transducer and analyses were performed during cumulative intravenous administration of β-methacholine as previously described [13]. The increase in respiratory overflow volume provoked by β-methacholine was represented as a percentage of the maximal overflow volume (100%) obtained by totally occluding the tracheal cannula. Data represent the mean ± SEM for groups of five mice. *$p < 0.05$ compared with mice given VV-HA-IL-12 and aerosolized OVA.*

(Tab. 2), which were similar to the profiles seen in mice exposed to aeroallergen but not given either of the vectors. In comparison, lung T cells from mice given VV or DNA encoding IL-12, and which were protected from allergic disease as described above, produced much lower levels of the type 2 cytokines but marked increases in levels of IFNγ production, indeed a 20-fold increase in the case of VV-HA-IL-12 (Tab. 2). Serum levels of OVA-specific antibodies of the type 2 cytokine-dependent IgE and IgG1 subclassess were also reduced in mice given VV encoding IL-12, while

Table 2 - Cytokine production by lung T cells from vector-treated allergic mice

Virus treatment	IFNγ (ng/ml ± SEM)	IL-4 (ng/ml ± SEM)	IL-5 (U/ml ± SEM)
VV-HA-X	9 ± 1	82 ± 12	6.8 ± 2.7
VV-HA-IL-12	272 ± 10**	25 ± 7**	0.3 ± 0.1*

*Lung cells were isolated, on day 31, from C57BL/6 mice which had been sensitized and treated with VV and aeroallergen (see Fig. 1). The cells were cultured for 3 days with anti-CD3 antibodies and cytokine levels in supernatants assayed by standard ELISA. Data represent the mean ± SEM for groups of five mice. *$p < 0.05$ and **$p < 0.01$ compared with mice given VV-HA-X.*

their OVA-specific IgG2a antibody levels were similar to those found in controls (Fig. 5).

Overall, it was clear that vector-directed IL-12 gene transfer in the lungs prevented the development of allergic airways disease and suppressed local production of the type 2 cytokines and subclasses of specific antibodies which have been strongly implicated in the pathogenesis of disease. Aeroallergen treatment of mice given control vector, not encoding IL-12, induced gross lung pathology associated with the activity of a local $CD4^+$ Th2-type cell population despite the VV infection, however this was not seen in animals given VV-HA-IL-12. T cells isolated from the latter secreted mainly IFNγ, with no evidence of eosinophilia and minimal morphological changes in their airways. The VV-HA-IL-12 construct nevertheless replicated sufficiently well to provide measurable levels of IL-12 in both the lungs and bloodstream for at least 5 days after infection. Others have shown that repeated administration of recombinant IL-12 or IFNγ protein inhibited allergic airways inflammation [28–30, 38, 39] and, in some cases, AHR, although regular or daily doses over long periods were usually required. However, our data clearly show both the efficacy and the safety of transient IL-12 expression following a single inoculum of either replicating (VV) or non-replicating (DNA) delivery vectors in selectively modulating allergic responses in mice whose specific immune responses were already committed to a Th2 phenotype.

Long-term protective and therapeutic effects of IL-12

The studies outlined above have clearly shown that vector-directed IL-12 suppresses allergic airways inflammation when constructs are administered to sensitized

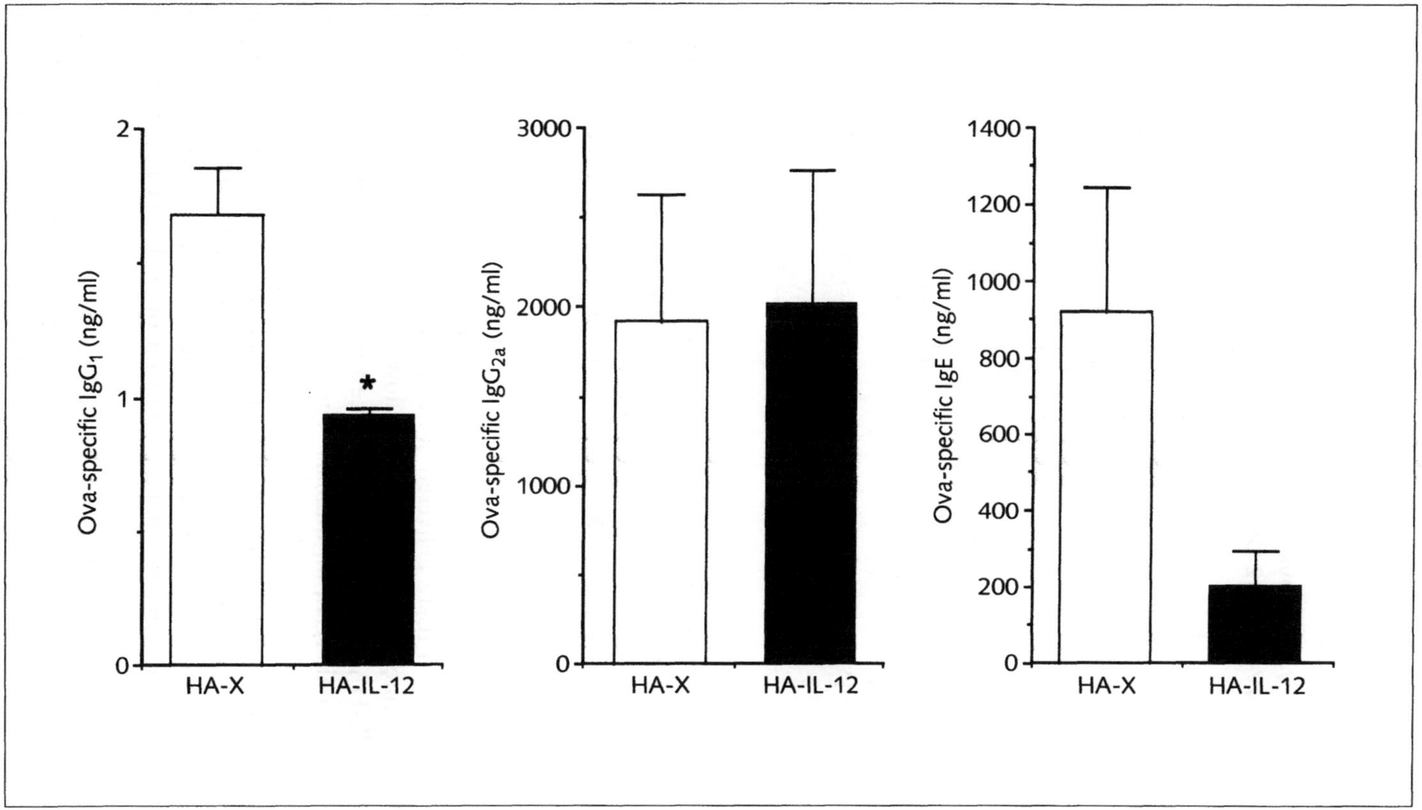

Figure 5

OVA-specific IgG1, IgG2a and IgE antibody levels on day 31 in serum from C57BL/6 mice sensitized and treated with virus and aeroallergen as described in Figure 2. Data represent the mean ± SEM for groups of five mice. $^{*}p < 0.05$ *compared with mice given VV-HA-X.*

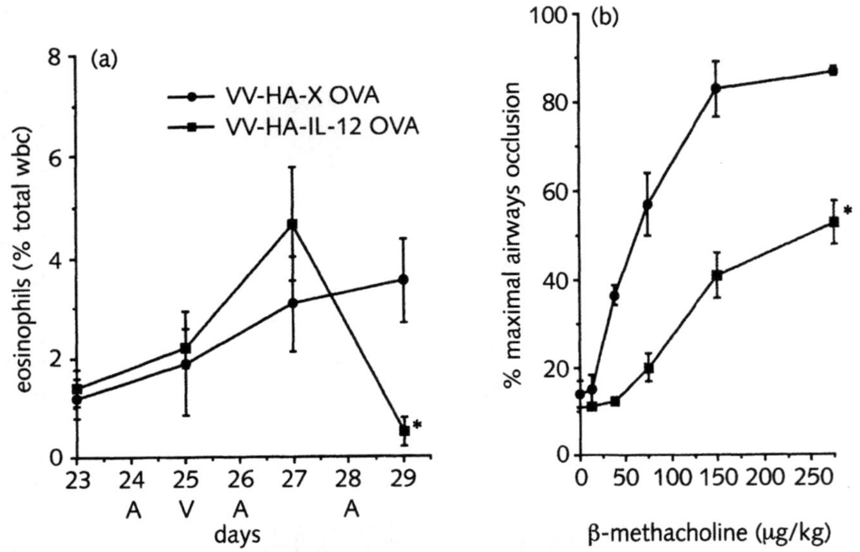

Figure 6
*(a) Eosinophil numbers in peripheral blood, and (b) airways hyperreactivity to β-methacholine on day 30, in C57Bl/6 mice. Mice were sensitized as described in Figure 2, and treated with aeroallergen (A) and given VV-HA-X or VV-HA-IL-12 (V) on the days indicated. Data represent the mean ± SEM for groups of five mice. *$p < 0.05$ compared with mice given VV-HA-X and aerosolized OVA.*

animals just prior to a subsequent course of exposure to aeroallergen. It is also important to establish that IL-12 delivered in this manner can provide longer term protection. When an interval of 4 weeks was allowed to lapse between intranasal administration of VV-HA-IL-12 to sensitized mice and the beginning of their course of treatment with aeroallergen, all animals remained fully protected against airways eosinophilic inflammation and AHR, demonstrating that our approach confers sustained protection against disease. It will be of great interest to determine both the degree to which the interval between delivery of VV-HA-IL-12 and challenge can be extended, and also the longer term protective effects of DNA vaccines given the persistent nature and sustained expression of IL-12 mediated by these vectors.

The therapeutic activity of vector-directed IL-12 (i.e. ability to reverse or suppress established airways inflammation) was also tested by treating mice at 1 day after either the initial or secondary aerosol treatments (days 25 or 27 in Fig. 1). In each case, the eosinophilic inflammation, AHR and airways disease which developed in aeroallergen-treated mice given the control vector were suppressed in mice given VV-HA-IL-12 (Fig. 6), suggesting that our approach has not only protective but also therapeutic potential for the treatment of allergic airways disease.

Immune mechanisms underlying the protective activity of vector-encoded IL-12

Since we had observed a marked enhancement of T cell expression of IFNγ in the lungs of mice given the IL-12 vectors, we reasoned that this factor might play an important role in mediating the protection against allergic airways disease afforded by IL-12 in our model. To explore this further, we used mice which lacked IFNγ function through disruption of the gene encoding the IFNγ receptor, IFNγ$R^{-/-}$ mice [40]. Sensitization and subsequent exposure to aeroallergen (see Fig. 1) led to the development of allergic airways disease in both IFNγ$R^{-/-}$ and control wild-type mice. However, whilst treatment of the latter with VV-HA-IL-12 was protective against disease, its effects in suppressing AHR (Fig. 7) and lung eosinophilia were abolished in the IFNγR mutants. Inhibition of blood eosinophilia was also reversed (Fig. 7), although not completely, and histological studies revealed airways disease which was less severe although still clearly discernible in these animals. Thus, it appears that IFNγ may play a central role in mediating the protective effects of vector-encoded IL-12 expression in our model, although at least some of the activity of IL-12 appears to be exerted independently of this factor.

In immunocompetent animals, the marked increases in local production of IFNγ observed following IL-12 gene transfer were probably mediated via enhancement of Th1-type lung T cell activity with a concomitant down regulation of expression of IL-4 and IL-5. These factors are strongly implicated in the pathogenesis of allergic asthma through their influence on IgE production, mast cell activity and eosinophil development [3–5]. Others have shown that daily exposure of mice to IFNγ aerosols over several days suppressed airways eosinophilia and specific IgE production in response to aeroallergen challenge [38, 39], probably via down regulation of local Th2 cell activity, although IFNγ may also directly influence the function of eosinophils, mast cells and inhibit IgE B cell switching [41–43]. Our studies, however, suggest that gene transfer of IFNγ is far less protective against allergic airways disease than IL-12 (unpublished), despite a recent report of suppression of some symptoms of disease mediated by intratracheal delivery of DNA encoding IFNγ [44]. IL-12, unlike IFNγ, may persist for many hours in body fluids and its production by cells carrying VV or DNA vectors could provide a continuous local stimulus for the secretion of IFNγ by the host. It is also possible that IL-12 may exert additional direct, IFNγ-independent inhibitory effects on IL-4 expression, Th2-driven immune responses and inflammatory cells [26–28].

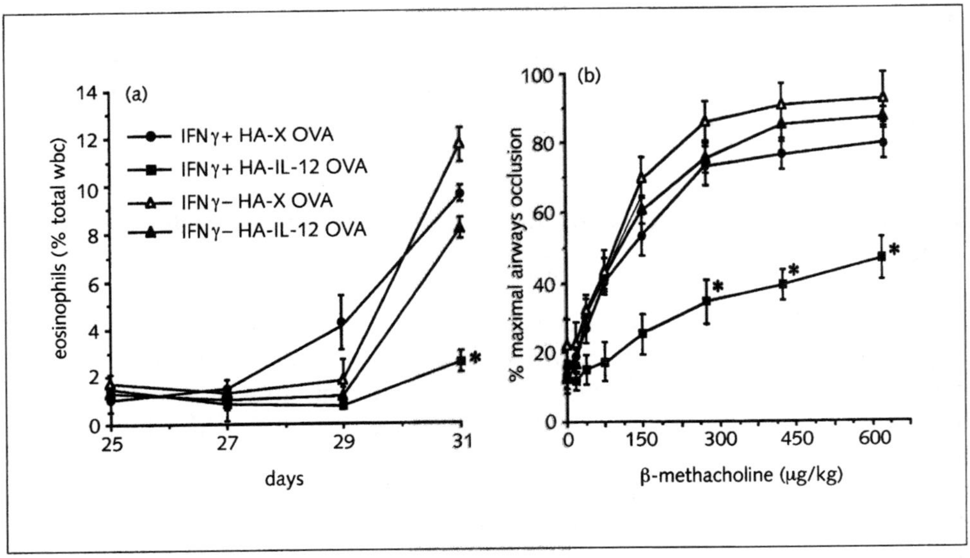

Figure 7
*(a) Eosinophil numbers in peripheral blood, and (b) airways hyperreactivity to β-methacholine on day 31, in 129/Sv/Ev wild-type (IFNγ⁺) and IFNγR⁻/⁻ (IFNγ⁻) mice. Mice were sensitized and treated with virus and aerosol as described in Figure 2. Data represent the mean ± SEM for groups of five mice. *p < 0.05 compared with IFNγ⁻ mice given VV-HA-IL-12 and aerosolized OVA.*

A synthesis of these findings suggests that IL-12 may have the capacity to inhibit multiple pathways contributing to allergic airways disease and AHR. One of the ways in which these effects might be mediated is via IFNγ-directed down regulation of the allergen-specific $CD4^+$ T cell phenotype and, therefore, IL-4 and IL-5 production. For example, in the present study, we have established our model in immunocompetent mice of both the C57Bl/6 and 129/Sv/Ev strains (wild-type controls for $IFN\gamma R^{-/-}$ mice). We had previously shown that allergic lung disease in C57Bl/6 mice is critically dependent upon antigen-induced eosinophil influx mediated by IL-5 [13], indeed these animals may be resistant to the induction of mast cell-dependent airways disease through their inability to produce mast cell protease 7 and secretory phospholipase A_2 [45]. In other strains, including 129/Sv/Ev mice, allergic airways disease and AHR can occur independently of eosinophilia and may be mediated by IgE-activated mast cell activity promoted by IL-4 [12]. We have demonstrated that IL-12 is protective in both C57Bl/6 and 129/Sv/Ev mice, even in the presence of circulating antigen-specific IgE antibodies. Further possible mechanisms underlying the activity of IL-12 in our model include a selective enhancement of Th1-type cell migration into pulmonary tissues and an inhibitory influence on the development and/or activity of inflammatory cells, mediated either directly or through up regulation of host IFNγ production.

Conclusions and prospects

Recent studies have provided convincing evidence that Th2-type immunity is the major component of the allergic asthmatic immune response. Thus, increased understanding of the regulation of Th2-type inflammatory immune responses, and of how such responses may be specifically inhibited, should facilitate the development of preventive measures and effective therapies against allergic airways disease. Further cytokines, particularly type 1 factors such as IL-12, are known to promote Th1 cell development, to inhibit Th2 cell development and to suppress Th2-driven immune responses. We have engineered the genes encoding murine IL-12 into rVV for use in a murine model of allergic airways disease in attempts to achieve sustained expression of IL-12 at appropriate sites and times and, hopefully, suppression of local type 2 cytokine secretion. A single intranasal inoculum of these constructs in sensitized mice prior to aeroallergen challenge was sufficient to confer protection against eosinophilic inflammation, lung damage and AHR in conjunction with a suppression of local $CD4^+$ T cell production of type 2 cytokines. Protection against airways disease lasted for at least 4 weeks and, in addition, VV-encoded IL-12 was highly effective in suppressing established allergic inflammation, demonstrating its therapeutic efficacy. The ability of IL-12 to stimulate host production of IFNγ appeared to be an important component of its protective effects, which were markedly attenuated in mice which lacked IFNγ function.

We have also developed non-replicating delivery vectors, including DNA vaccines, which have the potential advantages of (i) longer-term persistence in the host, and (ii) a capacity to be used for repeated immunisation in the same individual, due largely to the fact that they elicit little or no host immunity against vector components [46]. DNA vaccines encoding IL-12 genes sustained expression of this factor for at least 30 days in the lungs following a single intratracheal instillation. Furthermore, their protective efficacy against allergic airways inflammation and disease was as great as that mediated by our VV constructs. It will be of interest to determine the extent to which longer-term protective and therapeutic effects are mediated by these vectors given their persistent nature.

Recent reports from large scale epidemiological studies have suggested that exposure in early childhood to infectious agents which promote type 1 immune responses, such as measles virus or *Mycobacterium tuberculosis*, may inhibit the subsequent development of allergic disorders, including asthma, via immune deviation and suppression of type 2 responses [47, 48]. Such results require careful interpretation, given the complexity of the environmental and immunological contribution to asthma [49, 50] and evidence that severe bacterial or virus infection may actually trigger atopic episodes [51]. Nevertheless, attempts to inhibit allergen-specific Th2-mediated immune responses appear to represent an attractive approach to the prevention and/or treatment of allergic asthma. Such strategies, including IL-12 gene transfer, either with or without co-expression of genes encoding allergens, may also facilitate the establishment of specific protective type 1 immune responses, particularly in young individuals.

Acknowledgments
We thank Drs. Michel Aguet and Sui Huang (University of Zurich, Switzerland) for the 129/Sv/Ev wild-type and IFNγ$R^{-/-}$ mice, Dr. Stanley Wolf (Genetics Institute, Cambridge, MA) for providing the pED35 and pED40 plasmids, Dr. Giorgio Trinchieri (Wistar Institute, Philadelphia, PA) for the C15.6 mAb, Drs. Patricia Earl and Bernard Moss (National Institutes of Health, Bethesda, MD) for the pSC65 construct and Dr. Guna Karupiah (JCSMR, Canberra) for IFNγ ELISA reagents.

References

1 Leung DYM, Martin RJ, Szefler SJ, Sher ER, Ying S, Kay AB, Hamid Q (1995) Dysregulation of interleukin 4, interleukin 5 and interferon gamma gene expression in steroid-resistant asthma. *J Exp Med* 181: 33–40
2 Robinson DS, Hamid Q, Ying S, Tsicopoulos A, Barkans J, Bentley AM, Corrigan C, Durham SR, Kay AB (1992) Predominant TH2-like bronchoalveolar T-lymphocyte population in atopic asthma. *New Eng J Med* 326: 298–304
3 Geha RS (1992) Regulation of IgE synthesis in humans. *J Allergy Clin Immunol* 90: 143–150
4 Madden KB, Urban JF Jr, Ziltener HJ, Schrader JW, Finkelman FD, Katona IM (1991) Antibodies to IL-3 and IL-4 suppress helminth-induced intestinal mastocytosis. *J Immunol* 147: 1387–1391
5 Sanderson CJ (1992) Interleukin-5, eosinophils, and disease. *Blood* 79: 3101–3109
6 Garcia-Zepeda EA, Rothenberg ME, Ownbey RT, Celestin J, Leder P, Luster AD (1996) Human eotaxin is a specific chemoattractant for eosinophil cells and provides a new mechanism to explain tissue eosinophilia. *Nature Med* 2: 449–456
7 Azzawi M, Bradley B, Jeffery PK, Frew AJ, Wardlaw AJ, Knowles G, Assoufi B, Collins JV, Durham S, Kay AB (1990) Identification of activated T lymphocytes and eosinophils in bronchial biopsies in stable atopic asthma. *Am Rev Respir Dis* 142: 1407–1413
8 Bentley AM, Maestrelli P, Saetta M, Fabbri LM, Robinson DS, Bradley BL, Jeffery PK, Durham SR, Kay AB (1992) Activated T-lymphocytes and eosinophils in the bronchial mucosa in isocyanate-induced asthma. *J Allergy Clin Immunol* 89: 821–829
9 Kung TT, Stelts DM, Zurcher JA, Adams GK, Egan RW, Kreutner W, Watnick AS, Jones

H, Chapman RW (1995) Involvement of IL-5 in a murine model of allergic pulmonary inflammation: prophylactic and therapeutic effect of an anti-IL-5 antibody. *Am J Respir Cell Mol Biol* 13: 360–365

10 Nakajima H, Iwamoto I, Tomoe S, Matsumura R, Tomioka H, Takatsu K, Yoshida S (1992) $CD4^+$ T-lymphocytes and interleukin-5 mediate antigen-induced eosinophil infiltration into the mouse trachea. *Am Rev Respir Dis* 146: 374–377

11 Brusselle GG, Kips JC, Tavernier JH, Van Der Heyden JG, Cuvelier CA, Pauwels RA, Bluethmann H (1994) Attenuation of allergic airway inflammation in IL-4 deficient mice. *Clin Exp Allergy* 24: 73–80

12 Corry DB, Folkesson HG, Warnock ML, Erle DJ, Matthay MA, Wiener-Kronish JP, Locksley RC (1996) Interleukin 4, but not interleukin 5 or eosinophils, is required in an acute model of airway hyperrreactivity. *J Exp Med* 183: 109–117

13 Foster PS, Hogan SP, Ramsay AJ, Matthaei KI, Young IG (1996) Interleukin 5 deficiency abolishes eosinophilia, airways hyperreactivity, and lung damage in a mouse asthma model. *J Exp Med* 183: 195–201

14 Snapper CM, Paul WE (1987) Interferon-γ and B cell stimulatory factor-1 reciprocally regulate Ig isotype production. *Science* 236: 944–947

15 Mosmann TR, Coffman RL (1989) TH1 and TH2 cells: different patterns of lymphokine secretion lead to different functional properties. *Ann Rev Immunol* 7: 145–173

16 Yssel H, Schneider P, Spits H (1993) Production of IL-4 by human T cells and regulation of differentiation of T-cell subsets by IL-4. *Res Immunol* 144: 610–616

17 Manetti R, Parronchi P, Giudizi MG, Piccinni MP, Maggi E, Trinchieri G, Romagnani S (1993) Natural killer cell stimulatory factor (interleukin 12 [IL-12]) induces T helper type 1 (Th1)-specific immune responses and inhibits the development of IL-4-producing Th cells. *J Exp Med* 177: 1199–1204

18 Seder RA, Gazzinelli R, Sher A, Paul WE (1993) Interleukin 12 acts directly on CD4+ T cells to enhance priming for interferon gamma production and diminishes interleukin 4 inhibition of such priming. *Proc Natl Acad Sci USA* 90: 10188–10192

19 Hsieh CS, Macatonia SE, Tripp CS, Wolf SF, O'Garra A, Murphy KM (1993) Development of TH1 CD4+ T cells through IL-12 produced by Listeria-induced macrophages. *Science* 260: 547–549

20 Trinchieri G (1995) Interleukin-12: a proinflammatory cytokine with immunoregulatory functions that bridge innate resistance and antigen-specific adaptive immunity. *Ann Rev Immunol* 13: 251–276

21 Alfonso LC, Scharton TM, Vieira LQ, Wysocka M, Trinchieri G, Scott P (1994) The adjuvant effect of interleukin-12 in a vaccine against Leishmania major. *Science* 263: 235–237

22 Miller MA, Skeen MJ, Ziegler HK (1995) Nonviable bacterial antigens administered with IL-12 generate antigen-specific T cell responses and protective immunity against Listeria monocytogenes. *J Immunol* 155: 4817–4828

23 Wynn TA, Cheever AW, Jankovic D, Poindexter RW, Caspar P, Lewis FA, Sher A (1995)

An IL-12-based vaccination method for preventing fibrosis induced by schistosome infection. *Nature* 376: 594–596
24 Wynn TA, Reynolds A, James S, Cheever AW, Caspar P, Hieny S, Jankovic D, Strand M, Sher A (1996) IL-12 enhances vaccine-induced immunity to Schistosomes by augmenting both humoral and cell-mediated immune responses against the parasite. *J Immunol* 157: 4068–4078
25 Oswald IP, Caspar P, Jankovic D, Wynn TA, Pearce EJ, Sher A (1994) IL-12 inhibits Th2 cytokine responses induced by eggs of *Schistosoma mansoni*. *J Immunol* 153: 1707–1713
26 Wang ZE, Zheng S, Corry DB, Dalton DK, Seder RA, Reiner SL, Locksley RM (1994) Interferon gamma-independent effects of interleukin 12 administered during acute or established infection due to Leishmania major. *Proc Natl Acad Sci USA* 91: 12932–12936
27 Marshall JD, Secrist H, DeKruyff RH, Wolf SF, Umetsu DT (1995) IL-12 inhibits the production of IL-4 and IL-10 in allergen-specific human $CD4^+$ T lymphocytes. *J Immunol* 155: 111–117
28 Gavett SH, O'Hearn DJ, Li X, Huang SK, Finkelman FD, Wills-Karp M (1995) Interleukin 12 inhibits antigen-induced airway hyperresponsiveness, inflammation, and Th2 cytokine expression in mice. *J Exp Med* 182: 1527–1536
29 Kips JC, Brusselle GJ, Joos GF, Peleman RA, Tavernier JH, Devos RR, Pauwels RA (1996) Interleukin-12 inhibits antigen-induced airway hyperresponsiveness in mice. *Am Rev Respir Crit Care Med* 153: 535–539
30 Sur S, Lam J, Bouchard P, Sigounas A, Holbert D, Metzger WJ (1996) Immunomodulatory effects of IL-12 on allergic lung inflammation depend on timing of doses. *J Immunol* 157: 4173–4180
31 Mulligan RC (1993) The basic science of gene therapy. *Science* 260: 926–932
32 Sharma DP, Ramsay AJ, Maguire DJ, Rolph MS, Ramshaw IA (1996) Interleukin-4 mediates down regulation of antiviral cytokine expression and cytotoxic T-lymphocyte responses and exacerbates vaccinia virus infection *in vivo*. *J Virol* 70: 7103–7107
33 Ramsay AJ, Husband AJ, Ramshaw IA, Bao S, Matthaei KI, Koehler G, Kopf M (1994) The role of interleukin-6 in mucosal IgA antibody responses *in vivo*. *Science* 264: 561–563
34 Ramshaw IA, Ramsay AJ, Karupiah G, Rolph MS, Mahalingam S, Ruby JC (1997) Cytokines and immunity to viral infection. *Immunol Rev* 159: 119–135
35 Coupar BEH, Andrew ME, Boyle DB (1988) A general method for the construction of recombinant vaccinia viruses expressing multiple foreign genes. *Gene* 68: 1–10
36 Sambrook J, Fritsch EF, Maniatis T (eds) (1989) *Molecular cloning: a laboratory manual*. Cold Spring Harbor Laboratory Press.
37 Andrew ME, Coupar BEH, Ada GL, Boyle DB (1986) Cell-mediated immune responses to influenza virus antigens expressed by vaccinia virus recombinants. *Microb Pathog* 1: 443–452
38 Lack G, Bradley KL, Hamelmann E, Renz H, Loader J, Leung DYM, Larsen G, Gelfand

EW (1996) Nebulized IFN-γ inhibits the development of secondary allergic responses in mice. *J Immunol* 157: 1432–1439
39 Nakajima H, Iwamoto I, Yoshida S (1993) Aerosolized recombinant interferon-gamma prevents antigen-induced eosinophil recruitment in mouse trachea. *Am Rev Respir Dis* 148: 1102–1104
40 Huang S, Hendriks W, Althage A, Hemmi S, Bluethmann H, Kamigo R, Vilcek J, Zinkernagel R, Aguet M (1993) Immune response in mice that lack the interferon-γ receptor. *Science* 259: 1742–1745
41 Fujisawa T, Abu-Ghazaleh R, Kita H, Sanderson CJ, Gleich GJ (1990) Regulatory effects of cytokines on eosinophil degranulation. *J Immunol* 144: 642–646
42 Coleman JW, Morris AG (1991) Identification of a spleen cell-derived factor that inhibits sensitization of murine peritoneal mast cells as interferon-γ. *Int Arch Allergy Appl Immunol* 94: 179–180
43 Gauchat JF, Lebman DA, Coffman RL, Gascan H, De Vries J (1990) Structure and expression of germline e transcripts induced by interleukin-4 to switch to IgE production. *J Exp Med* 172: 463–473
44 Li X-M, Chopra RK, Chou T-Y, Schofield BH, Wills-Karp M, Huang S-K (1996) Mucosal IFN-γ gene transfer inhibits pulmonary allergic responses in mice. *J Immunol* 157: 3216–3219
45 Drazen JM, Arm JP, Austen KF (1996) Sorting out the cytokines of asthma. *J Exp Med* 183: 1–5
46 Ramsay AJ, Leong KH, Ramshaw IA (1997) DNA vaccination against virus infection and enhancement of antiviral immunity following consecutive immunisation with DNA and viral vectors. *Immunol Cell Biol* 75: 382–388
47 Shaheen SO, Aaby P, Hall AJ, Barker D, Heyes C, Shiell AW, Goudiaby A (1996) Measles and atopy in Guinea-Bisau. *Lancet* 347: 1792–1796
48 Shirakawa T, Enomoto T, Shimazu S, Hopkin J (1997) The inverse association between tuberculin responses and atopic disorder. *Science* 275: 77–79
49 Bochner BS, Undem BJ, Lichtenstein LM (1994) Immunological aspects of allergic asthma. *Ann Rev Immunol* 12: 295–335
50 Lynch NR, Hagel I, Perez M, Di Prisco MC, Lopez R, Alvarez N (1993) Effect of anthelmintic treatment on the allergic reactivity of children in a tropical slum. *J Allergy Clin Immunol* 92: 404–411
51. Lacour M (1994) Acute infections in atopic dermatitis: a clue for a pathogenic role of a Th1/Th2 imbalance. *Dermatology* 188: 255–257

Gene therapy for inflammatory diseases of the salivary glands

Philip C. Fox[1] *and Brian C. O'Connell*[2]

[1]Amarillo Biosciences Inc., 6509 Seven Locks Road, Cabin John, MD 20818, USA; [2]Department of Restorative Dentistry, School of Dental Science, Trinity College, Dublin, Ireland

Introduction

Chronic inflammatory diseases of the salivary glands are frequently associated with progressive destruction of secretory tissue and resulting salivary hypofunction. As salivary flow is compromised, patients experience oral dryness and difficulties with chewing, swallowing, and speaking. The absence of saliva is usually incompatible with normal oral health; diminished salivary flow results in mucosal inflammation, an increased incidence of oral infection, and a susceptibility to dental decay. The symptoms of salivary hypofunction are difficult to relieve by conventional therapies: patients often carry with them bottles of liquid, which they drink frequently to relieve their dryness. Salivary replacements (artificial saliva) meet with minimal patient acceptance. Secretogogues may transiently elevate salivary output, but have systemic side-effects which may be unacceptable and are appropriate for only a subset of patients with substantial remaining secretory parenchyma. Anti-inflammatory and disease-modifying anti-rheumatic drugs are of limited effectiveness in the prevention of disease progression and have not been shown to affect the exocrine inflammatory component or restore salivary flow.

The development of gene transfer technology in the past 5 years has offered new possibilities for the treatment of salivary gland diseases [1]. Some of the hypothetical advantages of gene-based therapies are: the possibility of reversing the disease process rather than symptomatic treatment, the ability to treat the salivary glands locally, and the potential for a single, or infrequent, therapeutic intervention. The position and the structure of the major salivary glands make them attractive targets for gene transfer. The ductal orifices may be visualized intraorally directly, and cannulated without surgery or even anesthetic. In sialography, the retrograde instillation of contrast medium into the salivary glands is routinely performed as a diagnostic procedure.

The currently available gene transfer vectors have different properties that determine their clinical range. For example, retroviruses may be the vector of choice for dividing cells that can be removed from the body, infected and amplified ex vivo,

Gene Therapy in Inflammatory Diseases, edited by C. H. Evans and P. D. Robbins

Table 1 - Comparison of experiments using different methods of gene transfer to rat major salivary glands in vivo

	Efficiency of gene transfer	Duration of expression	Genes expressed	Refs.
Adenovirus	++++	11 days[1]	β-gal, luciferase[2], 1-antitrypsin, E2F1, histatin 3, AQP1, AQP5, hGH[2]	[3, 4, 25, 28, 29]
Plasmid + adenovirus	++	5 days	luciferase, hGH	[5, 9]
Retrovirus	+	43 days[1]	β-gal	[8]
Liposomes	++	3 days[1]	hGH	[9]

[1]*Represents the last day of observation reported*
[2]*Unpublished observations*

and then replaced [2]. The complex three-dimensional structure of the salivary glands and their proximity to vital structures make them poor candidates for ex vivo transduction. Moreover, the salivary gland parenchyma consists of well-differentiated epithelial cells that divide very infrequently. Hence, the most likely approach for successful gene transfer to the salivary gland would take place *in situ* and would utilize a gene delivery system that does not require cell division. Because the glands consist of an extensively branched network of ducts, any gene transfer vector introduced via the ductal system can spread easily throughout the gland and contact every epithelial cell. The ability of a vector to contact each functional cell of the gland greatly increases the efficiency of gene transfer and reduces the amount of vector needed for treatment. This view has been supported by studies in experimental animals; Table 1 summarizes the results observed with various methods of gene transfer. In each case, the genetic material was delivered by retrograde ductal infusion. We have found that adenovirus-based gene transfer to the salivary gland is consistently efficient, though the major drawback is the limited duration of gene expression [3–5]. In rats, the salivary glands appear to be particularly effective at clearing adenovirus when compared to other commonly studied organs such as liver, lung, brain or muscle [6]. A potentially complicating factor is that it has also been demonstrated that administration of adenoviral vectors can cause an inflammatory response in a dose-dependent manner [6]. Although the inflammatory response may be controlled, this issue would have to be considered carefully if a chronically inflamed gland were to be the target for virus-based gene transfer. This has been shown to be an issue in an animal model of inflammatory arthritis treated with an adenovirus vector encoding a soluble TNFα receptor [7]. The introduction of viral antigens to the glands necessarily complicates any anti-inflammatory strategy.

Other viral vectors transduce salivary gland cells with low efficiency, though adeno-associated virus seems to persist longer *in vitro* than adenovirus (unpublished observation). To date, it has not been shown that any vector can readily integrate into the chromosomes of normal salivary gland cells *in vivo* [8]. In contrast to the viral vectors, liposome-based gene transfer to the glands may have the advantage of low immunogenicity. Nonetheless, lipid-mediated gene transfer is fairly inefficient and gene expression is transient [9]. Thus, further developments in gene delivery systems will be needed before safe, effective, and stable gene transfer to the salivary glands becomes clinically practical.

Human salivary glands

There are three pairs of major salivary glands in humans: parotid, submandibular, and sublingual. They are composed of two basic components; acinar and ductal cells. The acini comprise 80% of the glandular parenchyma, the ducts 15–20%, with the remainder made up of vessels, nerves and connective tissue. The acinar cells are of the serous type in the parotid gland, the mucous type in the sublingual, and a mixture of serous and mucous in the submandibular gland. This difference in acinar type contributes to the differences in the composition of the secretions between the glands. Water transport and the majority of salivary protein production and secretion take place in the acinar region [10]. A markedly hypotonic primary saliva is secreted into the lumen of the acini. This secretion is transported into the oral cavity through a branching duct system, composed of several distinct cell types. The ducts are salt-resorbing and the modified secretion which reaches the mouth is isotonic. There also are some proteins produced and secreted by the ductal cells.

A major challenge in the development of gene delivery systems to the salivary glands is to increase their cell specificity. The vectors currently available do not permit selective targeting of salivary acinar or ductal cells (Fig. 1), though it may be feasible to induce cell-specific expression through the use of acinar or ductal cell-specific promoter elements.

The parotid gland saliva enters into the oral cavity via a main excretory duct, termed Stensen's duct, which opens on the buccal mucosa approximately opposite the maxillary molar teeth. The submandibular and sublingual glands frequently secrete through a common main duct, Wharton's duct, which enters the oral cavity under the tongue in the anterior floor of the mouth. The sublingual glands also may secrete separately through several short ducts entering in the floor of the mouth. In addition to the paired major salivary glands, there are numerous minor salivary glands located just below the mucosal surface throughout the oral cavity and the hypopharynx [11].

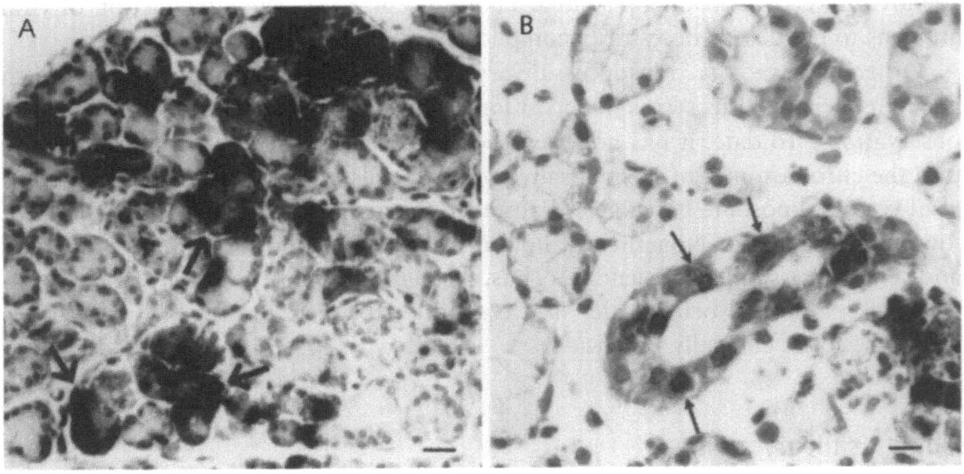

Figure 1
Adenovirus mediated gene transfer to rat submandibular gland in vivo. *The glands received AdRSV gal vector by retrograde ductal infusion. After 48 h the tissue was removed and reacted with X-gal, then processed and sectioned. (A) The dark staining demonstrates functional β-galactosidase expression in acini (large arrows; bar = 25 μm). (B) Ductal cells also expressed exogenous β-galactosidase (small arrows; bar = 11 μm).*

Salivary glands secrete fluid primarily in response to muscarinic-cholinergic stimuli. Protein secretion is mediated mainly by α- and β-adrenergic signaling. In response to maximal stimulation, such as that provided by eating, salivary function may increase 10–20-fold over basal (resting) flow rates. These elevated secretion rates can be maintained for extended periods of time (> 1 h); however, it is estimated that maximal stimulated flow is required only about 10% of the day. This stimulated flow is composed primarily of major gland secretions. The remainder of the time, a low, resting flow is maintained, which may be mainly of minor gland origin. In a 24-h period, 1–1.5 liters of saliva is secreted in humans.

Saliva is a complex fluid. In addition to serum-derived electrolytes, there are many (> 40) proteins, including several families of salivary glycoproteins [12]. As noted earlier, these play critical roles in the protection of oral and upper airway hard and soft structures and in support of oral functions. In the absence of adequate salivary function, individuals suffer serious compromises in oral and systemic health [13]. Individuals also experience increased mucosal sensitivity, mucosal ulcerations, and oral pain.

Salivary function may be altered by a number of factors. The most common causes include the effects of pharmaceuticals, anti-neoplastic therapies, and systemic diseases [14]. There are hundreds of drugs which induce symptoms of dry mouth (xerostomia) and a smaller number which have been demonstrated to reduce significantly the output of saliva. Most prominent in this latter group are anti-cholinergics, anti-hypertensives, anti-psychotics, and anti-depressants. Treatment of head and neck cancers with external beam radiotherapy or internal radionuclides, such as ^{131}I therapy for thyroid cancers, can lead to severe and permanent salivary hypofunction. Graft-versus-host disease induced by bone marrow transplantation can result in an immune-mediated salivary gland dysfunction and surgical ablation of head and neck cancers may compromise salivary function as well. There are many systemic diseases which can affect salivary performance. In particular, Sjögren's syndrome, an autoimmune exocrinopathy which will be discussed in detail below, can markedly affect salivary gland function through the progressive loss of secretory cells due to an immune-mediated chronic inflammatory infiltrate of the glands. Other systemic diseases with possible salivary involvement include cystic fibrosis, thyroid disease, metabolic disorders, and HIV (and other viral) infections.

Sjögren's syndrome

Sjögren's syndrome has a distinct histopathologic pattern of expression in the salivary glands [15]. There is a chronic, progressive inflammatory mononuclear cell infiltrate in a peri-ductal, peri-vascular cell distribution (Fig. 2). This infiltrate is composed predominantly (80%) of T cells, with a CD4:CD8 ratio of approximately 3:1. One sees a loss of acinar tissue, which becomes more profound as the condition progresses, with relative preservation of the ductal structures. In this latter regard, exocrine histopathology shares features with irradiation-induced salivary gland damage. The morphology of the gland in Sjögren's syndrome is demonstrated well by sialography, which shows dilated but intact ducts and an absence of normal acinar morphology [16].

The cause of Sjögren's syndrome is not known and the mechanisms responsible for the exocrine pathology are incompletely understood. Recently, it has been shown that both the infiltrating cells and the gland epithelial cells are immunologically active, producing numerous cytokines and other immune mediators [17–19]. Interestingly, the cells of healthy salivary glands also express many of the same cytokines, suggesting that they play a role in normal gland homeostasis. It is likely that a shift in the relative proportions of different cytokines is important in the development of exocrine pathology in Sjögren's syndrome. Another factor which has been noted recently which may play a role in the salivary gland pathology in Sjögren's syndrome is induction of inappropriate programmed cell death (apoptosis) [20, 21]. It has been suggested that expression of Fas and Fas ligand on salivary epithelial cells may lead to death of these cells, while lack of Fas on infiltrating lymphocytes could allow prolonged survival of these activated inflammatory cells.

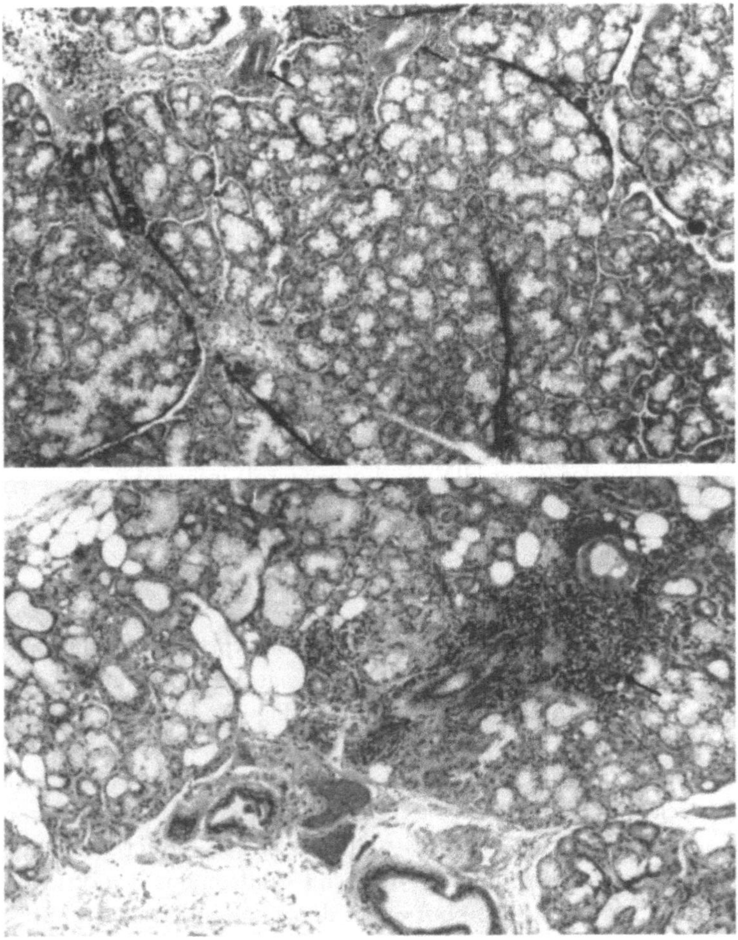

Figure 2
Human labial minor salivary glands. (A) Normal tissue from a healthy volunteer. The section is composed predominantly of acinar cells, with scattered ducts (arrows). (B) Tissue from a patient with primary Sjögren's syndrome. In contrast to A, note the loss of acinar cells, duct dilatation and the presence of focal, peri-ductal mononuclear cell infiltration (arrow).

While a full description of the sequence of events which leads to the marked secretory hypofunction of the exocrine glands in Sjögren's syndrome remains to be provided, it would appear that there are a number of promising therapeutic targets for gene-based treatments.

Gene transfer approaches for salivary gland disease

Because DNA-based therapies can involve a multitude of genes having very different functions, it is possible to suggest several therapeutic approaches to salivary gland diseases that use similar technology. Where restoration of salivary function is the primary concern, it may be possible to increase the fluid permeability of nonfunctional salivary tissue. If there has been extensive destruction of functional tissue then one might focus on the regeneration of salivary cells. However, the ultimate goal of gene therapy, as for any therapy, should be to prevent disease progression and to reverse the underlying disease process.

We have proposed a model in which fluid secretion might be increased from a damaged salivary gland. This model involves the transfer of a gene that encodes aquaporin, a membrane water channel [4, 22]. It has long been observed that chronic inflammation of the salivary glands leads preferentially to destruction of the fluid-secreting acinar cells. In other words, the water-impermeable ductal cells are to some degree spared, and the ducts often persist long after salivary function has been severely compromised. It is theoretically possible to convert the ductal cells into fluid secreting cells by changing the properties of the cell membrane. In its simplest form, membrane water permeability can be increased by the introduction of water channels into the membrane. In the past few years, a family of water channels, termed aquaporins, has been identified and cloned. However, in order for a ductal cell to become a secretory cell there must also be a driving force for water to flow from the basolateral to the luminal side of the cell. At this point it is not clear if salivary ductal cells would be capable of generating an osmotic gradient that would result in a luminal flow of water through water channels, without further modification of the membrane. If necessary, it may be possible to express ion transporters in the ductal cell membrane that will actively contribute to the movement of water through the cells. Nonetheless, using an irradiated gland model of salivary hypofunction in rats, it was demonstrated that the transfer of the aquaporin-1 gene alone was capable of restoring salivary flow to normal [4]. It remains to be seen if this approach will be useful for the treatment of salivary hypofunction caused by inflammatory diseases in humans. With the present gene transfer systems, it is feasible to deliver more than one gene to a cell, but the challenge for salivary glands will be to extend the duration of expression.

Because chronic inflammation of the salivary gland leads to the ablation of acinar cells, it may be desirable to use gene transfer techniques in order to enhance the regeneration of the salivary gland. As with many other differentiated tissues, the glands appear to lose their capacity to regenerate themselves as they age. However, the normal gland is able to maintain a functional cell population by replacing dead cells. The preponderance of data suggests that the replacement of parenchymal cells occurs by mitosis of all the major cell types, and not by the proliferation of a single pluripotent cell [23]. This is significant in the consideration of a gene transfer approach to regeneration because each salivary cell – and particularly each acinar cell – is a target for modification. This is a far simpler task than trying to assure gene transfer to a small number of stem cells. Ideally, it would be desirable to recapitulate the normal development of a salivary gland in order to accomplish cellular regeneration, but far too little is known about salivary gland development to attempt this. An alternative strategy has been to release salivary cells from the G_0/G_1 phase of the cell cycle and then allow them to proceed to complete cell division. There has been one attempt to initiate this process by the transfer of the gene encoding E2F1 to salivary cells *in vitro* and *in vivo* [24, 25]. E2F is a potent transcriptional regulator that can force cells to move from a resting state into S-phase. When E2F1 was expressed in salivary cells by an adenoviral vector, it had exactly this effect (Fig. 3). However, the cells seemed to accumulate in S-phase and did not progress to G_2/M. In order to overcome the cell's natural protection against uncontrolled division, it would be necessary to use at least one more gene product to effect mitosis. At any rate, this strategy would have to be considered carefully from a safety standpoint. Any attempt to override the cell cycle checkpoints by gene transfer would have to be very well controlled and reversible.

When salivary gland inflammatory disease has not progressed to cause severe tissue destruction, the preferred strategy may be to reverse the inflammatory process and prevent further damage. This would be the case in the majority of glands affected by Sjögren's syndrome. It is known that the inflammatory infiltrate in Sjögren's syndrome consists primarily of TH1 type $CD4^+$ cells. This cell population produces many pro-inflammatory cytokines and promotes class I responses and cytotoxic T cell responses. In other similar diseases it has been demonstrated that switching a predominantly TH1 cell population to a TH2 cell type was helpful in attenuating the inflammatory response, leading to significant clinical improvement. Specifically, the local production of IL-4 and IL-10 in a diabetic mouse model was able to suppress the TH1 cell-mediated response and lessen the severity of disease [26]. Adenoviral vectors are available that express many of these TH2 cytokines, so it should be possible to test the hypothesis that their expression will lead to improvement of salivary gland inflammatory disease. There are several murine models of Sjögren's syndrome. In particular, NOD.B10 mice manifest a salivary inflammatory condition that resembles the presentation of Sjögren's syndrome in humans, both histologically and functionally [27]. The use of viral vectors in the glands of mice is now feasible and may be useful for proof-of-concept experiments. Delivery of viral vectors encoding IL-4 or IL-10 might induce a switch in the cellular infiltrate to a more TH2 type, thereby deceasing inflammation and allowing improved secretory function. If successful in the murine model, this could be applied to humans. As stated previously, we will need to see substantial improvements in gene transfer vectors before they will be safe and effective for routine clinical applications.

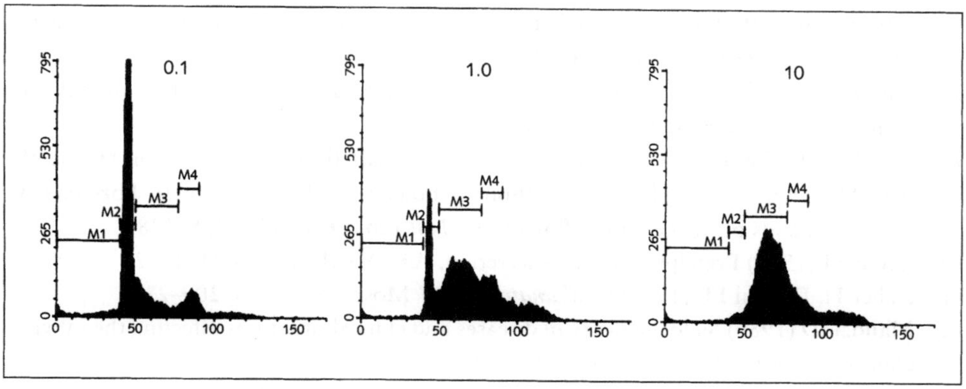

Figure 3
Overexpression of E2F1 in salivary epithelial cells overcomes the G_1/S cell cycle checkpoint. Synchronized HSG cells were infected with AdE2F1 at 0.1, 1 or 10 pfu/cell. Forty-eight hours after infection the cells were harvested and prepared for cell cycle analysis. The histograms show that increasing E2F1 expression shifts cells from the resting state (M2 gate) into S phase (M3 gate) in a dose-dependent manner.

References

1 Baum BJ , O'Connell BC (1995) The impact of gene therapy on dentistry. *J Am Dent Assoc* 126: 179–189
2 Blaese RM, Culver KW, Chang L, Anderson WF, Mullen C, Nienhuis A, Carter C, Dunbar C, Leitman S, Berger M et al (1993) Treatment of severe combined immunodeficiency disease (SCID) due to adenosine deaminase deficiency with CD34⁺ selected autologous peripheral blood cells transduced with a human ADA gene. Amendment to clinical research project, Project 90-C-195, January 10, 1992. *Hum Gene Ther* 4: 521–527
3 Mastrangeli A, O'Connell B, Aladib W, Fox PC, Baum BJ , Crystal RG (1994) Direct *in vivo* adenovirus-mediated gene transfer to salivary glands. *Am J Physiol* 266: G1146–G1155
4 Delporte C, O'Connell BC, He X, Lancaster HE, O'Connell AC, Agre P , Baum BJ (1997) Increased fluid secretion after adenoviral-mediated transfer of the aquaporin-1 cDNA to irradiated rat salivary glands. *Proc Natl Acad Sci USA* 94: 3268–3273
5 O'Connell BC, Ten HK, Lazowski KW, Tabak LA , Baum BJ (1995) Facilitated DNA transfer to rat submandibular gland *in vivo* and GRP-Ca gene regulation. *Am J Physiol* 268: G1074–G1078
6 Adesanya MR, Redman RS, Baum BJ , O'Connell BC (1996) Immediate inflammatory responses to adenovirus-mediated gene transfer in rat salivary glands. *Hum Gene Ther* 7: 1085–1093
7 Le CH, Nicolson AG, Morales A, Sewell KL (1997) Suppression of collagen-induced

arthritis through adenovirus-mediated transfer of a modified tumor necrosis factor receptor gene. *Arthritis Rheum* 40: 1662–1669
8 Barka T, Van der Noen HM (1996) Retrovirus-mediated gene transfer into salivary glands *in vivo*. *Hum Gene Ther* 7: 613–618
9 Goldfine ID, German MS, Tseng H-C, Wang J, Bolaff JL, Chen J-W, Olson DC, Rothman SS (1997) The endocrine secretion of human insulin and growth hormone by exocrine glands of the gastrointestinal tract. *Nat Biotechnol* 15: 1378–1382
10 Baum BJ (1993) Principles of saliva secretion. *Ann NY Acad Sci* 694: 17–23
11 Sicher H, DuBrul EL (1975) *Oral anatomy*. CV Mosby, St. Louis, 209–216
12 Mandel ID (1980) Sialochemistry in diseases and clinical situations affecting the salivary glands. *Crit Rec Clin Lab Sci* 12: 321–365
13 Fox PC, van der Ven PF, Sonies BC, Weiffenbach JM, Baum BJ (1985) Xerostomia: evaluation of a symptom with increasing significance. *J Am Dent Assoc* 110: 519–525
14 Fox PC (1996) Differentiation of dry mouth etiology. *Adv Dent Res* 10: 13–16
15 Daniels TE, Fox PC (1992) Salivary and oral components of Sjögren's syndrome. *Rheum Dis Clin N Am* 18: 571–589
16 Rabinov K, Weber AL (1985) *Radiology of the salivary glands*. GK Hall Medical Publishers, Boston, 231–234
17 Fox RI, Kang H, Ando D, Abrams J, Pisa E (1994) Cytokine mRNA expression in salivary gland biopsies of Sjögren's syndrome. *J Immunol* 152: 5532–5539
18 Ohyama Y, Nakamura S, Matsuzaki G, Shinohara M, Fujimura T, Yamada A, Itoh K, Nomoto K (1996) Cytokine messenger RNA expression in the labial glands of patients with Sjögren's syndrome. *Arthritis Rheum* 39: 1376–1384
19 Sun D, Emmert-Buck MR, Fox PC (1998) Differential cytokine mRNA expression in human labial minor salivary glands in primary Sjögren's syndrome. *J Autoimmunity* 28: 125–137
20 Ogawa N, Dang H, Kong L, Anaya JM, Liu GT, Tala N (1997) Lymphocyte apoptosis and apoptosis-associated gene expression in Sjögren's syndrome. *Arthritis Rheum* 39: 1875–1885
21 Manganelli P, Quaini F, Andreoli AM, Lagrasta C, Pilato FP, Zuccarelli A, Monteverdi R, D'Aversa C, Olivetti G (1997) Quantitative analysis of apoptosis and bcl-2 in Sjögren's syndrome. *J Rheumatol* 24: 1552–1557
22 Delporte C, O'Connell BC, He X, Ambudkar IS, Agre P , Baum BJ (1996) Adenovirus-mediated expression of aquaporin-5 in epithelial cells. *J Biol Chem* 271: 22070–22075
23 Denny PC, Ball WD , Redman RS (1997) Salivary glands: a paradigm for diversity of gland development. *Crit Rev Oral Biol Med* 8: 51–75
24 Lillibridge CD, O'Connell BC (1997) In human salivary gland cells, overexpression of E2F1 overcomes an interferon-gamma- and tumor necrosis factor-alpha-induced growth arrest but does not result in complete mitosis. *J Cell Physiol* 172: 343–350
25 O'Connell B, Lillibridge L, Ambudkar I, Kruse D (1998) Somatic gene transfer to salivary glands. *Ann NY Acad Sci* 842: 171–180

26 Sarvetnick N (1996) Mechanisms of cytokine-mediated localized immunoprotection. *J Exp Med* 184: 1597–1600

27 Robinson CP, Yamachika S, Brayer J, Peck AB, Humphreys-Beher MG (1998) A novel NOD-derived model for the study of primary Sjögren's syndrome. *Arthritis Rheum* 41: 150–156

28 O'Connell BC, Xu T, Walsh TJ, Sein T, Mastrangeli A, Crystal RG, Oppenheim FG , Baum BJ (1996) Transfer of a gene encoding the anticandidal protein histatin 3 to salivary glands. *Hum Gene Ther* 7: 2255–2261

29 Delporte C, Redman RS, Baum BJ (1997) Relationship between the cellular distribution of the alpha(v)beta3/5 integrins and adenoviral infection in salivary glands. *Lab Invest* 77: 167–173

Gene therapy for management of lupus: Correction of Fas and Fas ligand-induced apoptosis in murine disease – therapeutic rationale and strategies

Huang-Ge Zhang[1], *Martin Fleck*[2], *Hui-Chen Hsu*[1], *Carl K. Edwards III*[3], *David T. Curiel*[4], *Tong Zhou*[1] *and John D. Mountz*[1,5]

[1]University of Alabama at Birmingham, Department of Medicine, 701 South 19th Street, LHRB 473, Birmingham, AL 35294, USA; [2]University of Regensburg Medical Center, Department of Internal Medicine, 93042 Regensburg, Germany; [3]Amgen, Inc., One Amgen Center Drive, Thousand Oaks, CA 91320-1789, USA; [4]Gene Therapy Program, University of Alabama at Birmingham, 1824 6th Avenue South, WTI 620, Birmingham, AL 35294, USA; [5]Veterans Administration Medical Center, 700 South 19th Street, Birmingham, AL 35233, USA

Introduction

Identification of mutations of *fas* and *fas* ligand (*fasL*) in murine models of autoimmune disease have provided an important experimental tools for the analysis of tolerance and autoimmune disease. Mutations of *fasL* and *fas* are not a common cause of autoimmune disease in humans although a mutation of the *fas* gene has been associated with autoimmune lymphoproliferative syndrome [1–5] and we have described a mutation of the *fasL* gene in one patient with systemic lupus erythematosus (SLE) [6]. Furthermore, accumulating evidence suggests that dysregulation of apoptosis or altered levels of expression of FasL and Fas play an important role in the pathogenesis of diseases associated with immune regulation [6–11]. Fas apoptosis appears to be the primary mechanism for elimination of autoreactive T cells outside the thymus. FasL regulation is tightly controlled and specific cells and transcription factors have been identified that play a role in this process. Further investigations of Fas/FasL regulation should allow development of strategies to restore T-cell tolerance in autoimmune situations. In this chapter, we shall describe potential applications of gene therapy to develop strategies to overcome these defects.

Defective Fas and Fas ligand apoptosis genes in *lpr/lpr* and *gld/gld* mice

In 1991, the *fas* gene was assigned to mouse chromosome 19 in a region homologous with the long arm of human chromosome 10 [12, 13]. By comparing the composite linkage map of mouse chromosome 19, these investigators [14] further observed that the Fas locus is closely mapped to the homozygous *lpr* gene that was previously reported by Watanabe et al [14]. In 1992, Watanabe-Fukunaga et al. [14] first report-

Gene Therapy in Inflammatory Diseases, edited by C. H. Evans and P. D. Robbins

ed that the *lpr* gene is a mutation of a cell surface receptor gene, *fas*. Analysis on the expression of Fas gene and function of Fas antigen in *CBA-lpr*^{cg} mice successfully lead to the identification of the *lpr* gene as a point mutation of an cytoplasmic apoptosis signaling region of *fas* gene [14]. In 1993, four groups of investigators, including us, reported that Fas mutation in MRL-*lpr/lpr* mice was caused by a different mutation in the extracellular domain of the Fas gene that is due to the integration of an approximately 5.4 kbp fragment of endogenous retrovirus, called early transposon element (ETn), in the second intron region of *fas* [15–18]. The insertion of ETn in *fas* locus caused a premature termination and alternative splicing of *fas* transcript signal in *lpr* mice. The expression of Fas gene in the thymus of *lpr* mice is lower than that of normal mice. Furthermore, a small amount of mutant form of Fas gene is present in the thymus of lpr mice includes splicing of part of ETn sequences into the *fas* transcript.

C3H-*gld/gld* and C3H-*lpr/lpr* developed a nearly identical lymphoproliferative autoimmune disease suggesting a similar molecular basis for the defect in these mice [19]. The existence of Fas ligand was proposed to be due to similarities of phenotype and oncogene expression comparing C3H-*lpr/lpr* and C3H-*gld/gld* mice. The interaction between Fas and Fas ligand was studied by numerous investigators using bone marrow transplants, the most comprehensive [20] predicted that the mutant gene in gld mice was a cytokine that interacted with the mutated gene product present in *lpr* mice.

When Fas was found to be mutated in *lpr/lpr* mice, a Fas fusion protein was used to screen for cells expressing high levels of Fas ligand [21, 22]. Fas ligand was first cloned in 1993 and was shown to be mutant in *gld/gld* (generalized lymphoproliferative disease) mice in 1994 [23, 24].

Analysis of full-length *fas* ligand cDNA clones from C3H-*gld/gld* mice revealed a single discordance at base pair 889. This mutation is predicted to result in a phenylalanine to leucine substitution in the last strand of FasL protein. The three-dimensional structure of the Fas ligand based on the tumor necrosis factor α (TNFα) crystal structure predicts that mouse FasL AA position 274 forms part of a hydrophobic interface critical for Fas ligand trimer formation [25]. Based on the effect of the phenylalanine-to-leucine substitution in the structure of lysozyme, this substitution would create a space that would be filled by H_2O molecules, thereby decreasing the hydrophobicity of the FasL monomer interfaces and decreasing the stability of trimer formation and thus greatly decreases the ability of FasL to induce Fas-mediated apoptosis (Wu et al., unpublished observations).

Activation-induced cell death (AICD) as a mechanism to maintain self-tolerance

The primary apoptosis role of Fas/FasL is the deletion of autoreactive T cells in the periphery and downregulation of the immune response [26–37]. Fas is expressed in activated mature T cells [38], and the prolonged activation of T cells leads the cells to be susceptible to the cytolytic activity of anti-Fas antibody [39, 40]. These results suggest a role of Fas-mediated apoptosis in the induction of peripheral tolerance and/or in the antigen-stimulated suicide of mature T cells [41]. The interaction of FasL with Fas plays an important role in the downregulation of the immune response through several mechanisms including induction of cell death after T-cell activation Activation-Induced Cell Death (AICD). T-cell tolerance is due to both anergy induction and deletion via apoptosis. Deletion can occur by both autocrine (suicide), including AICD, or paracrine (murder) responses (Fig. 1). It is important to note that anergy and apoptosis can be distinct outcomes of partial activation, and anergy is not simply a prelude to apoptotic cell death. For example, activation of two T cell clones, both reactive with influenza hemagglutinin peptide A (HA) led to anergy for one clone and Fas/FasL apoptosis, or suicide, for the other clone [41]. For both clones, partial activation lead to a blunted intracellular calcium flux and failure to proliferate in response to further challenge with professional APCs. Furthermore, there was no difference in affinity for peptide, or difference in Bcl-2, bcl-x, or bax expression. Although the mechanisms responsible for the different patterns of behavior of these two clones are not well defined, it was proposed that subtle differences in TCR:CD3 signaling or differences in other apoptosis proteins were important.

Peripheral T cell tolerance can be induced by multiple mechanisms in which activation-induced antigen-specific T cells (ASTC) apoptosis plays an important role. This concept can be demonstrated by the following experiment by Zhang et al. [41]. TCR-transgenic cells against class I Ld were adoptively transferred into severe-combined immunodeficient (SCID) mice which express the Ld antigen (Ag) on all nucleated cells, and the fate of transferred antigen-specific T cells(ASTC) was followed *in vivo*. It was found that, after encountering Ag *in vivo*, the number of ASTC increased 10–15-fold followed by a decline in number to a value that was still above the starting value, which could be abrogated by blocking CD28, suggesting an important role played by the co-stimulatory signal. ASTC that disappeared from the periphery by AICD and the remaining ASTC moderately downregulated both TCR and CD8 on their cell surface and were unresponsive when cultured with Ld^+ cells. Interestingly, despite unresponsiveness, ASTC were still susceptible to apoptosis when transferred into a secondary host that provided a new source of Ag and APCs.

Correction of murine autoimmune disease using transgene strategy and gene therapy

The identification of *fas* or *fas* ligand defect in *lpr* and *gld* mice provided a clear rational to target these genes for therapeutic intervention. Two therapeutic

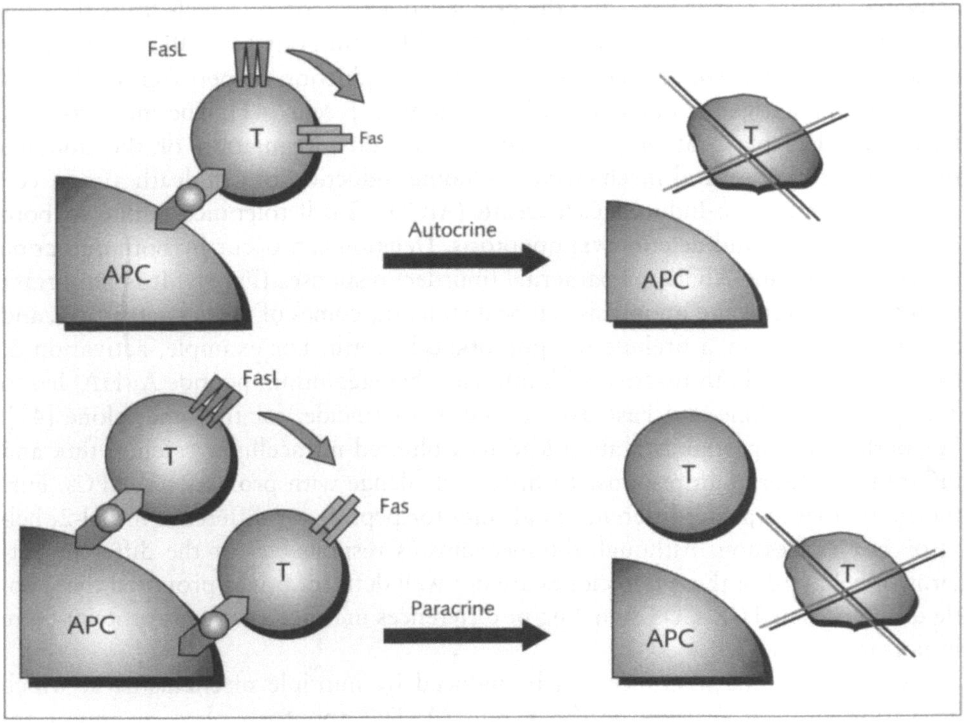

Figure 1
A schematic presentation of Fas/FasL-mediated apoptosis.
Deletion of lymphocytes by Fas/FasL-mediated apoptosis can occur as both autocrine (suicide), including AICD, or paracrine (murder) responses. (A) The suicide response proposes that the activation of T cells results in production of Fas and FasL in the same cell. These molecules then interact with each other and leads to the killing of the same effector and target cell. (B) The paracrine response proposes that the soluble FasL released from an activated lymphocyte can interact with target cells which express Fas on their surface. This engagement therefore does not kill the effector cells, but deletes the Fas-bearing by-stander cells.

approaches will be discussed in this section (Fig. 2). The first approach is to replace the defective Fas in *lpr* mice using an intact *fas* transgene that is directed by the CD2 promoter and enhancer to maintain the expression of Fas in T cells of transgenic mice. The second approach is to deliver intact *fasL* into APCs using gene therapy with adenovirus as the delivery vector to induce T cell tolerance and apoptosis.

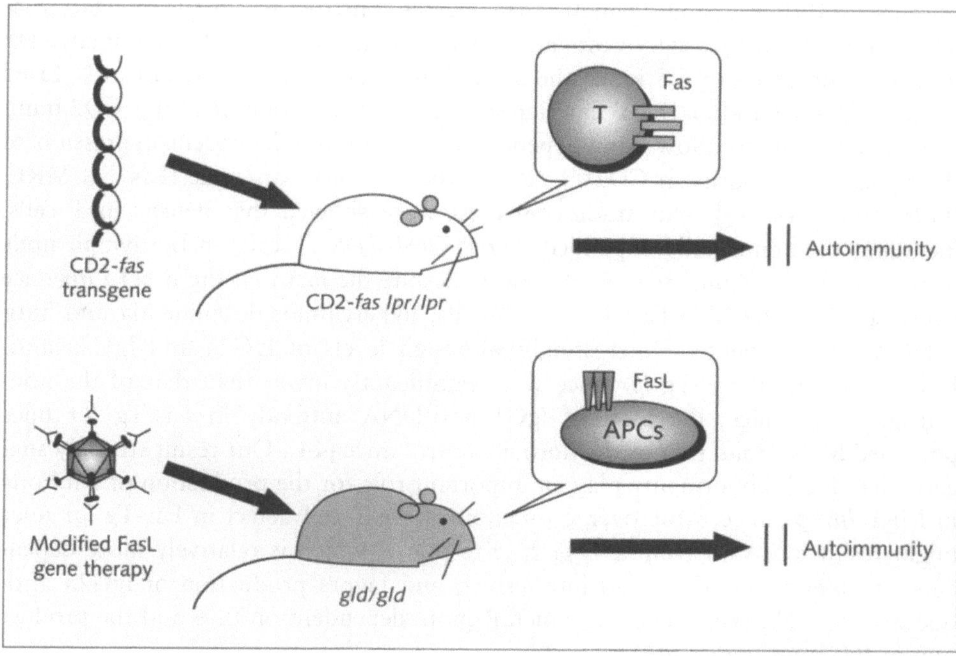

Figure 2
Correction of defective apoptosis using Fas transgene or FasL gene therapy.
*(Upper panel) Our data demonstrated that restoration of Fas expression in CD2-*fas *transgenic mice inhibited many aspects of autoimmunity and defects in AICD. There was decreased lymphoproliferation and autoantibody production in Fas-Tg* lpr *mice. Furthermore, the abnormally expanded* $CD4^-CD8^-B220^+$ *T cells were eliminated. In normal mice, the age-associated decline in AICD was also prevented by this transgene strategy (lower panel). We recently constructed an adenovirus system capable of expressing FasL. We propose that using modified tropism to immune cells, the lymphoproliferative autoimmune disease in* gld/gld *mice can be corrected without significant toxic effect such as hepatotoxicity. The folk (Y) on the adenovirus fiber-knob indicates ligands that alter tropism, such as mannose modification to increase infection via the mannose receptor on APC.*

CD2-*fas* transgenic *lpr* mice: elimination of autoantibody production in CD2-*fas* transgenic *lpr* mice

To determine whether defective Fas expression is responsible for the lymphoproliferative autoimmune disease in *lpr* mice, we developed a transgene strategy using a CD2 promoter and enhancer to maintain Fas expression in T cells of MRL-*lpr*/*lpr* mice [42, 43] (Fig. 2, upper panel). The CD2-*fas* construct was made by ligation of a full-length murine *fas* cDNA into an EcoRI site in front of exon 1 of a human CD2 minigene consisting of 5.5 kb of the 5' flanking sequence, exon 1, intron 1, fused exons 2-5, and 2.1 kb of the 3' flanking sequence. The 3' sequence of this CD2 minigene is sufficient to allow copy-dependent, integration-independent expression of the transgene primarily in $CD2^+$ T cells of the CD2-*fas* transgenic (Fas-Tg) MRL-*lpr*/*lpr* mice [44, 45]. Our studies on these mice showed that defects in T cells, including the abnormally expanded $B220^+$ $CD4^-CD8^-$ T cells in the lymph node were successfully eliminated. Furthermore, despite the fact that the Fas-Tg *lpr* mice expressed no detectable Fas RNA in B cells, hypergammaglobulinemia and anti-dsDNA were prevented. Interestingly, although levels of IgG2a and IgG2a anti-DNA antibody in Fas-Tg *lpr* mice were significantly lower than that of the non-transgenic *lpr* mice, the level of IgG1 anti-DNA antibody in Fas-Tg *lpr* mice remained higher than that of the normal control mice [44]. Our result strongly suggests that T cell abnormality play an important role for the production of antibody in MRL-*lpr*/*lpr* mice. Moreover, correction of the T cell defect in Fas-Tg *lpr* mice might result in a shift from a TH1-type response, which is relatively more dependent on interleukin (IL)-2 and interferon-γ and favors production of IgG2a antibodies, to a TH2-type response, which is more dependent on IL-4 and the production of IgG1 antibodies [46].

Use of FasL gene therapy to induce T cell tolerance and apoptosis

One major disadvantage of using a transgene strategy is that this technique cannot be applied to treatment of human SLE. A more feasible approach therefore is to use gene therapy to correct the autoimmune defect. Gene mapping studies and polymorphic associations indicate several genetic factors predispose to development of SLE including complement deficiencies [47–49], MHC alleles [50], T cell receptor polymorphisms [51, 52], TNF polymorphisms [53], and Fc receptor polymorphisms [54]. Genetic defects in Fas, observed in human patients with autoimmune lymphoproliferative syndrome [1–5], and Fas ligand, observed in one patient with lymphadenopathy and SLE [6], are a rare genetic cause of SLE. However, there is evidence that SLE is associated with defective apoptosis, and that increased apoptosis can ameliorate autoimmunity independent of the underlying cause. We therefore have focused on Fas ligand apoptosis gene therapy for applications to autoimmune diseases such as SLE.

A number of trials in both humans and animal models have demonstrated that biological gene therapies directed at the immune system can be useful in the treatment of autoimmune disease [55, 56]. Among the currently developed gene therapy vectors, adenovirus has been shown to transfer genes efficiently and to result in high expression of the reporter genes [57–58]. The major limitation is the immune response to the gene therapy, leading to elimination of infected cells in 2–4 weeks [59–66]. However, short term therapy may be sufficient for restoration of tolerance and decrease of self-reactive and inflammatory responses in SLE.

Adenovirus can be targeted to APCs or T cells, and gene expression may be regulated by promoter elements, such as lysozyme for expression in APC or CD3 for expression in T cells [61–61]. The major difficulty of Fas Ligand gene therapy is toxicity, especially in the liver. Therefore, we propose to use cell therapy as a strategy to overcome the toxicity problem and to apply this technique to correct FasL gene defect in *gld* mice (Fig. 2, lower panel). Our cell therapy study showed that transplantation of APCs that express Fas ligand can induce apoptosis of T cells that express Fas, resulting in antigen-specific T cell tolerance and suggest a novel function for APCs in the induction of T cell apoptosis. Furthermore, we observed that this response is mediated at the cell level and that an immune response to cells can be prevented by FasL production by these cells, suggesting a novel immunointervention strategy for adenovirus gene therapy in which FasL gene therapy can be used to confer immune privilege.

Construction of an adenovirus producing FasL

Adenovirus gene therapy is limited by induction of an immune response to the virus or gene-therapy product protein. APCs lead to Ag processing and presentation to T cells which can be highly immunogenic or tolerogenic depending on co-stimulatory molecules and production of other cytokines, such as FasL. T-cell tolerance after an immune response to adenovirus is also maintained by AICD of the T cells mediated by Fas/FasL interactions. Recently, it has been shown that FasL can create immune-privileged sites and prevent graft rejection by inducing apoptosis in the T cells although excessive tissue necrosis by FasL may lead to an inflammatory response, influx of neutrophils and acute graft rejection [67–69]. We surmised that APCs, such as macrophages, that express FasL might directly induce apoptosis of T cells that express Fas as cell therapy resulting in an adenovirus-specific T-cell tolerance without toxic effects of FasL. We have produced a FasL expressing recombinant adenovirus, denoted as Ad/LoxpFasL recombinant virus utilizing the Loxp and Cre system to assure the control of FasL expression only in the presence of co-infection with Ad/Cre in 293 cells [70–72] (Fig. 3). There was high expression of FasL mRNA only in cells infected with Ad/LoxpFasL + Ad/Cre, but not in cells infected with Ad/LoxpFasL or in a macrophage control. The co-infection of both Ad/LoxpFasL and Ad/Cre are necessary to excise Loxp to allow transcription of FasL under the CMV promoter in the adenovirus. Ad/LoxpFasL without Ad/Cre does not induce toxicity in the 293 cells .

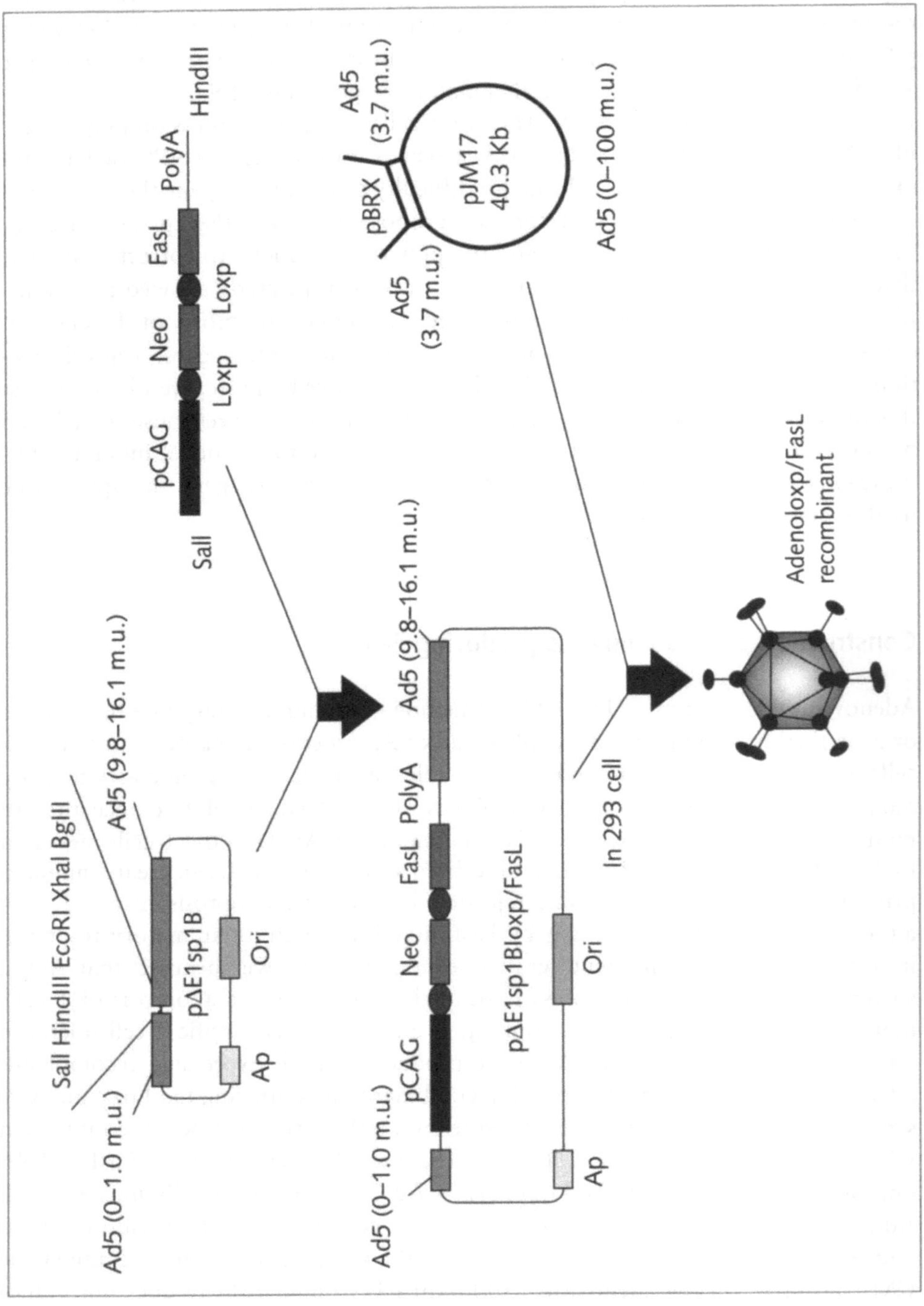
Sall HindIII EcoRI XhaI BglII
Ad5 (9.8–16.1 m.u.)
Ad5 (0–1.0 m.u.)
pΔE1sp1B
Ori
Ap
Sall
pCAG
Loxp
Neo
Loxp
FasL
PolyA
HindIII
Ad5 (3.7 m.u.)
pBRX
Ad5 (3.7 m.u.)
pJM17
40.3 Kb
Ad5 (0–100 m.u.)
Ad5 (0–1.0 m.u.)
pCAG
Neo
FasL
PolyA
Ad5 (9.8–16.1 m.u.)
pΔE1sp1Bloxp/FasL
Ori
Ap
In 293 cell
Adenoloxp/FasL
recombinant

Co-infection of Ad/LoxpFasL + Ad/Cre results in high levels of FasL capable of inducing apoptosis of A20 target cells

We then tested the cell lysing effect produced by the transfected cells. The Ad/Loxp-FasL was infected into APCs from *lpr/lpr* mice with and without Ad/Cre. Nineteen clones of resultant cells lines infected with Ad/LoxpFasL without Ad/Cre or with Ad/LoxpFasL with Ad/Cre were analyzed for the ability to lyse A20 target cells using the ^{51}Cr release assay. There was very high lysis of the A20 target cells by APC infected with Ad/LoxpFasL + Ad/Cre whereas there was no cytotoxicity using APC + Ad/LoxpFasL alone. These results show that Ad/LoxpFasL is not leaky and does not express FasL without the addition of Cre. Also, these results demonstrate that functional FasL is produced upon co-infection of both viruses into the Fas-deficient macrophage cell line from *lpr/lpr* mice. FasL activity in Ad/LoxpFasL + Ad/Cre infected macrophages were compared with that of macrophages transfected by electroporation with PMA-activated T cells. The macrophages infected by the adenovirus exhibited at least a 50–100-fold higher FasL activity compared to the others. High levels of FasL expression by the macrophages were sustained for at least 7 days of *in vitro* culture. These results indicate that the adenovirus can deliver the FasL gene into the primary-cultured macrophages and leads to high levels of FasL expression.

APCs transfected with FasL can induce apoptosis and specific T cell tolerance to antigens *in vitro* and *in vivo*

To determine whether APCs that express FasL can induce antigen-specific T-cell tolerance, an APC line was derived by short-term culture of peritoneal macrophages from Fas mutant B6-*lpr/lpr* mice. As expected, these cells did not express Fas, but expressed MHC class II IA^b , MHC class I H-2D^b antigens, Mac-1 and Fc-g receptor. Significant levels of the B7 co-stimulatory molecule were expressed on 50% of the cells. This cell line was transfected with a eukaryotic

Figure 3
Production of pΔE1sp1Bloxp/FasL.
We recently constructed an Ad/LoxpFasL recombinant virus utilizing the Loxp and Cre system to assure the control of FasL expression in APCs in the presence of co-infection with Ad/Cre. This is a 10.4 kb shuttle vector containing the fragment of adenovirus from 0 map unit to 1 map unit followed by the 0.7 kb CMV promoter. This was followed by 2 Loxp sites separated by a 2 kb stuffer fragment plus a 0.3 kb bovine growth hormone polyA tail. The full-length 0.9 kb FasL was cloned downstream from the stuffer fragment which was followed by an SV40 polyA tail and by the 9.8–16.1 map units of adenovirus.

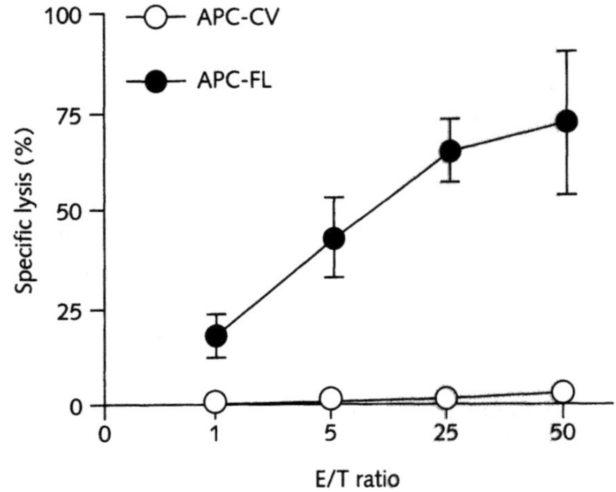

Figure 4
Specific lysis of A20 target cells by FasL expressing APCs.
*Peritoneal resident macrophages from B6-*lpr/lpr *mice were isolated and cultured in RPMI-1640-12% FCS. Macrophages were transfected with a pcDNAIII expression vector containing a full length murine FasL cDNA (APC-FL), or empty vector (APC-CV), using a standard DEAE-Dextran method. Transfected macrophages were selected with 0.5 mg/ml of G418. The selected macrophages were mixed with [^{51}Cr]-labeled, FasL-sensitive A20 cells at the indicated ratios and, after an 8 h incubation, the specific release was determined. This* in vitro *study demonstrated that the infected effector cells resulted in high levels of FasL capable of inducing apoptosis of A20 target cells. A similar APC "cell therapy" system may be useful for specific APC-gene therapy to induce tolerance by deletion of APCs which express self-peptides that drive an autoimmune response.*

expression vector (pcDNAIII) containing the full-length murine FasL and selected using G418. APCs transfected with FasL (APC-FL), but not control vector (APC-CV), exhibited high FasL activity (Fig. 4). APC-FL cells were capable of presenting alloantigen and induced a proliferative response if the responding T cells were obtained from MRL-*lpr/lpr* mice, which do not express Fas. However, presentation of antigen by APCs that expressed FasL to T cells that expressed Fas antigen, obtained from MRL-+/+ mice, abrogated the proliferative response. Thus, presentation of antigen by APCs that express FasL induced tolerance of the Fas-positive responding T cells.

Reduction of lymphadenopathy by local injection of FasL gene therapy into *gld/gld* mice

To determine if the Fas ligand lymphoproliferative autoimmune disease in gld/gld could be reversed by gene therapy, an adenovirus-FasL gene therapy construct was made. Using a Lox/Cre system two adenoviruses, one with Lox/FasL and another with Ad/Cre, could be grown separately and used to co-infect cells resulting in high expression of FasL in infected cells. The two adenoviruses were co-injected into lymph nodes of C3H-*gld/gld* mice. FasL activity was determined 5 days later by the ability of the transfected macrophages to induce apoptosis in the A20 cytotoxicity assay. There was high cytotoxicity activity by T cells from lymph nodes transfected with the Ad/LoxpFasL adenovirus. There was an approximate 5-fold decrease in the mean number of lymph node cells in the Ad/LoxpFasL adenovirus infected mice compared to control infected mice (Fig. 5). The main effect was a decreased number of $CD3^{+}B220^{+}CD4^{-}CD8^{-}$ T cells (Fig. 5). These results demonstrate: (1) a novel adenovirus/FasL gene therapy approach is feasible, and (2) this gene therapy approach can be used to reverse lymphoproliferative autoimmune disease in C3H-*gld/gld* mice. It is noteworthy that Ad/LoxpFasL adenovirus plus the Ad/CRE adenovirus did not induce significant apoptosis of the liver and lung after local injection into the lymph node. These results suggest that local therapy with the Ad/Loxp-FasL adenovirus plus the Ad/CRE adenovirus might be feasible. These results shed new insights into the function of the $CD3^{+}$ $B220^{dull}$ T cells and are consistent with observations that T cells are important to eliminate alloreactive T cells after T cell transfer [73], and the population of cells surviving AICD exhibit high Fas and FasL expression [74].

Sjögren's syndrome and autoimmune disease in *lpr/lpr* and *gld/gld* mice induced by murine cytomegalovirus infection

The spectrum of post-infection autoimmune disease includes vasculitis, endocarditis, hepatitis, pneumonitis, arthritis, and glomerulonephritis [75–86]. Defective apoptosis has been proposed to be related to the development of chronic autoimmune diseases. This was analyzed in *lpr/lpr* and *gld/gld* mice during murine cytomegalovirus (MCMV) infection. Mice were infected i.p. with MCMV strain Smith (10^5 p.f.u.). A persistent inflammation (> day 100) of the salivary glands resembling histological features of the Sjögren's Syndrome was found only in *lpr/lpr* mice, despite the lack of infectious virus. These results suggest that Fas mediated apoptosis is not necessary for the clearance of MCMV infected cells. However, Fas-mediated apoptosis is necessary for the downmodulation of the immune response and defective Fas-mediated apoptosis can lead to a post-infection chronic inflammatory response which may trigger autoimmune disease.

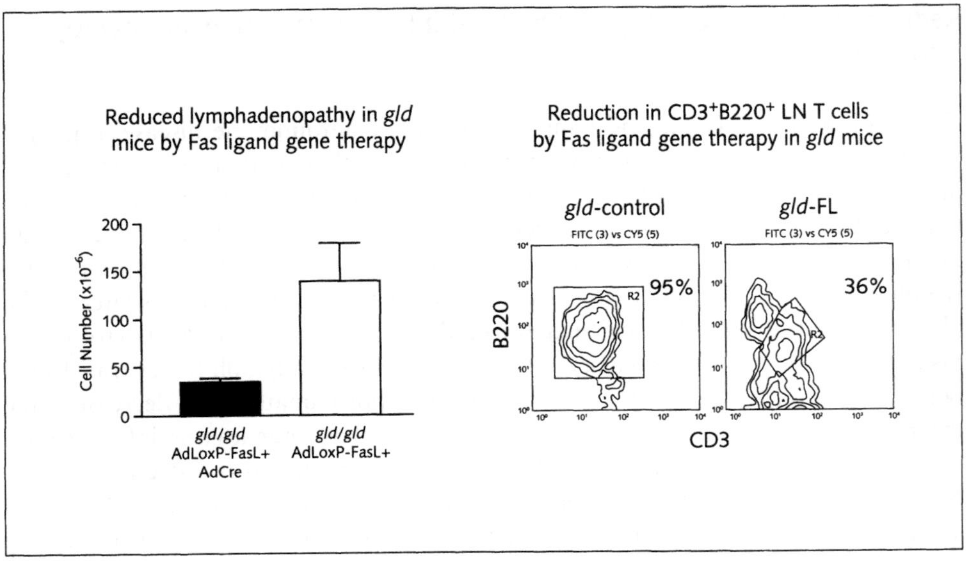

Figure 5
Decreased lymphoproliferative disease of Ad/LoxpFasL adenovirus infected gld/gld *mice. Single cell suspensions of lymph node cells were produced from gld/gld mice 7 d after infection with either the Ad/LoxpFasL adenovirus plus the Ad/CRE adenovirus, or the Ad/Loxp-FasL adenovirus alone as a control. Left panel: Analysis of the number of lymph nodes cells 7 days after direct injection of Ad/LoxpFasL adenovirus plus the Ad/CRE adenovirus locally into the lymph nodes. The results represent the mean ± SEM. Right panel: Flow cytometry analysis of B220 and CD3 expression 7 days after direct injection of Ad/LoxpFasL adenovirus plus the Ad/CRE adenovirus locally into the lymph node. The values are representative of five mice treated separately.*

Ad/Fas ligand gene therapy for MCMV induced chronic inflammation

Mouse cytomegalovirus (MCMV) results in a chronic inflammatory response in Fas ligand deficient *gld/gld* mice. After 100 days, viable virus is cleared from the salivary gland. However, the salivary gland develops persistent inflammation consisting of foci of lymphocytes which are primarily clustered between the ducts and glandular tissue. Since these mice have a mutation in Fas ligand, neither these lymphocytes nor the salivary tissue can express Fas ligand. In this regard, there is some question as to whether Fas ligand is necessary for development of Sjögren's Syndrome and anti-inflammatory infiltrate. In the present model, the infiltrate seen in association with adenovirus induced Sjögren's Syndrome is independent from production of Fas ligand.

Lymphocytes require activation to become susceptible to Fas-mediated apoptosis. Therefore, it is not clear if Fas ligand can induce apoptosis of inactivated infiltrating lymphocytes within a site of inflammation. Although some lymphocytes in inflammatory sites are activated, the majority of lymphocytes are thought to be bystanders or, at least, not specifically activated by antigen.

A third consideration for Fas ligand gene therapy is the potential for Fas ligand to induce damage of the tissue as well as the inflammatory cells. This has become an important issue related to the observation that although Fas ligand appears to induce apoptosis of inflammatory cells in the vicinity of the beta islets thereby allowing transfer of islet graphs, it is also been established that high induction of Fas ligand in insulin promoter/Fas ligand transgenic mice induces apoptosis of islet cells and that NOD/*lpr*/*lpr* mice do not develop insulitis. Together these experiments point out the important issue that Fas ligand can be important for down regulation of an immune response, but can also cause further damage of target tissue in the vicinity of this response.

To determine if mouse Fas ligand could induce apoptosis, the two-virus system was used for local injection directly into salivary gland of Fas ligand deficient *gld*/*gld* mice 100 days post MCMV infection. The MCMV Sjögren's syndrome model in Fas L deficient *gld*/*gld* mice was analyzed after injection of Ad/LoxpFasL + Ad/Cre. Groups of mice received Ad/LoxpFasL + Ad/Cre (1×10^9 PFU each) virus in 0.1 cc media. The local injections were carried out by making a small incision over the parotid salivary gland allowing direct visualization of the salivary gland. Preliminary experiments using trypan blue indicated that this volume and technique allowed a relatively good distribution of injected fluid throughout the target salivary gland. Thus, these experiments will allow for direct evaluation of whether the combined virus can be used for local treatment of an autoimmune inflammatory disease, and if the virus can produce Fas ligand in this site. The mice were sacrificed 10 days after salivary gland injection. For Fas ligand expression, an anti-mouse Fas L antibody (Santa Cruz, CA) which uses a primary antibody followed by secondary FITC-conjugated avidin to reveal the pattern of staining.

There was a significant decrease in the anti-inflammatory response without apparent injury to salivary gland tissue (Fig. 6). This was determined by analysis of at least five sections from each mouse in the chronic phase (post 100 days) MCMV infection, receiving Ad/LoxpFasL + Ad/Cre gene therapy. There was a significant reduction of both the inflammatory infiltrate that was seen only in the injected salivary gland but not adjacent control salivary gland or adjacent lymph node. There were foci of FasL expression indicated by specific binding of the fluorescent labeled antibody. The expression was not continuous, indicating that Ad/LoxpFasL + Ad/Cre was either not taken up by all cells or was not expressed in all cells. It is known that uptake of adenovirus in mice depends on the presence of the mouse cytomegalovirus adenovirus receptor (MCAR). Together these results indicate that local injection of Ad/LoxpFasL + Ad/Cre can be efficacious in treatment of chronic inflammatory diseases.

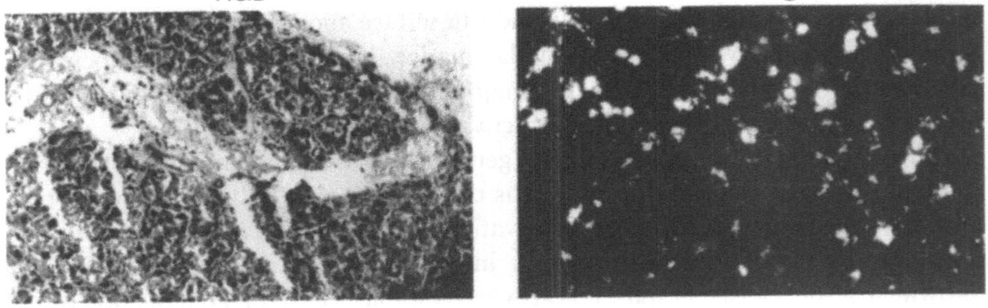

Figure 6
Ad/Fas ligand gene therapy for MCMV induced chronic inflammation.
The MCMV Sjögren's Syndrome model in FasL deficient gld/gld *mice was analyzed after injection of Ad/FasL + Ad/Cre. Groups of mice received Ad/LoxpFasL + Ad/Cre (1×10^9 PFU each) virus in 0.1 cc media. The local injections were carried out by making a small incision over the parotid salivary gland allowing direct visualization of the salivary gland. Fas ligand expression was determined using an anti-mouse FasL antibody (Santa Cruz, CA). Photography was carried out at 320× magnification using a fluorescent microscope. There was a significant decrease in the inflammatory response without apparent injury to salivary gland tissue, as determined by analysis of at least five sections from each mouse in the chronic phase (post 100 days) of MCMV infection, after receiving Ad/LoxpFasL + Ad/Cre gene therapy.*

Soluble TNF-R as a modulator of adenovirus inflammation and autoimmune disease

Rationale for use of soluble TNF-R as a modulator of adenovirus inflammation

TNFα is one of the principal mediators of inflammation in the chronic phase of autoimmune disease, as well as a mediator of cell death after adenovirus gene therapy [87–90]. Neutralization of TNF with TNF inhibitors, such as sTNF-RI, greatly reduces tissue injury and cell death [91–96]. Adenovirus takes advantage of TNF as an immune mediator to promote expression of several immunosubversive proteins supporting its escape from immunosurveillance. The interaction of TNF with its receptor is a strong virulence factor for inflammation and elimination of viral infections. The E3 gp19k protein not only prevents CTL recognition of Ad infected fibroblasts by sequestering MHC class I proteins in the endoplasmic reticulum, but also E3 proteins 10.4k, 14.5k and 14.7k function to protect infected cells from TNFα cytolysis. Ad mutants that lack the E3 genes encoding these proteins have been shown to exhibit greatly induced pulmonary infiltration after intranasal inoculation into C57BL/10SnJ mice. Therefore, neutralization of TNF may be beneficial to decrease chronic inflammation as well as prolong transgene expression.

Inhibition of TNFα decreases inflammation and prolongs adenovirus gene expression in lung

The effect of treatment with TNF-bp, a polyethyleneglycol linked dimer of sTNFRI on inflammation of the lung and viral clearance after intransal administration of AdCMVlacZ (1×10^{10} p.f.u.) was evaluated. Three days after intranasal administration, there was a moderate inflammatory infiltrate in the lungs of control (CT)-treated C57BL/6-+/+ mice, which peaked at day 7, and was nearly resolved by day 30 (Fig. 7A). In contrast, 3 days after administration of AdCMVlacZ, there was no evidence of an inflammatory infiltrate in the lungs of TNFbp treated C57BL/6-+/+ mice and only minimal evidence of infiltrates were observed from day 3 through day 30. We next determined the expression of the *lacZ* adenovirus gene-therapy product (Fig. 7B). The results indicated that the expression of β-gal in control-treated C57BL/6-+/+ mice reached its highest levels by day 7, but was considerably reduced by day 21 and remained at low levels through day 30 (Fig. 7B). The expression of the β-gal in TNF-bp-treated C57BL/6-+/+ mice also peaked at day 7, but, in contrast to the control-treated mice, the expression of β-gal remained high in the lung through day 30. These results indicate that there is greatly decreased inflammatory disease and prolonged gene expression in AdCMVlacZ virus-infected mice treated with TNF-bp compared with vehicle-treated mice. These results indicate that TNFα is a key factor in the pathogenesis of inflammation in AdCMVlacZ-virus infected mice. Thus, TNF-bp PEG-linked dimer may be therapeutically useful in reducing the inflammatory response to adenovirus gene therapy.

Conclusion

The discovery of mutations in *fas* and *fasL* genes in *lpr* and *gld* mice has changed the direction of research into the pathogenesis and the therapy of autoimmune disease. The most striking revelation from the *lpr* and *gld* lesson is that these two molecules are important regulators of apoptosis. As we have discussed in this chapter, this concept has lead researchers to understand many of the important mechanisms associated with the development of T cells and the establishment of self-tolerance. Furthermore, research conducted in the last five years has shed great light on the mechanisms of Fas-mediated apoptosis by identifying many Fas/FasL-associated apoptosis regulating molecules. These studies not only demonstrated the essence

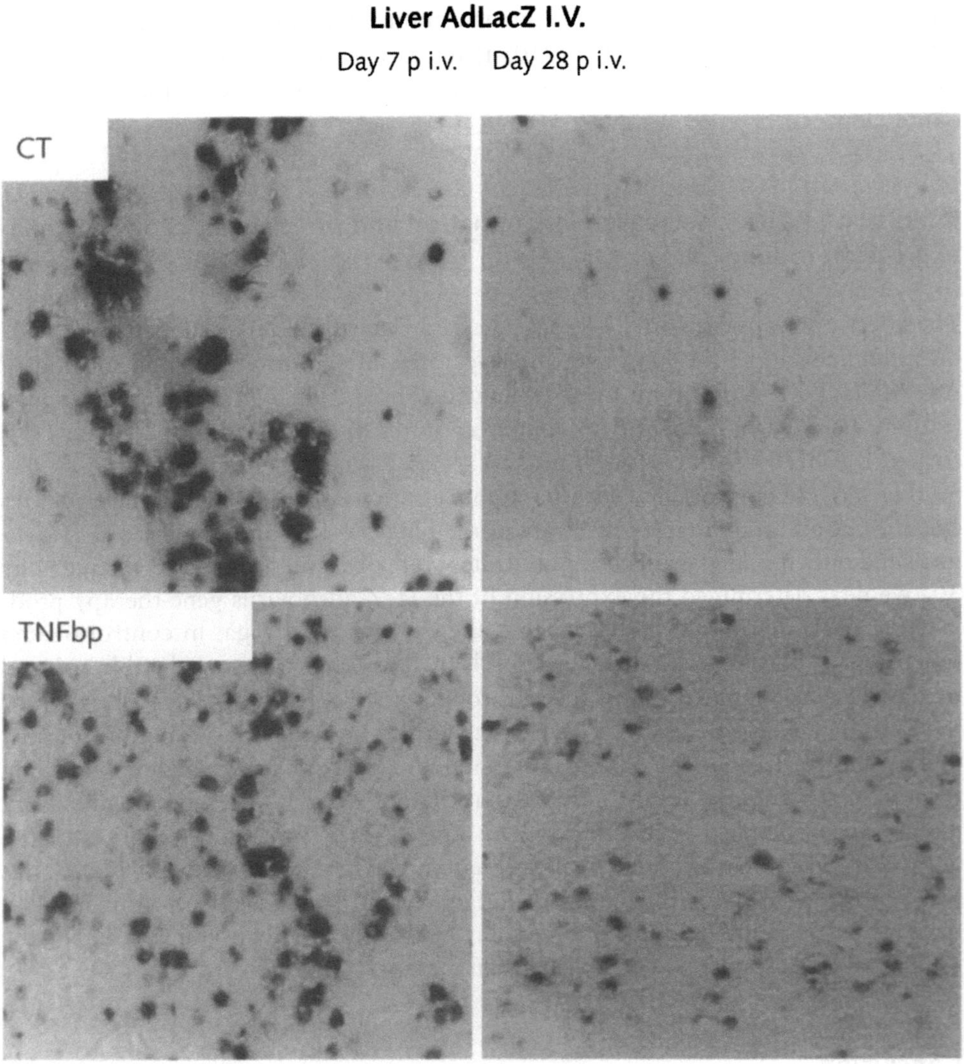

Figure 7
Pulmonary inflammatory infiltration and β-gal expression after intranasal administration of AdCMVlacZ. Lung tissue from control-treated (CT) C57BL/6-+/+ mice, C57BL/6-+/+ mice treated with TNF-bp, and were examined 7 and 28 days after intranasal administration of AdCMVlacZ (1 × 10^{10} p.f.u.). Tissue frozen sections were prepared for analysis of β-gal staining (Magnification × 320).

and complexity of gene regulation, but also provided many of the candidate genes that could be involved in the pathogenesis of autoimmune disease. Finally, the *lpr* and *gld* mice have provided two precise targetable therapeutic animal models for experiments on transgenes and gene therapy. Therefore, although mutations in Fas and FasL are rare in humans, we believe the studies that we described in this chapter may set a good example for future studies in diseases caused by a single gene defect and help develop therapeutic intervention for these diseases.

Acknowledgment
This work was supported in part by a Veterans Administration Merit Review Award; Veterans Administration Career Development Award; NO-1 AR-62224, P50 AI23649, R01-AR42547, R01-AI42900 from National Institutes of Health, a grant from Sankyo Co., Ltd., and a grant from Amgen, Inc., Boulder, Colorado. The production of transgenic mice at UAB was supported by National Cancer Institute grant CA13148, to the University of Alabama at Birmingham Comprehensive Cancer Center. H.-C. H. is a recipient of the postdoctoral fellowship from the Arthritis Foundation. T. Z. is a recipient of an Arthritis Foundation Investigator Award. H.-G. Zhang is supported by Grant No. T32 AR07450. We thank Ms. Judy White for secretarial expertise.

References

1 Fisher GH, Rosenberg FJ, Straus SE, Dale L et al (1995) Dominant interfering Fas gene mutations impair apoptosis in a human autoimmune lymphoproliferative syndrome. *Cell* 81: 935–946
2 Rieux-Laucat F, LeDeist F, Hivroz C, Roberts IA et al (1995) Mutations in Fas associated with human lymphoproliferative syndrome and autoimmunity. *Science* 263: 1347–1349
3 Fuss IJ, Strober W, Dale JK et al (1997) Characteristic T helper 2 T cell cytokine abnormalities in autoimmune lymphoproliferative syndrome, a syndrome marked by defective apoptosis and humoral autoimmunity. *J Immunol* 158: 1912–1618
4 Sneller MC, Wang J, Dale JK et al (1997) Clinical, immunologic, and genetic features of an autoimmune lymphoproliferative syndrome associated with abnormal lymphocyte apoptosis. *Blood* 89: 1341–1348
5 Drappa J, Vaishnaw AK, Sullivan KE et al (1996) Fas gene mutations in the Canale-Smith syndrome, an inherited lymphoproliferative disorder associated with autoimmunity. *New Eng J Med* 335: 1643–1649
6 Wu J, Wilson J, He J, Xiang L, Schur PH, Mountz JD (1996) Fas ligand mutation in a patient with systemic lupus erythematosus and lymphoproliferative disease. *J Clin Invest* 98: 1107–1113

7 Mountz JD, Wu J, Cheng J, Zhou T (1994) Autoimmune disease. A problem of defective apoptosis. *Arthritis Rheum* 37: 1415–1420

8 Elkon KB (1994) Apoptosis in SLE – too little or too much? *Clin Exp Rheumatol* 12: 553–559

9 Rose LM, Latchman DS, Isenberg DA (1994) Bcl-2 and Fas, molecules which influence apoptosis. A possible role in systemic lupus erythematosus? *Autoimmunity* 17: 271–278

10 Ohsako S, Hara M, Harigai M, Fukasawa C, Kashiwazaki S (1995) Expression and function of Fas antigen and bcl-2 in human systemic lupus erythematosus lymphocytes. *Clin Immunol Immunopath* 73: 109–114

11 Mysler E, Bini P, Drappa J, Ramos P, Friedman SM, Krammer PH, Elkon KB (1994) The apoptosis-1/Fas protein in human systemic lupus erythematosus. *J Clin Invest* 93: 1029–1034

12 Watanabe T, Sakai Y, Miyawaki S, Shimizu A, Koiwai O, Ohno K (1991) A molecular genetic linkage map of mouse chromosome 19, including the lpr, Ly-44, and Tdt genes. *Biochemical Genetics* 29: 325–335

13 Inazawa J, Itoh N, Abe T, Nagata S (1992) Assignment of the human Fas antigen gene (FAS) to 10q24.1. *Genomics* 14: 821–822

14 Watanabe-Fukunaga R, Brannan CI, Copeland NG, Jenkins NA, Nagata S (1992) Lymphoproliferation disorder in mice explained by defects in Fas antigen that mediates apoptosis. *Nature* 356: 314–317

15 Adachi M, Watanabe-Fukunaga R, Nagata S (1993) Aberrant transcription caused by the insertion of an early transposable element in an intron of the Fas antigen gene of lpr mice. *Proc Natl Acad Sci USA* 90: 1756

16 Chu J-L, Drappa J, Parnassa AP, Elkon KB (1993) The defect in *Fas* mRNA expression in MRL/*lpr* mice is associated with insertion of the retrotransposon, *ETn*. *J Exp Med* 178: 723

17 Kobayashi S, Hirano T, Kakinuma M, Uede T (1993) Transcriptional repression and differential splicing of Fas mRNA by early transposon (ETn) insertion in autoimmune lpr mice. *Biochem Biophy Res Comm* 191: 617–624

18 Wu J, Zhou T, He J, Mountz JD (1993) Murine autoimmune disease due to integration of an endogenous retrovirus in an apoptosis gene. *J Exp Med* 178: 461–468

19 Mountz JD, Mushinski JF, Mark GE, Steinberg AD (1985) Oncogene expression in autoimmune mice. *J Mol Cell Immunol* 2: 121–131

20 Allen RD, Marshell JD, Roths JB and Sidman CD (1990) Differences defined by bone marrow transplantation suggest that *lpr* and *gld* are mutations of genes encoding an interacting pair of molecules. *J Exp Med* 172: 1367–1375

21 Suda T, Okazaki T, Naito Y,et al (1995) Expression of the Fas ligand in cells of T cell lineage. *J Immunol* 154: 3806–3813

22 Suda T and Nagata S (1994) Purification and characterization of the Fas-ligand that induces apoptosis. *J Exp Med* 179: 873–879

23 Takahashi T, Tanaka M, Brannan CI, Jenkins NA, Copeland NG, Suda T, Nagata S

(1994) Generalized lymphoproliferative disease in mice, caused by a point mutation in the Fas ligand. *Cell* 76: 969–976
24 Lynch DH, Watson ML, Alderson MR, Baum PR, Miller RE, Tough T, Gibson M, Davis-Smith T, Smith CA, Hunter K, Bhat D, Din W, Goodwin RG, Seldin MF (1994) The mouse Fas-ligand gene is mutated in gld mice and is part of a TNF family gene cluster. *Immunity* 1: 131–136
25 Peitsch MC, Tschopp J (1995) Comparative molecular modeling of the Fas-ligand and other members of the TNF family. *Mol Immunol* 32: 761–772
26 Kabelitz D, Pohl T, Pechhold K (1993) Activation-induced cell death (apoptosis) of mature peripheral T lymphocytes. *Immunol Today* 14: 338–339
27 Trauth BC, Klas C, Peters AM et al (1989) Monoclonal antibody-mediated tumor regression by induction of apoptosis. *Science* 245: 301–305
28 Lowin B. Hahne M. Mattmann C, Tschopp J (1994) Cytolytic T-cell cytotoxicity is mediated through perforin and Fas lytic pathways. *Nature* 370: 650–652
29 Klas C, Debatin KM, Jonker RR et al (1993) Activation interferes with the APO-1 pathway in mature human T cells. *Intl Immunol* 5: 625–630
30 Bossu P, Singer GG, Andres P, Ettinger R, Marshak-Rothstein A, Abbas AK (1993) Mature CD4+ T lymphocytes from MRL-lpr mice are resistant to receptor-mediated tolerance and apoptosis. *J Immunol* 151: 7233–7239
31 Van Parijs L, Ibraghimov A, Abbas AK (1996) The roles of costimulation and Fas in T cell apoptosis and peripheral tolerance. *Immunity* 4: 321–328
32 Ju ST, Panka DJ, Cui H, Ettinger R, el-Khatib M, Sherr DH, Stanger BZ, Marshak-Rothstein A (1995) Fas(CD95)/FasL interactions required for programmed cell death after T-cell activation. *Nature* 373: 444–448
33 Alderson MR, Tough TW, Davis-Smith T, Braddy S, Falk B, Schooley KA,Goodwin RG, Smith CA, Ramsdell F, Lynch DH (1995) Fas ligand mediates activation-induced cell death in human T lymphocytes. *J Exp Med* 181: 71–77
34 Dhein J, Walczak H,Baumler C, Debatin KM, Krammer PH (1995) Autocrine T-cell suicide mediated by APO-1/(Fas/CD95). *Nature* 373: 438–441
35 Brunner T, Mogil RJ, LaFace D, Yoo NJ, Manboubl A, Echeverre F, Martin J, Force WR, Lynch DH, Ware CF, Green DR (1995) Cell-autonomous Fas (CD95)/Fas-ligand interaction mediates activation-induced apoptosis in T-cell hybridomas. *Nature* 373: 441–444
36 Green DR and Scott DW (1994) Activation-induced apoptosis in lymphocytes. *Curr Opin Immunol* 6: 476–483
37 Dhein J, Walczak H, Baumler C, Debatin KM, Krammer P H (1995) Autocrine T-cell suicide mediated by APO-1/(Fas/CD95). *Nature* 73: 438–441
38 Rathmell JC, Cooke MP, Ho WY, Grein J, Townsend SE, Davis MM, Goodnow CC (1995) CD95 (Fas)-dependent elimination of self-reactive B cells upon interaction with CD4+ T cells. *Nature* 376: 181–184
39 Scott DW, Grdina T, Shi YT (1996) Cells commit suicide, but B cells are murdered. *J Immunol* 156: 2352–2356

40 Hargreaves RG, Borthwick NJ, Montani MS, Piccolella E, Carmichael P, Lechler RI, Akbar AN, Lombardi G (1997) Dissociation of T cell anergy from apoptosis by blockade of Fas/Apo-1 (CD95) signaling. *J Immunol* 158: 3099–3107

41 Zhang L (1996) The fate of adoptively transferred antigen-specific T cells *in vivo*. *Eur J Immunol* 26: 2208–14

42 Palmiter RD, Brinster RL (1986) Transgenic mice. *Annu Rev Genet* 20: 465–499

43 Mountz JD, Zhou T, Johnson L (1990) Production of transgenic mice and application to immunology and autoimmunity. *Am J Med Sic* 300: 322–329

44 Wu J, Zhou T, Zhang J, He J, Gause WC, Mountz JD (1994) Correction of accelerated autoimmune disease by early replacement of the mutated *lpr* gene with the normal Fas apoptosis gene in the T cells of transgenic MRL-*lpr*/*lpr* mice. *Proc Natl Acad Sci USA* 91: 2344–2348

45 Greaves DR, Wilson FD, Lang G, Kioussie D (1989) Human CD2 3'-flanking sequences confer high-level, T cell-specific, position-independent gene expression in transgenic mice. *Cell* 56: 979–986

46 Street RE, Mossman TR (1991) Functional diversity of T lymphocytes due to secretion of different cytokine patterns. *FASEB J* 5: 171–177

47 Sullivan KE, Petri MA, Schmeckpeper BJ, McLean RH, Winkelstein JA (1994) Prevalence of a mutation causing C2 deficiency in systemic lupus erythematosus. *J Rheum* 21: 1128–1133

48 Moulds JM, Reveille JD, Arnett FC (1996) Structural polymorphisms of complement receptor 1 (CR1) in systemic lupus erythematosus (SLE) patients and normal controls of three ethnic groups. *Clin Exp Immunol* 105: 302–305

49 Truedsson L, Alper CA, Awdeh ZL, Johansen P, Sjoholm AG, Sturfelt G (1993) Characterization of type I complement C2 deficiency MHC haplotypes. Strong conservation of the complotype/HLA-B-region and absence of disease association due to linked class II genes. *J Immunol* 151: 5856–5863

50 Goldstein R, Sengar DP (1993) Comparative studies of the major histocompatibility complex in French Canadian and non-French Canadian Caucasians with systemic lupus erythematosus. *Arthritis Rheuma* 36: 1121–1127

51 Desai-Mehta A, Mao C, Rajagopalan S, Robinson T, Datta SK (1995) Structure and specificity of T cell receptors expressed by potentially pathogenic anti-DNA autoantibody-inducing T cells in human lupus. *J Clin Invest* 95: 531–541

52 Huang Q, Morris D, Dunckley H, Grennan D, Manolios N (1997) Lack of linkage between anti-nuclear antibody or clinical features of systemic lupus erythematosus (SLE) and TCR-A/Vbeta loci in families of subjects with SLE. *Lupus* 6: 527–532

53 Chen CJ, Yen JH, Tsai WC, Wu CS, Chiang W, Tsai JJ, Liu HW (1997) The TNF2 allele does not contribute towards susceptibility to systemic lupus erythematosus. *Immunology Lett* 55: 1–3

54 Wilson AG, Gordon C, di Giovine FS, de Vries N, van de Putte LB, Emery P, Duff GW (1994) A genetic association between systemic lupus erythematosus and tumor necrosis factor alpha. *Eur J Immunology* 24: 191–195

55 Strand V (1997) Approaches to the management of systemic lupus erythematosus. *Curr Opin Rheuma* 9: 410–420

56 Müller-Ladner U, Gay RE, Gay S (1997) Cellular pathways of joint destruction. *Curr Opin Rheuma* 9: 213–220

57 Bakker AC, Joosten LA, Arntz OJ, Helsen MM, Bendele AM, van de Loo FA, van den Berg WB (1997) Prevention of murine collagen-induced arthritis in the knee and ipsilateral paw by local expression of human interleukin-1 receptor antagonist protein in the knee. *Arthritis Rheuma* 40: 893–900

58 Müller-Ladner U, Roberts CR, Franklin BN, Gay RE, Robbins PD, Evans CH, Gay S (1997) Human IL-1Ra gene transfer into human synovial fibroblasts is chondroprotective. *J Immunol* 158: 3492–3498

59 Evans CH, Robbins PD (1996) Pathways to gene therapy in rheumatoid arthritis. *Curr Opin Rheuma* 8: 230–234

60 Otani K, Nita I, Macaulay W, Georgescu HI, Robbins PD, Evans CH (1996) Suppression of antigen-induced arthritis in rabbits by ex vivo gene therapy. *J Immunol* 156: 3558–3562

61 Harris CE, Agarwal S, Hu P, Wagner E, Curiel DT (1993) Receptor-mediated gene transfer to airway epithelial cells in primary culture. *Am J Resp Cell Mol Biol* 9: 441–447

62 Deshane J, Cabrera G, Grim JE, Siegal GP, Pike J, Alvarez RD, Curiel DT (1995) Targeted eradication of ovarian cancer mediated by intracellular expression of anti-erbB-2 single-chain antibody. *Gyn Oncology* 59: 8–14

63 Michael SI, Huang CH, Romer M U, Wagner E, Hu PC, Curiel DT (1993) Binding-incompetent adenovirus facilitates molecular conjugate-mediated gene transfer by the receptor-mediated endocytosis pathway. *J Biol Chem* 268: 6866–6869

64 Gao L, Wagner E, Cotten M, Agarwal S, Harris C, Romer M, Miller L, Hu PC, Curiel D (1993) Direct *in vivo* gene transfer to airway epithelium employing adenovirus-polylysine-DNA complexes. *Human Gene Therapy* 4: 17–24

65 Curiel DT (1993) Adenovirus facilitation of molecular conjugate-mediated gene transfer. *Progress Med Virol* 40: 1–18

66 Schwarzenberger P, Spence SE, Gooya JM, Michiel D, Curiel DT, Ruscetti FW, Keller JR (1996) Targeted gene transfer to human hematopoietic progenitor cell lines through the c-kit receptor. *Blood* 87: 472–478

67 Griffith TS, Brunner T, Fletcher SM, Green DR, Ferguson TA (1995) Fas ligand-induced apoptosis as a mechanism of immune privilege. *Science* 270: 1189–1192

68 Lau HT, Yu M, Fontana A, Stoeckert CJ Jr (1996) Prevention of islet allograft rejection with engineered myoblasts expressing FasL in mice. *Science* 273: 109–112

69 Allison J, Georgiou HM, Strasser A, Vaux DL (1997) Transgenic expression of CD95 ligand on islet b cells induces a granulocytic infiltration but does not confer immune privilege upon islet allografts. *Proc Natl Acad Sci USA* 94: 3943–3947

70 Choulika A, Guyot V, Nicolas JF (1996) Transfer of single gene-containing long terminal repeats into the genome of mammalian cells by a retroviral vector carrying the cre gene and the loxP site. *J Virology* 70: 1792–1798

71 Wang P, Anton M, Graham FL, Bacchetti S (1995) High frequency recombination between loxP sites in human chromosomes mediated by an adenovirus vector expressing Cre recombinase. *Somatic Cell Mol Gen* 21: 429–441

72 Sakai K, Mitani K, Miyazaki J (1995) Efficient regulation of gene expression by adenovirus vector-mediated delivery of the CRE recombinase. *Biochem Biophys Res Comm* 217: 393–401

73 Cheng J, Liu C, Yang P, Zhou T, Mountz JD (1997) Increased lymphocyte apoptosis in Fas ligand transgenic mice. *J Immunol* 159: 674–684

74 Mountz JD, Zhou T, Eldridge J, Berry K, Blüthmann H (1990) Transgenic rearranged T cell receptor gene inhibits lymphadenopathy and accumulation of $CD4^{-}CD8^{-}B220^{+}$ T cells in *lpr/lpr* mice. *J Exp Med* 172: 1805–1817

75 Newkirk MM, Watanabe Duffy KN, Leclerc J, Lambert N, Shiroky JB (1994) Detection of cytomegalovirus, Epstein-Barr virus and herpes virus-6 in patients with rheumatoid arthritis with or without Sjogren's syndrome. *British J Rheum* 33: 317–322

76 Davis-Poynter NJ, Lynch DM, Vally H, Shellam GR, Rawlinson WD, Barrell BG, Farrell HE (1997) Identification and characterization of a G protein-coupled receptor homolog encoded by murine cytomegalovirus. *J Virol* 71: 1521–1529

77 Polic B, Jonjic S, Pavic I, Crnkovic I, Zorica I, Hengel H, Lucin P, Koszinowski UH (1996) Lack of MHC class I complex expression has no effect on spread and control of cytomegalovirus infection *in vivo*. *J Gen Virol* 77 : 217–225

78 Skarstein K, Wahren M, Zaura E, Hattori M, Jonsson R (1995) Characterization of T cell receptor repertoire and anti-Ro/SSA autoantibodies in relation to sialadenitis of NOD mice. *Autoimmunity* 22: 9–16

79 Cauli A, Yanni G, Pitzalis C, Challacombe S, Panayi GS (1995) Cytokine and adhesion molecule expression in the minor salivary glands of patients with Sjögren's syndrome and chronic sialoadenitis. *Ann Rheum Dis* 54: 209–15

80 Newkirk MM, Shiroky JB, Johnson N, Danoff D, Isenberg DA, Shustik C, Pearson GR (1996) Rheumatic disease patients, prone to Sjögren's syndrome and/or lymphoma, mount an antibody response to BHRF1, the Epstein-Barr viral homologue of BCL-2. *British J Rheum* 35: 1075–1081

81 Fleck M, Kern ER, Zhou T, Wintersberger W, Edwards III CK, Mountz JD (1997) A new model for Sjögren's Syndrome and autoimmune disease in *lpr* mice induced by murine Cytomegalovirus infection. *Arthritis Rheum* 40

82 Skarstein K, Holmdahl R, Johannessen AC, Goldschmidt T, Jonsson R (1995) Short-term administration of selected anti-T-cell receptor V beta chain specific MoAb reduces sialadenitis in MRL/lpr mice. *Scand J Immunol* 42: 529–534

83 Ahlfors E, Jonsson R, Czerkinsky C (1996) Experimental T cell-mediated inflammatory reactions in the murine oral mucosa. II. Immunohistochemical characterization of resident and infiltrating cells. *Clin Exp Immunol* 104: 297–305

84 Tanaka K, Koga Y, Lu YY, Zhang XY, Wang Y, Kimura G, Nomoto K (1994) Murine cytomegalovirus-associated pneumonitis in the lungs free of the virus. *J Clin Invest.* 94: 1019–1025

85 Yuhasz SA, Dissette VB, Cook ML, Stevens JG (1994) Murine cytomegalovirus is present in both chronic active and latent states in persistently infected mice. *Virol* 202: 272–280

86 Collins T, Pomeroy C, Jordan MC (1993) Detection of latent cytomegalovirus DNA in diverse organs of mice. *J Infect Dis* 168: 725–729

87 Wold WS (1993) Adenovirus genes that modulate the sensitivity of virus-infected cells to lysis by TNF. *J Cell Biochem* 53: 329–335

88 Kolls JK, Lei D, Nelson S, Summer WR, Greenberg S, Beutler B (1995) Adenovirus-mediated blockade of tumor necrosis factor in mice protects against endotoxic shock yet impairs pulmonary host defense. *J Infec Dis* 171: 570–575

89 Day DB, Zachariades NA, Gooding LR (1994) Cytolysis of adenovirus-infected murine fibroblasts by IFN-gamma-primed macrophages is TNF- and contact-dependent. *Cell Immunol* 157: 223–238

90 Ranheim TS, Shisler J, Horton TM, Wold LJ, Gooding LR, Wold WS (1993) Characterization of mutants within the gene for the adenovirus E3 14.7-kilodalton protein which prevents cytolysis by tumor necrosis factor. *J Virol* 67: 2159–2167

91 Haak-Frendscho M, Marsters SA, Mordenti J, Brady S, Gillett NA, Chen SA, Ashkenazi A (1994) Inhibition of TNF by a TNF receptor immunoadhesin. Comparison to an anti-TNF monoclonal antibody. *J Immunol* 152: 1347–1353

92 Fisher CJ Jr, Agosti JM, Opal SM, Lowry SF, Balk RA, Sadoff JC, Abraham E, Schein RM, Benjamin E (1996) Treatment of septic shock with the tumor necrosis factor receptor: Fc fusion protein. The Soluble TNF Receptor Sepsis Study Group. *NEJM* 334: 1697–1702

93 Teng MN, Turksen K, Jacobs CA, Fuchs E, Schreiber H (1993) Prevention of runting and cachexia by a chimeric TNF receptor-Fc protein. *Clin Immunol Immunopath* 69: 215–222

94 Suffredini AF, Reda D, Banks SM, Tropea M, Agosti JM, Miller R (1995) Effects of recombinant dimeric TNF receptor on human inflammatory responses following intravenous endotoxin administration. *J Immunol* 155: 5038–5045

95 Kolls J, Peppel K, Silva M, Beutler B (1994) Prolonged and effective blockade of tumor necrosis factor activity through adenovirus-mediated gene transfer. *PNAS* 91: 215–219

96 Adams LB, Mason CM, Kolls JK, Scollard D, Krahenbuhl JL, Nelson S (1995) Exacerbation of acute and chronic murine tuberculosis by administration of a tumor necrosis factor receptor-expressing adenovirus. *J Inf Dis* 171: 400–405

97 Kolls JK, Lei D, Nelson S, Summer WR, Greenberg S, Beutler B (1995) Adenovirus-mediated blockade of tumor necrosis factor in mice protects against endotoxic shock yet impairs pulmonary host defense. *J Inf Dis* 171: 570–575

Gene therapy for multiple sclerosis

Michael K. Shaw[1], Richard DalCanto[2] and C. Garrison Fathman[2]

[1]Wayne State University School of Medicine, 540 E. Canfield, Detroit, MI 48201, USA;
[2]Stanford University School of Medicine, Department of Medicine, Division of Immunology and Rheumatology, Stanford, CA 94305-5111, USA

Introduction

Recent advances in the field of immunology have increased our understanding of the pathology and regulation of autoimmune diseases. This knowledge is allowing the scientific community to consider the treatment of these diseases using new modalities of immunotherapy. The classic forms of therapy for autoimmune disease are directed at general suppression of the immune response. In contrast, newer forms of therapy are aimed at specific cells or cytokines that contribute to or regulate the aberrant immune response.

Cytokine therapy, the administration of cytokines to modulate an immune response, is one of the more promising of these directed therapies. Recent clinical trials with systemic administration of interferon-β (IFNβ) have demonstrated the immunomodulatory effects of this cytokine on the relapse rate in multiple sclerosis (MS) patients [1]. Further enthusiasm for cytokine immunotherapy comes from research in animal models of autoimmune disease. In one animal model for MS, experimental autoimmune encephalomyelitis (EAE), systemic administration of IFNβ as well as other anti-inflammatory cytokines such as interleukin (IL)-4 or transforming growth factor-β (TGFβ) have shown therapeutic potential [2–4].

Although treatments with anti-inflammatory cytokines hold therapeutic potential, the side-effects inherent in their systemic administration are severe, limiting their utility [5]. Optimally, these side-effects could be limited by delivering the cytokine only to the site or sites of inflammation. Unfortunately, thus far, no practical methods have been developed to affect the local delivery of cytokines to the multiple sites of pathology in multifocal autoimmune diseases such as MS.

Recent work in our laboratory and others suggests that gene therapy techniques may now be employed to this end [6, 7]. These therapies take advantage of the fact that the very cells that cause autoimmune disease can be used as delivery vehicles to shuttle regulatory cytokines to the multiple sites of inflammation. Gene therapy techniques are employed to rapidly and stably modify these disease causing cells (after they are removed from an animal) so that they secrete regulatory cytokines,

Gene Therapy in Inflammatory Diseases, edited by C. H. Evans and P. D. Robbins

such as interleukin (IL)-4 or IL-10, which are able to downregulate the autoimmune response. These cells, when transferred back to animals undergoing an episode of autoimmune disease, provide relief from clinical symptoms. These experiments suggest that cytokine gene therapy may provide a specific intervention for a multifocal disease process such as MS.

Introduction to gene therapy

In general, gene therapy entails the introduction of specific, functional genes into cells for therapeutic or preventive purposes. Early gene therapy trials centered on the replacement of defective or missing genes in genetic disease [8]. More sophisticated therapies are now being developed in which gene therapy techniques may be used for several purposes including: (1) destroying malignant cells in neoplastic disease [9]; (2) immunization against infectious diseases [10]; (3) modification of immune responses [11]; or (4) repair of single base pair mutations [12].

Gene therapy techniques are rapidly evolving. Presently, therapeutic genes are introduced into cells *in vitro* and the treated cells are then re-introduced into the patient or experimental animal. In newer therapeutic protocols, gene therapy methods are being developed which could allow therapeutic genes to be introduced directly, *in vivo*. Methodologies are also being developed to target specific cell types for gene delivery [13], and new vectors are being created which allow for the selective temporal expression of the gene products [14].

Presently, a variety of methods are utilized to introduce the genes of choice into target cells with varying degrees of success. The simplest methods employ the direct introduction to target cells of naked plasmid DNA via transfection or injection (i.e. using a gene gun) [15]. Although effective *in vitro*, it is difficult to envision these methods being employed *in vivo* for deep tissue targets. Other protocols entail encapsulating the plasmid DNA into liposomes for *in vivo* delivery [12, 16]. The method of choice at the present however appears to be gene delivery mediated by viral transduction of target cells using retroviral and non-retroviral systems (herpes virus and adenovirus systems).

Viral delivery

All virally mediated gene delivery systems use modified versions of naturally occurring viruses to deliver genetic material. These systems take advantage of the fact that a portion (sometimes a large portion) of the viral genome can be deleted and replaced with a therapeutic package of genes without affecting viral infectivity. The gene of choice is simply cloned into the viral genome, which is contained in an expression plasmid. This plasmid is then introduced into a viral tissue culture system, where it is packaged into non-replicative virions. Simple, efficient packaging systems have been developed which allow the production of high titre virus stocks encoding for nearly any foreign genetic material in a matter of days [17].

Besides speed, viral systems have several advantages over other gene therapy systems. Viral vectors are able to infect many different cell types and the virions can be modified to target specific receptor bearing cells [18]. Lastly, viral transduction, using retroviruses, allows for stable expression of the foreign gene, owing to the integration of reverse transcribed viral DNA into the target cells DNA [19].

Introduction to MS and its animal model EAE

Multiple sclerosis is one of the most thoroughly studied autoimmune diseases. It is a demyelinating disease of the central nervous system which affects an estimated 300 000 Americans. Disease prevalence is higher in females with nearly twice as many woman affected, with disease onset occurring between the ages of 20–40 [20]. The disease has an uneven geographical extent and occurs mainly in North America, Japan, Northern Europe and Australia, with a notable propensity to affect those living in higher latitude, temperate regions [21].

Both genetic and environmental factors have been implicated in disease pathogenesis, although the influence of each factor on disease incidence is difficult to access. The most clearly defined genetic association is with HLA DR genes, particularly DR6 in Japanese MS patients and DR2/DQw1 in North American patients [22]. Other evidence for a genetic component of MS comes from twin studies which show a concordance of disease among identical twins, although the relatively low prevalence of disease precludes a determination of the precise gene(s) involved [23].

Of the various proposed environmental factors affecting disease, infectious agents are most often stipulated on the basis of data from epidemiology and migration studies. Recently, herpes simplex virus [24] joined the list of potential viral initiators of MS [25]. To date though, no single infectious agent has been clearly implicated as playing a role in the initiation of MS.

Although the precipitating event(s) leading to the development of multiple sclerosis is unknown, the pathology is most consistent with an immunologic etiology. The disease remains poorly studied in humans, however, owing to a number of factors; the disease organ is inaccessible, the genetics of disease are not readily manipulated and therapies cannot be readily tested. With this in mind, animal models of this disease have been developed which allow the testing of therapeutics. The best studied model for MS is the induced autoimmune disease, experimental autoimmune encephalomyelitis (EAE). Sharing many of the pathologic and clinical features of MS, EAE is the source of much of our current knowledge of the autoimmune processes in MS (for review see [26]).

Experimental autoimmune encephalomyelitis

EAE is an induced, T cell mediated disease of the central nervous system. EAE is most often studied in rodents where the disease can be induced by immunization with central nervous system components such as myelin basic protein or proteolipid protein [27, 28]. The disease manifests clinically with an ascending paralysis, which in severe cases can lead to death. Associated symptoms include weightloss, incontinence and blindness. Depending on the precise model used, clinical symptoms may occur in a chronic form, or a relapsing remitting form, which more closely resembles the human disease. Pathologically, the disease manifests with a multifocal central nervous system inflammation with resulting mononuclear cell infiltration and subsequent demyelination of motor neurons.

Although the inflammatory process in the central nervous system includes the infiltration of many cell types, the key cell type implicated in the initiation of disease processes is the $CD4^+$ T lymphocyte. Numerous studies have demonstrated the presence of antigen specific $CD4^+$ T cells at the site of disease pathology [29]. Furthermore, mice in which $CD4^+$ T cells have been depleted, or in which the CD4 function has been blocked with monoclonal antibodies, do not develop EAE [30]. The most convincing illustration of the role of $CD4^+$ T cells in EAE comes from adoptive transfer studies, where it has been shown that the injection of naïve mice with antigen specific $CD4^+$ T cell populations or more convincingly, transfer of clonal populations of $CD4^+$ T cells, can lead to the development of EAE [31, 32].

The events precipitated by these $CD4^+$ T cells have yet to be precisely determined, but it can be speculated that their effector function relates closely to the profile of cytokines that they secrete. A growing body of evidence indicates that "encephalitogenic" T cells are of the Th1 subtype, that is they secrete pro-inflammatory cytokines such as IL-2, IFNγ and TNFα. The most striking evidence of this fact is that most T cell clones capable of transferring disease are of the Th1 type, Th2 clones rarely transfer disease [33]. In addition, during the effector phase of disease induction, pro-inflammatory cytokines can be detected *in vivo*, in the spinal cord of experimental animals [34]. Lastly, as is seen in non-autoimmune models of Th1 T cell regulation, this autoimmune disease appears to be regulated by the effect of Th2 cytokines (for review see [35]).

Regulation of EAE

While the induction phase of EAE is clearly due to the effects of $CD4^+$ T cells, it has recently been discovered that $CD4^+$ T cells also play a role in the natural regulation of disease. Investigators were led to this finding from observations made of disease course in both the rat and mouse models of EAE. As discussed earlier, disease course in the rodent models occurs in a number of patterns. For instance, MBP immunization of Lewis rats leads to acute paralytic disease, from which most animals spontaneously recover. Rats recovering from disease are refractory to subsequent attempts to re-induce EAE.

In mice, adoptive transfer of MBP-specific T cells leads to a relapsing remitting form of EAE. In this model, episodes of disease are followed by spontaneous recovery with periods of little or no clinical or pathological symptoms. In both of these models, the spontaneous remissions that occur suggest a naturally occurring mechanism for the regulation of the inflammatory processes. Elucidation of the regulatory pathways is underway, but the $CD4^+$ T cell is again implicated. It appears that $CD4^+$, Th2 type T cells are the putative regulatory cells, and that the disease process is controlled by the secretion of anti-inflammatory cytokines.

A number of experimental approaches have implicated regulatory Th2 like T cells in disease regulation. In general these experiments show that it is possible to prevent EAE by skewing the T cell response from a pathogenic Th1 type to a protective Th2 phenotype. First, modulation of autoimmune responses by the systemic administration of anti-inflammatory cytokines such as IL-4, IL-10 or TGFβ has shown therapeutic potential in MS and in animal models of MS [2–4]. Targeting of autoantigen to B cells by coupling it to anti-immunoglobulin antibody results in the induction of Th2 T cells and results in protection from disease [36]. Protective oral administration of antigen is associated with the production of regulatory T cells producing IL-4 and TGFβ [37]. Finally, blocking of the co-stimulatory molecule B7.1, which results in a predominant Th2 T cell response, is an effective therapeutic for EAE [38). These experiments, in which the cytokine milieu is altered to affect disease, so-called "cytokine deviation", form the basis of a therapy for MS using gene therapy techniques.

Gene therapy for multiple sclerosis

Systemic administration of anti-inflammatory cytokines has been shown to be an effective therapeutic in both MS and EAE. Theoretically, the effect of this administration is due to the modulation of pathogenic T cells. Although effective, side-effects inherent in the systemic administration of cytokines necessitate their local delivery. An alternative approach would be to use antigen-specific T lymphocytes as delivery vehicles to target the modulatory cytokines. These cells could be modified using gene transfer techniques to secrete anti-inflammatory cytokines and then re-injected into a patient with active disease. The modified cells would be expected to home to sites of inflammation, secrete the cytokines locally and potentially dampen the immune attack. The feasibility of this approach has been recently demonstrated by our laboratory [5] and by Tuohy and colleagues [6]. The studies described below summarize the results of tissue-specific delivery of modulatory cytokines to the CNS of mice with EAE.

Treatment with IL-4

To test the concept of site specific delivery of cytokines by genetically modified T cells, we employed the murine model of EAE. A transformed encephalitogenic, MBP-specific T cell, G1.15H, was used in our studies as the "delivery vehicle." Although deleterious to the host in long-term experiments, these transformed cells are highly transducible and thus circumvent the problem of low transduction efficiency of murine primary T cell lines. Adoptive transfer of the unmodified G1.15H to naïve mice verified its EAE inducing and thus CNS homing capabilities.

The first cytokine tested in our experimental design was IL-4 since this cytokine had been demonstrated to be a mediator in EAE regulation as evidenced by its role in the natural recovery from disease [39], experimental protection from disease after oral tolerance induction [37] and after immunization with altered peptide ligands of MBP [40]. After transduction with an IL-4 encoding retrovirus and drug selection, ELISA confirmed the cell line to secrete IL-4. Subsequent limiting dilution cloning of these transduced cells yielded individual clones secreting distinct levels of IL-4, between 1 and 8 pg/ml of IL-4/10^5 cells. EAE was induced in experimental animals by immunization with MBP in complete Freund's adjuvant with concurrent injection of b-pertusis as co-adjuvant. Using this protocol, we are able to induce EAE with a consistent onset time of 15–16 days. Ten days after immunization to induce disease, the mice were given transduced or control (mock transduced) cells to test for therapeutic efficacy.

As expected, adoptive transfer of 10^6 transduced T cells secreting high levels of IL-4 (approximately 8 pg/ml/10^5 cells) ameliorated clinical EAE. Disease onset for the IL-4 treatment group was delayed by 2 days and the average disease score was significantly lower than control mice receiving untransduced cells or PBS. Transfer of cells secreting lower levels of IL-4 also had therapeutic effect on clinical disease though to a lesser extent (data not presented).

We next demonstrated that amelioration of disease was due to local and not systemic delivery of IL-4 using several experimental approaches. The first concern was that the effect on disease was due simply to high serum levels of IL-4 since the transferred cells consistently produced the cytokine. To check the extent of this problem, mice that received T cells transduced to express IL-4 were bled at various time points after cell transfer and serum IL-4 was determined by ELISA. No cytokine was detected in the serum until day 24-post transfer, well after initial recovery from disease. Even at this point serum IL-4 levels were still relatively low, ranging from 1.19 pg/ml to 2.53 pg/ml. This finding indicates that disease remission was not due to high systemic levels of IL-4.

In a second experimental approach, we verified the presence of transduced T cells in the CNS at the time of disease amelioration by testing spinal cord tissue from treated animals for retroviral specific IL-4 expression by RT-PCR analysis. Retroviral IL-4 transcription could be detected in the CNS of treated animals 15 days after transfer of transduced T cells. In a related experiment, T cells were transduced with a vector to express β-galactosidase (LacZ) a genetic marker that can be easily detected in histological sections by simple staining techniques. These cells were used in adoptive transfer experiments similar to the IL-4 transductants. Ten days after immunization, the cells were transferred to animals. At the peak of disease onset animals receiving genetically modified cells were sacrificed and histological sections of their spinal cords were examined for the presence of LacZ expressing cells in collaboration with Dr. Mauro DalCanto at Northwestern University. Similar to the PCR results, transduced T cells could be detected in EAE lesions in the CNS (data not presented).

A third experimental approach confirmed that amelioration of disease was dependent on T cell homing to the CNS. We reasoned that T cells transduced to express IL-4 that could not recognize CNS antigens would be ineffective at delivering IL-4 to the CNS. To test this hypothesis, additional transfer experiments were performed, using as controls, transduced T cells expressing IL-4 but lacking antigen-specific TCR expression. In this experiment, a TCR negative variant of the IL-4-secreting, disease ameliorating clone was used as a control. This line had significantly less effect on the disease course when compared to its TCR expressing counterpart.

TGFβ treatment

IL-4 is just one of a number of cytokines implicated in the regulation of EAE. Other Th2 type cytokines include IL-10 and TGFβ. We further tested the efficacy of our therapeutic approach by using these cytokines singly in place of IL-4. Retroviral vectors incorporating the fluorescence activated cell sorter (FACS) selectable marker green fluorescent protein (GFP) were used in these studies. Coordinate expression of either IL-10 or TGFβ and GFP was assured by cloning the cytokine gene upstream of the GFP gene and an internal ribosome entry site (IRES) element. Using these vectors the MBP specific T cell line was transduced and individual clones selected for both cytokine gene expression and TCR expression (or lack thereof) by FACS.

Preliminary experiments using TGFβ transduced T cells indicate that this cytokine is not an effective modulatory molecule when delivered locally. On the contrary, transfer of 10^7 TGFβ expressing cells to MBP immunized animals exacerbated disease severity compared to control animals (Fig. 1). Further experiments are needed to assess the TCR-specific homing pattern of these cells, and to determine the mechanism by which TGFβ transduced T cells aggravate clinical disease.

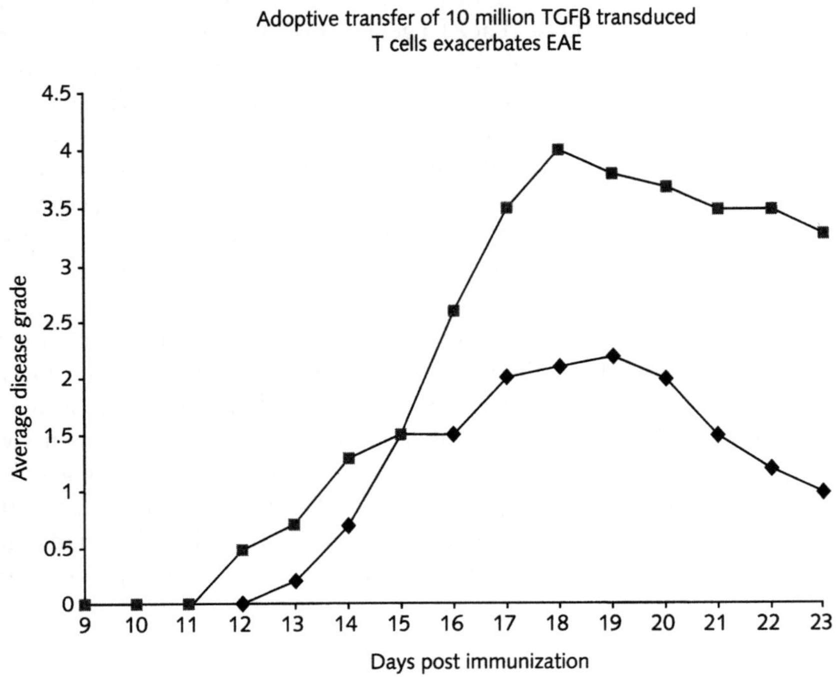

Figure 1
Adoptive transfer of TGFβ transduced T cells exacerbates disease. MBP immunized mice received 10^6 untransduced cells (diamonds) or 10^6 TGFβ transduced cells (squares) intravenously on day 10 post immunization. Data represents mean disease scores.

IL-10 treatment

Experiments to test the treatment of EAE with cells modified to secrete IL-10 have provided mixed results in our laboratory. In initial studies T cells transduced with IL-10 produced low levels of secreted IL-10 (10–20 pg/ml/10^5 cells). These cells were ineffective modulators of EAE when used in the adoptive transfer model described above. Later attempts to produce IL-10 secreting T cell clones were more successful and the results of adoptive transfer experiments differed also. These experiments indicated that cells secreting higher levels of IL-10 could ameliorate disease (Fig. 2).

Confirming these conclusions were experiments by Tuohy and co-workers who also demonstrated that antigen-specific T cells modified to secrete IL-10 can modu-

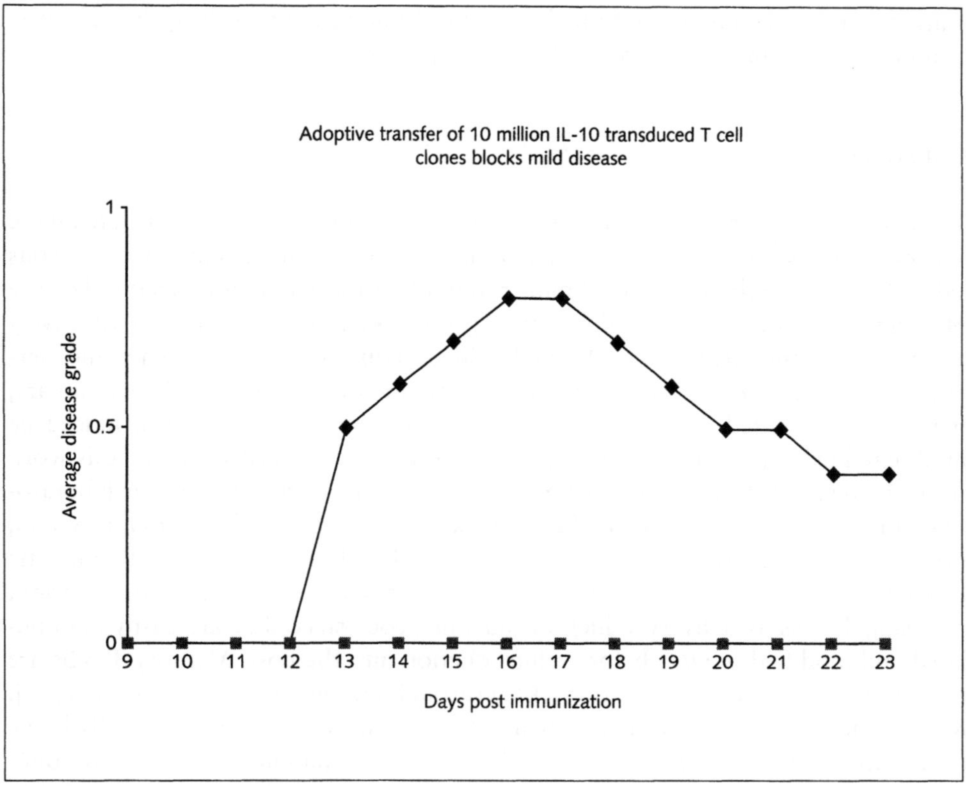

Figure 2
Adoptive transfer of 10^7 IL-10 transduced T cells blocks mild EAE. $(PL/J \times SJL/J)_{F1}$ mice were immunized with guinea pig MBP and then treated on day 10 with intravenous injection of 107 untransduced cells (diamonds) or 10^7 IL-10 transduced cells (squares) secreting high amounts of IL-10 (200 pg/ml/10^5 cells). Data represent mean disease scores.

late disease course [6]. Tuohy's group produced a primary T cell line and clones derived from this line that are specific for the PLP peptide 139–151. These cells were modified to secrete high levels of IL-10 in an antigen inducible manner. This was accomplished by placing IL-10 gene expression under the control of an IL-2 promoter system. The IL-2 promoted IL-10 gene was transfected into T cells and cytokine secreting cells selected. One clone was examined that produced high levels of IL-10 (approximately 2000 pg/ml/5 × 10^5 cells). Upon adoptive transfer, this clone was able to inhibit the onset of EAE in PLP immunized mice. Moreover, transfer of the clone to animals in which clinical signs of EAE had already developed accelerated recovery and reduced mean maximal disease scores. Histological examination of treated animals confirmed the clinical findings in that demyelination was diminished in animals receiving IL-10 secreting cells.

Conclusions

The majority of approaches taken to control autoimmune disease concentrate on the general suppression of the aberrant immune response. This results in deleterious side-effects due to the systemic administration of anti-inflammatory agents. The use of antigen-specific T cells, modified to express regulatory cytokines, to selectively target anti-inflammatory molecules to the site of pathology represents a unique therapeutic approach to the treatment of autoimmune disease. Although preliminary, the results presented here indicate that the autoimmune processes can indeed be modulated using this therapeutic approach. More work is needed to take this work from the research bench to the patient's bedside. Current research in our laboratory is concentrating on improving the transduction efficiency of the retroviral system, targeting the retrovirus specifically to activated T cells and testing the therapeutic efficacy of using other anti-inflammatory cytokines either alone or in combination.

Using T cells as delivery vehicles is advantageous since they are easily manipulated and modified *in vitro* before reintroduction into the host. Memory T cells are thought to have long lifespans, trafficking throughout the body for many years [41]. More importantly, the antigen-specificity of T cells allows them to specifically home to multiple depots of antigen in the body such as at inflammatory sites of autoimmune disease. This has been demonstrated in the murine model of EAE where MBP-specific T cells have been shown to traffic to the CNS, both during the induction phase of disease as well as during relapses in a relapsing- remitting model of EAE [42, 43].

Although a number of gene therapy techniques are available for inserting the therapeutic genes into the antigen-specific T cells of choice, we believe that retroviral systems hold many advantages over other methods. Retroviral gene therapy results in long-term, stable expression of gene products due to insertion of the retroviral genome into the host cells. As well, retroviral systems allow for large numbers of cells to be modified and selected in a short period of time, usually days. This is compared to other methods such as transfection, which require rare recombinational events, and thus months, to gain stable expression. Lastly, retroviral modification is technically simple, requiring only knowledge of simple molecular biology and tissue culture techniques to perform.

Although gene therapy holds great promise for many human diseases, it is still too early to predict the extent and timetable of its success for any particular disease such as multiple sclerosis. If these preliminary findings hold true then the future of this therapeutic approach can only benefit from advances in gene therapy research under development.

References

1 IFNB MS Study Group (1995) Interferon beta-1β in the treatment of multiple sclerosis: Final outcome of the randomized controlled trial. *Neurology* 45: 1277–1285

2 Inobe JI, Chen Y, Weiner H (1996) *In vivo* administration of IL-4 induces TGF-beta-producing cells and protects animals from experimental autoimmune encephalomyelitis. *Annal NY Acad Sci* 778: 390–392

3 Johns, LD, Flanders KC, Ranges GE, Sriram S (1991) Successful treatment of experimental allergic encephalomyelitis with transforming growth factor-beta 1. *J Immunol* 147: 1792–1796

4 Racke MK, Dhib-Jalbut S, Cannella B, Albert PS, Raine CS, McFarlin D (1991) Prevention and treatment of chronic relapsing experimental allergic encephalomyelitis by transforming growth factor-beta 1. *J Immunol* 146: 3012–3017

5 Steinman L(1996) A few autoreactive cells in an autoimmune infiltrate control a vast population of nonspecific cells: a tale of smart bombs and the infantry. *Proc Natl Acad Sci USA* 93: 2253–2256

6 Shaw MK, Lorens JB, Dhawan A, DalCanto R, Tse HY, Tran AB, Bonpane C, Eswaran SL, Brocke S, Sarvetnick N, Steinman L, Nolan GP, Fathman CG (1997) Local delivery of interleukin 4 by retrovirus-transduced T lymphocytes ameliorates experimental autoimmune encephalomyelitis. *J Exp Med* 185: 1711–1714

7 Mathisen PM, Yu M, Johnson JM, Drazba JA, Tuohy VK (1997) Treatment of experimental autoimmune encephalomyelitis with genetically modified memory T cells. *J Exp Med* 186: 159–164

8 Blaese RM, Culver KW, Miller AD, Carter CS, Fleisher T, Clerici M, Shearer G, Chang L, Chiang Y, Tolstoshev P et al (1995) T lymphocyte-directed gene therapy for ADA-SCID: initial trial results after 4 years. *Science* 270: 475–480

9 Dranoff G (1997) Strategies for cancer gene therapy. *Cancer Chemother Biol Response Modif* 17: 328–348

10 Xu L, Sanchez A, Yang Z, Zaki SR, Nabel EG, Nichol ST, Nabel GJ (1998) Immunization for Ebola virus infection. *Nature Med* 4: 37–42

11 Schmidt-Wolf G, Schmidt-Wolf IGH (1995) Cytokines and gene therapy. *Immunol Today* 25: 1137–1140

12 Kren BT, Bandyopadhyay P, Steer CJ (1998) *In vivo* site-directed mutagenesis of the factor IX gene by chimeric RNA/DNA oligonucleotides. *Nature Med* 4 (3): 285–290

13 Cosset FL, Morling FJ, Takeuchi Y, Weiss RA, Collins MK, Russell SJ (1996) Retroviral retargeting by envelopes expressing an N-terminal binding domain. *J Virol* 69 (10): 6314–6322

14 Hofmann A, Nolan GP, Blau HM (1996) Rapid retroviral delivery of tetracycline-inducible genes in a single autoregulatory cassette. *Proc Natl Acad Sci USA* 93: 5185–5190

15 Yang N-S, Sin WH (1995) Gene gun and other non-viral approaches for cancer gene therapy. *Nature Med* 1: 481–483

16 Croxford JL, Triantaphyllopoulos K, Podhajcer OL, Feldmann M, Baker D, Chernajovsky Y (1998) Cytokine gene therapy in experimental allergic encephalomyelitis by injection of plasmid DNA-cationic liposome complex into the central nervous system. *J Immunol* 160: 5181–5187
17 Pear WS, Nolan GP, Scott ML, Baltimore D (1993) Production of high-titer helper-free retroviruses by transient transfection. *Proc Natl Acad Sci USA* 90: 8392–8396
18 Gunzburg WH, Fleuchaus A, Saller R, Salmons B (1996) Retroviral vector targeting for gene therapy. *Cytokines Mol Ther* 2: 177–184
19 Kuby J (1997) The immune system in AIDS. In: *Immunology*. W.H. Freeman and Company, New York, 523–553
20 Bansil S, Cook SD, Rohowsky-Kochan C (1995) Multiple sclerosis: immune mechanism and update on current therapies. *Ann Neurol* 37 (1): S87–S101
21 Kurtzke JF (1977) Geography in multiple sclerosis. *J Neurol* 215 (1): 1–26
22 Voskuhl RR, Goldstein AM, Simonis T, Davey RJ, McFarland HF (1996) DR2/DQw1 inheritance and haplotype sharing in affected siblings from multiple sclerosis families. *Ann Neurol* 39: 804–807
23 Ebers GC, Bulman DE, Sadovnick AD, Paty DW, Warren S, Hader W, Murray TJ, Seland TP, Duquette P, Grey T et al (1986) A population-based study of multiple sclerosis in twins. *N Engl J Med* 315: 1638–1642
24 Soldan SS, Berti R, Salem N, Secchiero P, Flamand L, Calabresi PA, Brennan MB, Maloni HW, McFarland HF, Lin HC, Patnaik M, Jacobson S (1997) Association of human herpes virus 6 (HHV-6) with multiple sclerosis: increased IgM response to HHV-6 early antigen and detection of serum HHV-6 DNA. *Nature Med* 3: 1394–1397
25 Dalgleish AG (1997) Viruses and multiple sclerosis. *Acta Neurol Scand Suppl* 169: 8–15
26 Swanborg RH (1995) Experimental autoimmune encephalomyelitis in rodents as a model for human demyelinating disease. *Clin Immunol Immunopathol* 77: 4–13
27 Kies MW (1965) Chemical studies on an encephalitogenic protein from guinea pig brain. *Ann NY Acad Sci* 122: 161–168
28 Yamamura T, Namikawa T, Endoh M, Kunishita T, Tabira T (1986) Experimental allergic encephalomyelitis induced by proteolipid apoprotein in Lewis rats. *J Neuroimmunol* 12: 143–153
29 Burns J, Rosenzweig A, Zweiman B, Moskovitz A, Lisak R (1984) Recovery of myelin basic protein reactive T cells from spinal cords of Lewis rats with autoimmune encephalomyelitis. J *Immunol* 132: 2690–2692
30 Brostoff SW, Mason DW (1984) Experimental allergic encephalomyelitis: successful treatment *in vivo* with a monoclonal antibody that recognizes T helper cells. *J Immunol* 133: 1938–1942
31 Ben-Nun A, Lando Z (1983) Detection of autoimmune cells proliferating to myelin basic protein and selection of T cell lines that mediate experimental autoimmune encephalomyelitis (EAE) in mice. *J Immunol* 130: 1205–1209
32 Zamvil SS, Nelson PA, Mitchell DJ, Knobler RL, Fritz RB, Steinman L (1985) Encephal-

itogenic T cell clones specific for myelin basic protein. An unusual bias in antigen recognition. *J Exp Med* 162: 2107–2124

33 Kalman B, Alder H, Lublin FD (1995) Characteristics of the T lymphocytes involved in experimental allergic encephalomyelitis. *J Neuroimmunol* 61: 107–116

34 Issazadeh S, Ljungdahl A, Hojeberg B, Mustafa M, Olsson T (1995) Cytokine production in the central nervous system of Lewis rats with experimental autoimmune encephalomyelitis: dynamics of mRNA expression for interleukin-10, interleukin-12, cytolysin, tumor necrosis factor alpha and tumor necrosis factor beta. *J Neuroimmunol* 61: 205–212

35 Olsson T (1995) Cytokine-producing cells in experimental autoimmune encephalomyelitis and multiple sclerosis. *Neurology* 45 (6): S11–S15

36 Saoudi A, Simmonds S, Huitinga I, Mason D (1995) Prevention of experimental allergic encephalomyelitis in rats by targeting autoantigen to B cells: evidence that the protective mechanism depends on changes in the cytokine response and migratory properties of the autoantigen-specific T cells. *J Exp Med* 182: 335–344

37 Chen Y, Kuchroo VK, Inobe J, Hafler DA, Weiner HL (1994) Regulatory T cell clones induced by oral tolerance: suppression of autoimmune encephalomyelitis. *Science* 265: 1237–1240

38 Kuchroo VK, Das MP, Brown JA, Ranger AM, Zamvil SS, Sobel RA, Weiner HL, Nabavi N, Glimcher LH (1995) B7-1 and B7-2 costimulatory molecules activate differentially the Th1/Th2 developmental pathways: application to autoimmune disease therapy. *Cell* 80: 707–718

39 Karpus WJ, Gould KE, Swanborg RH (1992) $CD4^+$ suppressor cells of autoimmune encephalomyelitis respond to T cell receptor-associated determinants on effector cells by interleukin-4 secretion. *Eur J Immunol* 22: 1757–1763

40 Gaur A, Boehme SA, Chalmers D, Crowe PD, Pahuja A, Ling N, Brocke S, Steinman L, Conlon PJ (1997) Amelioration of relapsing experimental autoimmune encephalomyelitis with altered myelin basic protein peptides involves different cellular mechanisms. *J Neuroimmunol* 74: 149–158

41 Jamieson BD, Ahmed R (1989) T cell memory. Long-term persistence of virus-specific cytotoxic T cells. *J Exp Med* 169: 1993–2005

42 Cross AH, Cannella B, Brosnan CF, Raine C (1990) Homing to central nervous system vasculature by antigen-specific lymphocytes. I. Localization of 14C-labeled cells during acute, chronic, and relapsing experimental allergic encephalomyelitis. *Lab Invest* 63: 162–170

43 Skundric DS, Kim C, Tse HY, Raine CS (1993) Homing of T cells to the central nervous system throughout the course of relapsing experimental autoimmune encephalomyelitis in Thy-1 congenic mice. *J Neuroimmunol* 46: 113–121

Gene therapy for type I diabetes mellitus

Nick Giannoukakis[1], Massimo Trucco[2] and Paul D. Robbins[1]

[1]Department of Molecular Genetics and Biochemistry, University of Pittsburgh School of Medicine, Pittsburgh, PA 15261, USA; [2]Division of Immunogenetics, Children's Hospital of Pittsburgh, University of Pittsburgh School of Medicine, W1246 Biomedical Science Tower, Pittsburgh, PA 15261, USA

Introduction

Insulin-dependent diabetes mellitus (IDDM) or type I diabetes mellitus, is the outcome of a progressive and selective immune-mediated destruction of the insulin-producing β cells of the pancreatic islets of Langerhans. While evidence of a T lymphocyte involvement in the immunopathogenesis of the disease is demonstrated by histologic analysis of the pancreata from children at the onset of the disease and confirmed in animal models like the non-obese diabetic (NOD) mouse or the Bio-Breeding (BB) rat, the mechanisms which trigger the immunologic invasion of the islets still eludes our complete understanding. IDDM is one of the multifactorial-type diseases with a strong genetic component predisposing certain individuals. The genetic susceptibility has been very well documented with the highest risk conferred upon individuals carrying particular alleles at different HLA class II loci [1–4]. Other loci have subsequently been identified using whole genome scanning approaches in affected sib-pair linkage analyses; however, the association of many of these loci to IDDM has recently been questioned [5–8]. It must be borne in mind that the genetic transmission of susceptibility alleles at loci linked to and/or associated with IDDM need not result in disease, although the risk of developing IDDM is increased compared to individuals not carrying such alleles. The involvement of a non-genetic environmental component in disease onset, was inferred from earlier genetic analyses where the susceptibility attributable to genetics was found to be less than 50% [3].

Many different environmental triggers have been considered during the last 20 years including proteins present in cow's milk [9] as well as viral agents to which children are frequently exposed before or after their immune system has completely developed [10–12]. What is clear is that the initial trigger involves or activates an inflammatory infiltration of the islets (insulitis) with a progressive accumulation of T lymphocytes, macrophages and B-lymphocytes, all of which contribute to the eventual destruction of the insulin-producing β cells while sparing the other cells of the endocrine pancreas [4, 13].

Gene Therapy in Inflammatory Diseases, edited by C. H. Evans and P. D. Robbins

Insulitis: The cellular and molecular constituents of islet inflammation

Macrophages

The insulitic infiltrate is mainly composed of T lymphocytes and macrophages. Macrophages are derived from the monocyte lineage and are very efficient antigen-presenting cells. They express class II MHC molecules which present exogenously-derived, internally-processed antigens to $CD4^+$ T cells. These, in turn, orchestrate an immune response by releasing cytokines like interleukin-2 (IL-2), tumor necrosis factor α (TNFα) and interferon γ (IFNγ). In response to IFNγ, macrophages upregulate the cell surface expression of class II MHC and increase the production of the proinflammatory cytokine IL-1β. Macrophages are believed to play a primary role in the development of IDDM, because they are the first cells found around the islets during the onset of insulitis, but more importantly because their depletion following silica particle injection into streptozotocin-induced diabetic BB rats and CD-1 mice completely prevented diabetes [14, 15]. Islets contain resident macrophages (about 10–15 per islet) which are known to express and secrete the proinflammatory cytokine IL-1 [16]. The activation of resident macrophages may represent a triggering event associated with IDDM onset. Further evidence in favor of the importance of macrophages in IDDM onset derive from studies examining microencapsulated islet xenografts in streptozotocin-induced diabetic mice [17]. In these studies, it was observed that 65% of the biosynthetic membrane was surrounded by macrophages whereas only 5% was surrounded in normal mice. Furthermore, in the diabetic mice, there was an altered morphology of the islets as well as a decrease in insulin secretion. These events could be reproduced by injections of recombinant IL-1β that is able to cross the biosynthetic polymer. Further studies show that IL-1β is not the only mediator of microencapsulated islet dysfunction, as antibodies against IL-1β failed to prevent the dysfunction [17]. However, there is a convincing body of data to support the pivotal role of macrophage-derived IL-1 during the onset of insulitis as a direct and/or indirect mediator of β cell dysfunction and destruction.

T lymphocytes

The importance of T lymphocytes in IDDM is based on the following observations: (1) T cells are detected in the mononuclear cell infiltrates in the islets at disease onset [18–21], (2) immunosuppressants delay the onset of IDDM [22, 23], (3) autoreactive T lymphocytes are detectable in IDDM patients [24], (4) IDDM can be transferred from a diabetic patient to an immunosuppressed non-diabetic recipient by bone marrow transplantation [25], and (5) IDDM can be adoptively transferred to normal mice using autoreactive T cells from genetically diabetic mice [26, 27]. Beta-cell-specific T cells have been demonstrated in newly-diagnosed IDDM patients either prediabetic or recent-onset [28–30] and are present in the islet infiltrate at disease onset [21, 31]. This infiltrate contains both $CD4^+$ as well as $CD8^+$ T cells. Such beta-cell-specific cells have also been observed in the circulation of healthy individuals, albeit in lower numbers and with less reactivity than in diabetics, indicating that other factors are required to trigger disease onset. In addition, most diabetogenic T cell clones are not limited to one particular antigen, but to a plethora of molecules that may not be beta-cell-specific such as glutamate decarboxylase (GAD) [32] which is expressed in other islet cells as well as in neurons [33]. It is worthwhile to note that of all known autoantigens, GAD65/67 has a six amino acid long segment that is homologous to a protein of the Coxsackie B virus [34]. This has raised the possibility that recognition of GAD epitopes may be due to molecular mimicry as a consequence of Coxsackie B virus infection, but recent studies indicate that this may not be the case [12].

From a few studies performed in the mouse, it appears that the predominant T lymphocyte subtype present in the autoimmune infiltrate is that of the $CD8^+$ class [35, 36]. An examination of the TCR type present on these autoreactive T cell clones indicated that the TCR variable segments,Vβ, were heterogeneous, reflecting the heterogeneity of these cells in the infiltrate. Although oligoclonality was suggested in some individuals by the finding of a predominant Vβ8 TCR [37, 38], other studies reported the predominant expression of TCR-Vβ7 that suggests the reaction to a superantigen [39, 40]. It has also been suggested that chronic insulitis can be a consequence of bacterial or viral infections and that it may be involved in the etiology of IDDM. However, only a minority of patients with chronic pancreatitis become insulin-dependent. In fact, there were no manifestations of autoimmunity in genetically predisposed individuals who were afflicted with pathogen-induced insulitis [41]. These results demonstrate that inflammatory islet cell damage is not necessarily autoimmune T cell-dependent, nor does chronic inflammation necessarily lead to insulin dependency. Furthermore, the T lymphocytes present in the insulitic infiltrate do not have to be actively engaged in beta-cell destruction, as proven in studies showing the presence of chronically activated T cells around the islets of non-diabetics [41] as well as non-activated T cells in the islets of recent-onset diabetics [42, 43]. Animal models of insulitis have indicated that, despite the presence of active T lymphocytes adjacent to beta-cells, this does not always lead to islet destruction [44].

The major autoreactive T lymphocyte type involved in the recognition of beta-cell antigens is the $CD4^+$ cell, while the predominant cell type found in the islet infiltrate is the $CD8^+$ cell [35, 36]. In the NOD mouse, it was shown that a diabetogenic T cell clone could by itself initiate the disease in an immunocompromised host [45]. In other studies, it was determined that diabetes in mice occurred in the absence of $CD4^+$ cells [46, 47], and in some instances, diabetes required combinations of both $CD4^+$ and $CD8^+$ T cells [46, 47]. Although these transfer studies do not indicate the spontaneous nature of autoimmune diabetes, and caution must therefore be used in their interpretation, they illustrate the importance of the T lymphocyte in the pathophysiology of the disease. Other studies have indicated a perturbation in the ratio of $CD4^+/CD8^+$ T cells in the peripheral blood of IDDM individuals [48–50]. In some studies the ratio declined with disease progression [48–50] and in patients investigated prior to IDDM onset, it was discovered that $CD8^+$ levels where elevated [51]. Despite these observations, the exact role of $CD4^+$ and $CD8^+$ cells in the pathophysiology of IDDM is not yet fully clarified.

The $CD4^+$ T helper cells (T_H) can be divided into two categories: T_H1 and T_H2. Their biological actions differ as a consequence of their different cytokine secretion profile upon activation. T_H1 cells are recognised on the basis of their production of IL-2 and IFNγ and are mostly associated with cellular immune responses (i.e. activation of $CD8^+$ cytotoxic cells). T_H2 cells, on the other hand, are mainly associated with the production of IL-4 and IL-10 and shift the immune response to predominantly humoral (i.e. activation of B lymphocytes, and antibody production). An inverse correlation has been described between humoral and cellular responses to the GAD67 autoantigen in diabetics which also suggested a selective activation of certain T_H subsets among different individuals [52]. The beta cell-specific humoral response has been associated with a slow progression of IDDM [52]. On the contrary, an inverse relationship between cellular and humoral responses to the GAD65 autoantigen and insulin has been described in high-risk relatives of diabetics as well as in new patients [53]. It is not completely clear whether T lymphocytes of the T_H2 type play a protective role in the pathogenesis of IDDM, but there are data strongly supporting T_H1 involvement.

In NOD mice, detectable amounts of IFNγ can be found concomitant with the insulitic infiltration and the initiation of the islet destruction. Also, monoclonal antibodies against IFNγ can prevent the autoimmune destruction of the islets [54, 55]. In a recent report aimed at dissecting, in the NOD mouse, the contribution of T_H1 versus T_H2 cells in the development of diabetes, although both cell types were expressing the same diabetogenic TCR, it was shown that the disease was clearly T_H1-mediated. In the same model, the T_H2 cells could not induce diabetes, nor were they able to prevent it by downregulating T_H1 cells [56].

Finally, the importance of regulatory and proinflammatory cytokines in the etiopathogenesis of IDDM has been demonstrated and it appears that IFNγ, TNFα, IL-4 and IL-10 have important effects on the exacerbation of insulitis, the initiation of the beta cell destruction, and the control of the cytotoxic response [57]. The destruction of β cells in a variety of murine models is delayed or prevented by T cells producing T_H2-type cytokines like IL-4, IL-10 and TGFβ [58]. IL-10 in particular, is a potent inhibitor of IFNγ production and macrophage function [59]. In a series of studies, it was shown that T cell-mediated destruction of β cells in the NOD mouse can be prevented by the transfer of suppressor T cell clones islolated from the insulitic infiltrate of NOD mice that do not develop IDDM [58, 60]. One of these clones, NY4.2, could also prevent the destruction of islet grafts into acutely-diabetic syngeneic mice. These clones secreted substantial amounts of IL-10 and TGFβ [58]. The most convincing evidence that IL-10 can prevent IDDM onset derives from studies using recombinant IL-10 (rIL-10). In adult NOD mice, IDDM onset is delayed and its incidence is significantly decreased when the mice were given rIL-10 [61]. Furthermore, the administration of a non-cytolytic IL-10/Fc fusion protein (the Fc portion prolongs the protein half-life) to NOD mice from 5–25 weeks of age, prevented diabetes. These mice remained disease-free long after the cessation of treatment [62]. In the islets of these mice, the expression of TNFα and IFNγ was inhibited. Moreover, the inability to adoptively transfer IDDM to these mice using non-treated NOD splenocytes, suggests the existence of IL-10-modulated suppressor T cells in the host [62]. Finally, daily injections of IL-10, subcutaneously, into prediabetic NOD mice delayed IDDM onset and incidence. In this study, the severity of insulitis was reduced to a predominant peri-insulitis and normoglycemia was maintained for a while. However, results obtained in transgenic mice with the IL-10 gene under the control of the insulin promoter, contradict the immunosuppressive effect of IL-10 in IDDM [63, 64]. A possible explanation of this could be that because insulin is expressed in the thymus [65, 66], and IL-10 suppresses the cell-surface expression of B7.1 and B7.2 co-stimulatory molecules on antigen-presenting dendritic cells [67] involved in thymic negative selection [68, 69], the absence of a co-stimulatory signal could result in failure of negative selection of autoreactive T cells thereby allowing them to survive and mature. IL-10 expression in islets will therefore not be able to generate the same effect.

It is conceivable that since each T_H1-type cytokine (e.g. TNFα and IFNγ) provides its own specific and unsubstitutable contribution to β cell destruction, by neutralising one cytokine, the whole process could be inhibited. It is also likely that the cytokines act synergistically and in a coordinated fashion. Blocking the expression and/or action of one may impact on the production/effects of the others and on the entire pathological process leading to IDDM. It is still a matter of speculation which are the factors that control the balance of T_H1 to T_H2 in IDDM. Factors which may lead to preferential development and predominance of T_H1 cells include the density of HLA/antigenic peptide complexes on the surface of antigen-presenting cells [70], TCR affinity/avidity for the HLA/peptide complex or the interaction and the strength of interaction of costimulatory molecules [71].

IDDM therapy: existing and experimental approaches

Currently, the only widely available treatment for IDDM is insulin injection. Various insulin formulations to control blood glucose levels are in use which can be short or long-lasting. Exogenous insulin administration also offers the additional benefit of retarding the development of diabetic complications like nephropathy and retinopathy. However, the risk of insulin-induced hypoglycemia and hyperinsulinemia-mediated atherogenesis and hypertension suggest that more precise means of controlling blood glucose in a physiologically-relevant manner are needed. Ideally, IDDM therapy should be able to reproduce the physiological secretion of insulin in response to glucose while also avoiding, or preventing autoimmune phenomena. Current advances in the engineering of β cell lines and non β-cells as glucose-sensing replacements of insulin production, offer promise for adult-onset, non-autoimmune diabetes [72]. The ideal solution for IDDM would be instead, to offer intact, immune privileged islets or insulin-secreting cells to diabetic recipients at a site where portal islet-hepatic hormonal contact is re-established. The most physiological solution is the transplantation of insulin-secreting tissue into diabetic recipients. The transplantation of entire pancreas is a procedure that has been successfully performed, alone or concurrent with kidney transplantation and of the more than 1000 grafts reported, 46% of the recipients became insulin-independent and exhibited normalisation of hemoglobin A_{1c} levels [73].

Recent advances in methodology of isolation of intact functional human and non-human islets from pancreas has resulted in clinical testing of islet transplantation instead of whole pancreas transplantation. Although there have been some successes with human allografts, where immunosuppressed recipients have remained insulin-independent for a number of years following islet transplantation via the portal vein, most of the patients failed to achieve insulin-independence [74]. Futhermore, immunosuppressive agents in clinical use today, which are used to prevent allograft rejection, especially glucocorticoids, cyclosporin A and FK-506 [75], are toxic and can cause malignancy as well as an induction of diabetes. Autografts have met with better success, but in the majority of cases, the availability of human donors remains an important obstacle [74]. Xenotransplantation is emerging as a potential option and aside from the ethical concerns as well as those for zoonosis, important immunologic hurdles remain to be surmounted [76–79]. Microencapsulated islets in synthetic polymers have been effective in some instances, but their long-term survival has met with obstacles, most likely involving fibrosis of the polymer, islet core damage and death due to ischemic oxygen deprivation and cytokine-induced damage [80–97]. Recent experimental strategies involving the genetic engineering of islets followed by transplantation to allogeneic rodent and non-human primate models have demonstrated that local modulation of the immune response may be sufficient to prevent allograft rejection as well as autoimmunity. Possible modulation and suppression of xenograft rejection by means of genetic engineering will be discussed in a later section.

Gene transfer to islets: Delivery vehicles

Islets consist of differentiated cells with limited mitotic-capability. Insulin-secreting β cells are found at the core of a typical islet surrounded by glucagon-producing α cells and somatostatin-synthesising δ cells. A small number of pancreatic polypeptide-producing cells (PP) are also present [98]. Islets have an extensive microcirculation as well as a rich innervation, both parasympathetic and adrenergic [98]. In general, β cells account for 50–80% of an islet. Because of their non-dividing nature, islet cells are not good targets for Moloney-based leukemia retroviral vectors, but are excellent targets for adenoviruses, both *in vitro* and *in vivo* [99, 100]. Recent data indicate that herpes simplex viruses (HSV) as well as HIV-1-based lentiviruses can infect human islets *in vitro* [101–104] (and manuscript submitted), and we have demonstrated that human islets can be infected with lentiviruses to nearly-identical levels as with adenoviruses (manuscript submitted). More importantly, adenoviral and lentiviral infection does not appear to affect the function of β cells *in vitro*, although nothing is known about viral effects on the other cell types [103, 105] (and manuscript submitted). Transgene expression from adenovirally-infected islets *in vivo* is transient, most likely because of the immune reaction mounted against the adenoviral proteins. Moreover, the episomal nature of adenoviral vectors precludes long-term therapeutic effects in islets, although these vectors are perfectly suitable for proof-of-principle experimentation. Recent developments in HSV vehicles leading to reduced or complete loss of toxicity, along with long-term, high level transgene expression and a large capacity for cloning of many genes, makes them good candidates for infecting non-dividing cells [106–109]. Lentiviral vectors also are promising in that they can be grown to relatively high titers with the recent availability of packaging cell lines [110], can stably infect non-dividing cells *in vivo*, and appear not to be immunogenic *in vivo* [101, 102]. Gene gun-mediated delivery of reporter genes as well as immunomodulatory cytokines has been attempted with varying levels of gene expression from plasmids, and there are data showing statistically-significant prolongation of *in vivo* islet survival following *in vitro* gene gun delivery [111–113], Finally, cationic lipids have been tested *in vitro* with some success in transfecting islets, but the level of transfection was considerably lower compared to viral infection [114]. Table 1 lists some of the vectors that have been tested for IDDM gene and cell therapy.

Genetic engineering of islets for the facilitation of transplantation as a therapy for IDDM

Although there are observations demonstrating that retrograde pancreaticobiliary injection of recombinant adenoviral particles is feasible and able to result in transgene expression [115–117], the fact that islets comprise only 2% of the pancreatic mass suggests that very little therapeutic effect can be expected. Clearly, *in vitro* genetic manipulation of islets followed by transplantation is a simpler process which results in the expression of a therapeutic transgene exclusively from islets and from virtually all cell types, provided the vector is designed for such a purpose. Recent

Table 1 - Gene transfer vehicles for use in IDDM gene and cell therapy

Gene transfer vehicle	Targets/Therapeutic objectives in animal models
E1, E3-deleted adenovirus	Islets; prolongation of graft survival
	Dendritic cells; tolerance induction to alloantigens
	Antigen-presenting cells; tolerance to vector proteins
HSV-1 amplicon	Islets; protection from apoptosis
HIV-1 lentivirus	Islets; prevention of IDDM
Retrovirus	Islet-infiltrating T lymphocytes; suppression of IDDM
	bone marrow cells; prevention of xenoreactive antibody production

attempts to facilitate islet transplantation in rodent and non-human primates, both allogeneic and xenogeneic following genetic modification have had mixed success. Most experimentation has been conducted in mice and rats. Furthermore, although attempts to suppress autoimmunity in the NOD mouse with the transplantation of genetically-modified islets expressing immunomodulatory transgenes has also met with mixed success, the possibility for improvement has countless alternatives and can use many combined approaches illustrated in the next and subsequent sections.

Interleukin-4

The identification of interleukin-4 (IL-4) and interleukin-10 (IL-10) as cytokines with immunosuppressive properties, as well as the cloning of a viral homologue of interleukin-10 (vIL-10) from Epstein-Barr virus, led to attempts to use recombinant forms of these cytokines as a means of preventing IDDM in NOD mice as well as to prolong islet allograft survival. Recombinant IL-4 administration to NOD mice was shown to prevent IDDM onset when the treatment was initiated at 2 weeks of age, prior to the manifestation of insulitis [118, 119]. The immunomodulatory role of IL-4 is supported by studies of oral tolerance, where IDDM prevented by oral insulin was associated with increased IL-4 levels in the mucosa as well as an IL-4-dependent shift from the T_H1-type to the T_H2-type immune response [118–120]. More recently, islets from transgenic NOD mice expressing IL-4 transplanted into a syngeneic host were spared autoimmune destruction, but were rejected in allogeneic recipients [121]. The relevance of IL-4 becomes questionable when taking into account studies where recombinant IL-4 administration to NOD mice receiving syngeneic islet transplants failed to prevent IDDM. Also, no protection from IDDM was conferred to alloxan-treated NOD mice receiving transplants of syngeneic islets infected with an adenoviral vector expressing IL-4 [122]. It is not known whether the failure to prevent IDDM was due to the failure of IL-4, a host response against the viral gene products, or to non-specific effects of alloxan treatment. In fact, very recently, Gallichan et al. have demonstrated that IL-4 expressed from a lentiviral vector in NOD-scid mouse islets transplanted into syngeneic hosts, can prevent insulitis of the graft following the introduction of diabetogenic splenocytes and, more interestingly, that the host pancreas was spared from the adoptive transfer of IDDM [123].

Interleukin-10

IL-10 prevents IFNγ production by T_H1-type T lymphocytes, downregulates class II MHC expression on antigen-presenting cells (APC), and prevents IL-12 production by APC [124]. However, IL-10 stimulates immunoglobulin production by B lymphocytes, stimulates $CD8^+$ cells, blocks T cell apoptosis and stimulates NK activity. In contrast, vIL-10 lacks the growth-promoting effects of IL-10 on some of these cell types which could lead to immunostimulation [125, 126]. Adenoviral as well as cationic lipid gene transfer of vIL-10 to mouse heart was able to prolong cardiac survival in allogeneic hosts by inhibiting donor-specific, humoral and anti-adenoviral antigen immune responses [127, 128]. Although no data exist supporting the prolongation of islet allograft survival or suppression of insulitis in appropriate animal models following the transplantation of IL-10 or vIL-10, Benhamou et al. have demonstrated that adenoviral gene transfer of vIL-10 to human islets *in vitro* leads to a significantly reduced allogeneic lymphocyte proliferation which is dependent on the level of vIL-10 produced [129]. In contrast, islets from transgenic mice expressing IL-10 under the control of the insulin gene promoter were not protected from allorejection nor were they spared from insulitis in a viral model of IDDM. In this model, mice expressing lymphocytic choriomeningitis virus (LCMV) antigens from islet β cells were primed with LCMV [130–132]. Finally, systemic production of IL-10, following the intramuscular injection of an episomal plasmid vector encoding the gene in young NOD mice, was able to prolong the time to overt diabetes, but did not have a significant effect on insulitis severity [133].

Transforming growth factor β

Transforming growth factor β (TGFβ), in addition to its effects on cell proliferation, extracellular matrix formation and wound healing, acts as an immunoregulatory cytokine which inhibits natural killer cell function, thymocyte proliferation, antibody production and the induction of T lymphocyte suppressor activity [134]. By virtue of its immunosuppressive effects, it has been used alone or in combination with IL-10 as a means of preventing IDDM and/or prolonging islet allograft survival. However, initial evaluation suggested that islets from transgenic mice expressing TGFβ were rejected as readily as non-transgenic islets in allogeneic recipients [135]. Moreover, these transgenic islets were not able to escape autoimmune destruction in IDDM occuring as a cross-reaction to LCMV. In contrast, intramuscular injection of a naked plasmid DNA expression vector encoding TGFβ1 to NOD mice, led to an improvement of insulitis as well as a decrease in the incidence of IDDM, both in cyclophasphamide-accelerated as well as in natural course models [136]. In addition, the levels of pancreatic IL-12 and IFNγ message were depressed in TGFβ1-producing NOD mice [136]. Finally, recent experiments, demonstrate that the transplantation of islets infected *in vitro* with adenoviral vectors encoding IL-10 and TGFβ into discordant xenogeneic recipients (dog-to-rat), can lead to significant prolongation of graft survival [137].

Inhibition of CD28-B7 co-stimulation

Long-term xenogeneic engraftment of islets with donor-specific tolerance to alloantigens was demonstrated by Lenschow et al. who exploited co-stimulation blockade [138]. Full activation of T lymphocytes requires a second signal in addition to the interaction between the T cell receptor (TCR) and the peptide/MHC class II complex on an antigen presenting cell. This second signal can be provided by the B7 molecules, B7-1 (CD80) and B7-2 (CD86), expressed at the surface of antigen presenting cells such as dendritic cells. B7 molecules interact with the CD28 protein at the surface of T cells which will result in its full activation. Blockade of the CD28-B7 interaction leads to T cell anergy or apoptosis [139]. Lenschow et al. achieved co-stimulation blockade by using a fusion protein whose extracellular domain derives from CTLA-4, a B7 counterreceptor and an IgG1 Fc portion to stabilise the protein. The fusion, CTLA-4Ig, effectively acts as a decoy for B7 molecules and prevents the B7-CD28 interaction. Administration of recombinant CTLA-4Ig to mice, prevented the rejection of human islets and induced long-term donor-specific tolerance [138]. Further experimentation with systemic administration of CTLA-4Ig protein demonstrated its effects on prolonging murine islet allograft survival [140], prolongation of the survival of microencapsulated rabbit and porcine neonatal islet xenografts in diabetic NOD mice [88, 141], and the prolongation of allograft islet survival as well as the promotion of donor-specific hyporesponsiveness *in vitro* in non-human primates [142]. Recently, gene transfer of CTLA-4Ig to islets *in vitro* followed by transplantation, has shown that its local expression can result in prolongation of allogeneic as well as xenogeneic graft survival. Gene gun-mediated delivery of CTLA-4Ig to mouse islets *in vitro* resulted in prolongation of graft survival in an allogeneic host [113]. Moreover, the co-transplantation of allogeneic murine islets with syngeneic myoblasts engineered to express CTLA-4Ig, led to prolongation of islet survival, however, there was no benefit when the myoblasts were allogeneic [143]. Although the prolongation of allo- and xenograft survival in some instances was significant in the context of local CTLA-4Ig secretion, it is becoming clear that it will be necessary to intervene on other pathways leading to islet-specific T cell anergy or elimination to completely prevent autoimmune attack as well as transplant rejection.

Apoptosis: activation and suppression

Following activation, T lymphocytes are subject to elimination regulated by apoptosis which is mediated by the interaction between Fas antigen (CD95/APO-1) and Fas ligand (FasL; CD95L) [144–146]. FasL is expressed in a variety of tissues which are characterised by an immune privilege such as the testis and the cornea of the eye [147, 148]. The immune privilege is thought to involve the elimination of Fas-positive infiltrating T lymphocytes following the interaction with tissue-expressed FasL [148]. FasL-expressing myoblasts were co-transplanted with islets in allogeneic murine hosts with significant prolongation of islet survival [149]. In contrast, FasL-expressing islet allografts underwent a neutrophil-mediated destruction in mice [150]. In other organ allografts however, FasL expression following gene transfer can confer prolongation of graft survival. Examples include FasL-expressing rat renal and liver allografts [151, 152]. Interestingly, the form of FasL was suggested to be important in determining whether the transplant would be protected or rejected. Soluble FasL variants appear to confer protection from apoptosis whereas cell-membrane bound molecules appear to result in apoptosis [153]. In fact, survival of allogeneic islets expressing soluble human FasL was significantly prolonged in rodents [112]. Very recently, FasL was shown to induce neutrophil infiltration by inducing the production of IL-1β [154]. This observation is interesting in that it suggests that blockade of the IL-1 signaling system, in conjunction with FasL expression may lead to long-term acceptance of allografts.

Another series of studies indicates that insulitis could be preceded by β cell apoptosis in the islets. In NOD mice, apoptosis has been detected as early as 3 weeks of age and could be Fas-dependent [155]. Fas is not normally expressed in islets, but IL-1β has been shown to stimulate its upregulation to the cell surface of β cells in mice and humans in a nitric oxide (NO)-dependent manner [156, 157]. Blockade of IL-1β binding to the signaling type I IL-1 receptor with naturally-occurring antagonist protein (IL-1 receptor antagonist protein; IRAP) or with recombinant soluble IL-1 receptor has resulted in protection from IL-1β-induced, Fas-triggered β cell damage [158–162]. In fact, systemic injections of IRAP into NOD mice could prevent autoimmune infiltration of syngeneic islet transplants as well as IDDM onset [160].

Interference with Fas-triggered apoptosis as well as associated or consequent pathways could also be exploited to protect islets and this has been demonstrated *in vitro*. Bcl-2 is a gene that prevents apoptosis including that induced following Fas activation [163]. *In vitro*, Bcl-2 expression from a replication-defective herpesvirus amplicon vector was shown to confer protection to β cells from apoptosis induced by a cocktail of proapoptotic cytokines (IL-1β, TNFα and IFNγ). HSV-Bcl-2-infected islets were not impaired in their ability to respond to glucose [104]. In addition, oxidant stress is an important factor for islet function, independently of apoptosis induction, both at the time of insulitis onset as well as in transplant survival. Benhamou et al. have shown that adenoviral gene transfer of catalase can reduce the oxidant stress in rodent and human islets *in vitro* [164]. Although none of these transgenes have been tested in appropriate animal models, it is likely that a combination of apoptosis blockade as well as immunosuppression might lead to the prevention of insulitis onset and the indefinite prolongation of islet allografts.

Cell therapy and tolerance induction

In 1994, Utsugi et al. isolated two autoreactive T lymphocyte clones from NOD mice with suppressor activity based on the prolongation of syngeneic islet graft survival and prevention of IDDM in the absence of any immunosuppression following T lymphocyte infusion into syngeneic mice [165]. One of the two clones identified, NY4.2, which is MHC class II-positive and $CD4^+$, was shown to protect against IDDM onset in young NOD mice and also prevented islet graft destruction in acutely diabetic syngeneic NOD mice when transfused a few days prior to transplantation. Characterisation of the cytokine-secretion profile of NY4.2 indicated that it secreted very high levels of TGFβ, IL-10 and IFNγ. The suppressor effect could be abrogated by an antibody directed against TGFβ, but not against IL-10 or IFNγ [58, 166]. Moritani et al. also demonstrated that the genetic engineering of NOD islet-specific $CD4^+$ T_H1 T cells with a retroviral vector encoding murine IL-10, resulted in a significant decrease of IDDM incidence and insulitis grade in syngeneic recipient mice with cyclophasphamide-accelerated diabetes (66% vs. 8% IDDM incidence) [60]. Whether the suppressor effects occur at the level of the islet or the periphery is currently unknown, and whether human islet-specific clones could ever be feasibly and routinely obtained for this type of therapy remains to be explored.

Donor-specific tolerance and acceptance of islet allograft survival as well as suppression of IDDM onset has been achieved by intrathymic injection of donor islet tissue and soluble donor antigens in rodents. In seminal work, Posselt et al. achieved a long-term prolongation of rat islet grafts in allogeneic recipients following a single injection of anti-lymphocyte serum and intrathymic injection of donor islets [167]. In addition, they also were able to achieve both tolerance to allogeneic islets as well as suppression of autoimmunity in spontaneously-diabetic BB rats [168].

IDDM was prevented in BB rats and in young NOD mice following intrathymic islet injection [168–172] although in another rat model of diabetes, this could not be reproduced [173]. Posselt et al. suggested that tolerance occurred as consequence of the deletion of islet-reactive thymocytes. In addition to islet allografts, Zeng et al. reported long-term islet xenograft tolerance following intrathymic injection of rat donor islets [174] to mice, although subsequent data suggests that no tolerance can be achieved in the same model unless both donor and islet passenger T cells are depleted prior to intrathymic injection [175]. Donor-derived spleen cells irradiated with ultraviolet light can also lead to tolerance of rat islet allografts in total body-irradiated and anti-lymphocyte serum-induced recipients following their intrathymic injection [176–178]. Tolerance to allogeneic islet grafts in rat models was also achieved using intrathymic injection of donor bone-marrow cells and was shown to be donor-specific and associated with thymic chimerism and attenuated donor-specific immunoreactivity *in vitro* [179]. Intrathymic injection of soluble class I MHC antigens from an allogeneic rat donor led to prolongation of islet allograft survival in the absence of any inductive or peri-transplant immunosuppressive treatment [180]. Recently, Singer et al. have demonstrated that IDDM in transgenic NOD mice expressing a non-diabetogenic class I MHC molecule in place of the diabetogenic I-Ab^{g7}, could be prevented [181]. Finally, intrathymic injection of insulin B-chain or GAD65 protein, two autoantigens in IDDM, into young NOD mice, was able to suppress IDDM onset [182]. If the mechanism of tolerance induction and suppression of autoimmunity occurs at the level of the thymus by the elimination of thymocytes that recognise donor antigen (islet-derived) or injected antigen, then it could be feasible by gene engineering approaches to inject vectors encoding autoantigens into the thymus of individuals at high genetic risk for developing IDDM or to inject vectors encoding soluble donor class I/class II MHC antigens into diabetic patients receiving islet transplants. In fact, recent results suggest that thymic gene delivery using adenoviral vectors is possible and can result in tolerance to the virus as well [183].

Another potential means of inducing donor-specific tolerance involves genetically-engineered dendritic cells (DC). DC are derived from $CD34^+$ hematopoietic progenitors and following antigen uptake from peripheral sites, migrate to secondary lymphoid organs and present antigen to naïve T cells. In fact, DC are the most potent APCs identified to date. Upon antigen capture, DC undergo maturation, particularly evident in changing of their phenotype. Mature DC express high levels of class II MHC and many co-stimulatory molecules like CD40, CD80, CD86 and adhesion proteins (ICAM-1/CD54, LFA-3/CD58) at the cell surface, and they secrete potent immunostimulatory cytokines like IL-12 [139]. Although considered potent immunostimulators, DC have recently been shown to possess tolerogenic characteristics under defined conditions. DC tolerogenicity has been observed by the suppression of T cell responses in T cell ontogeny, as well as allo-, tumor and autoimmunity [184]. The conditions that can yield tolerogenic DC include UV irradiation, as well as exposure to IL-10, TGFβ or CTLA4Ig. How a tolerogenic DC acts to suppress immunoreactivity is not completely understood, but may involve anergy, a shift to T_H2-type responses, apoptosis or the induction of regulatory cells [184]. Gene delivery to myeloid DC in culture has been achieved using adenoviral and retroviral vectors encoding CTLA-4Ig, TGFβ and vIL-10 [185] [186–188]. CTLA-4Ig-expressing DC exhibit a reduction in cell surface CD86, can induce alloantigen-specific T cell hyporesponsiveness and display enhanced survival in non-immunosuppressed, allogeneic hosts [188]. The *in vivo* presentation of alloantigens by donor or recipient DC in the absence of co-stimulation along with local production of immunosuppressive molecules like TGFβ, could likely promote the inhibition of anti-donor reactivity and promote tolerance induction without any major systemic immunosuppression. DC engineered to express vIL-10 following retroviral gene transfer produce high levels of vIL-10 *in vitro*, exhibit marked reduction in cell surface MHC and co-stimulatory molecule expression, decrease T cell allostimulation and promote the induction of T cell hyporesponsiveness [185]. Using genetically-engineered DC to manipulate anti-donor immunoreactivity may be a feasible approach to improved therapy of islet allograft rejection.

Xenotransplantation

If islet transplantation for IDDM therapy is to become a clinical reality, an immediate challenge is the availability of human cadaveric donor tissue. Islets from animals is an alternative but is associated with ethical and immunological hurdles. The risks associated with transmission of donor-resident micro-organisms and viruses and their effects on human health remain to be fully understood. Immunologically, xenogeneic tolerance may never become possible or necessary and therefore, accomodation of xenogeneic islets and the immunomodulation required to prevent chronic rejection need to be evaluated in greater detail. Porcine islets offer the best choice for humans as donor tissue based on a number of factors described elsewhere [74].

Discordant vascularised xenografts face an immediate hyperacute rejection that is complement-mediated following the binding of preformed, naturally-occuring antibodies against xenoantigens. Non-human primate recipients of porcine donor organs have exhibited xenoreactive antibody-mediated hyperacute rejection [189–191]. The xenoepitope has been defined in porcine tissues as an α-galactosyl oligosaccharide that is synthesised by a galactosyltransferase present in pig, but not in humans except in the gut-inhabiting flora [192, 193]. Complement-mediated lysis of porcine xenografts occurs within minutes by the classical pathway culminating in the formation of the membrane attack complex. Depletion of the circulating xenoreactive antibodies can prolong xenograft survival significantly as recent studies in pig-to-baboon renal transplantation indicate [191]. It is possible, however, that antibody-dependent pathways other than complement activation, such as the alternative pathway may be involved in hyperacute rejection. Consequently, strategies aimed to modulate the binding of proteins involved in the complement cascade can be beneficial in preventing hyperacute rejection. Transgenic pigs expressing regulators of complement activation, such as decay accelerating factor (DAF), membrane cofactor protein (MCP) and CD59 are currently under development with the objective of interfering with the activation of host-derived complement against vascularised xenografts [194]. In fact, there are reports demonstrating that porcine xenografts expressing DAF, DAF and CD59 and soluble CR1, a receptor that competes with membrane CR1 for binding to complement, can be protected from hyperacute rejection [195–197]. It is likely that gene transfer using viral delivery vehicles to express these proteins *in vitro* prior to transplantation may find use in xenogeneic islet transplantation in the future.

Enzymatic diversion of the α-galactosyl xenoepitope to the oligosaccharide whose terminal residues define the O antigen in human blood to which antibodies do not exist, can be achieved by expressing α-(1,2)-fucosyltransferase in xenogeneic cells [198]. In both pig and human the fucosyltransferase substrate is the same, therefore the porcine substrate will be remodelled to the non-antigenic H-epitope of the antigen defining the human universal donor O blood group. *In vitro*, it has been shown that as much as 80% of the oligosaccharide is in the fucosylated form following stable gene transfer [193, 198–200]. Identical levels of fucosylated oligosaccharide are observed in transgenic mice expressing the fucosyltransferase [193, 198, 200]. Recently, another means of inhibiting the production of anti-xenoepitope antibodies, involving molecular chimerism, has been described. Galactosyltransferase-deficient murine bone marrow-derived cells infected with a retrovirus encoding the porcine homologue were introduced into recipient mice, followed by transplantation with porcine tissue. No xenoreactive antibody was detectable nor were sera from the reconstituted mice able to kill porcine cells *in vitro* [201]. It may be feasible to use these technologies for islet xenotransplantation in the future.

Future prospects

Allogeneic or xenogeneic islet transplants may face other immune obstacles like antibody-dependent cell-mediated cytotoxicity, attack by natural killer cells which act in an MHC non-restricted fashion, and non-immune events like acute glucotoxicity, free radical and oxidation-mediated dysfunction and damage. Listed in Tables 2 and 3 are gene transfer and cell therapy strategies which have been examined as well as potential ones that could be exploited. Cell therapy-based approaches could facilitate tolerance to allo- or xenoantigen alone, or in conjunction with islet transplantation. Identification of thymic precursors from bone marrow may lead to their use as reservoirs for donor-specific antigen and/or autoantigen in inducing tolerance to transplanted islets or resulting in the prevention of IDDM in young individuals

Table 2 - Potential interactions and biochemical pathways that can be exploited to prevent IDDM and induce transplant tolerance

Interactions/Reactions/Processes	Potential modulator
Superoxide generation	Superoxide dismutase
Peroxides	Catalase
Apoptosis induction	bcl-2, bcl-x_L, crmA, dominant negative FADD
IL-1:IL-1R	IRAP, soluble (s)IL-1-IR-Ig, sIL-1-IIR-Ig
TNFα:TNFRI	sTNF-IR-Ig
Chemokine effects	Soluble receptors
Neutrophil activation	sCD18, sICAM-1, sLFA-3, sHLA-G
Adhesion molecules	Soluble chimeric Ig proteins: sLFA-3Ig, sCD48, sICAM-1, sICAM-2, sVCAM, soluble selectins
NK cells	sCD2Ig, MHC class I peptides
Fas:FasL	sFasIg, dominant negative Fas
IFNγ:IFNγR	sIFNγR-Ig

The soluble-Ig proteins referred to above indicate an extracellular ligand-binding domain fused in-frame to a carboxy-terminal immunoglobulin domain to render the molecule stable and to increase its half-life in vitro.

Table 3 - Cell therapy approaches for IDDM and tolerance induction

Cell type/modification	Therapeutic objective
Donor DC expressing CTLA-4Ig, IL-10, vIL-10, TGFβ, sCD40-Ig, FasL	Tolerance to donor antigens; prolongation of allograft survival
Islet-infiltrating lymphocytes expressing IL-10, TGFβ	Suppression of IDDM; shift of T_H1 to T_H2-type cytokine production in host
Intrathymic donor antigen injection	Tolerance to donor antigens, prevention of IDDM

at high genetic risk, based on early genetic testing. Recent advances in genetic engineering of antigen presenting cells could lead to ways of promoting donor-specific tolerance as well as suppression of autoimmunity. In fact, a recent study using antigen presenting cells expressing FasL and infected with adenovirus demonstrated that adenoviral-protein-specific T cells were eliminated in a Fas-FasL-dependent manner [202]. This approach could conceivably be exploited to infect antigen presenting cells like DC with autoantigen and FasL-encoding vectors for the prevention of IDDM. Finally, the need for regulatable and tissue-specific expression cessettes in non-immunogenic, stably-integrating vectors that can be selectively targeted to islets *in vivo*, may obviate the need for transplantation altogether. Whatever the approach, it is likely that gene therapy for IDDM will be patient-specific. A better understanding of the genetics, the trigger and the immunopathology of IDDM as well as the factors affecting allogeneic and xenogeneic tolerance is necessary for these approaches to find clinical use.

References

1 Todd JA, Bell JI, McDevitt HO (1987) HLA-DQ beta gene contributes to susceptibility and resistance to insulin-dependent diabetes mellitus. *Nature* 329 (6140): 599–604

2 Morel PA, Dorman JS, Todd JA, McDevitt HO, Trucco M (1988) Aspartic acid at position 57 of the HLA-DQ beta chain protects against type I diabetes: a family study. *Proc Natl Acad Sci USA* 85 (21): 8111–8115

3 Eisenbarth G (1991) Prediction and prevention strategies in type I diabetes. *Mt Sinai J Med* 58 (4): 274–279

4 Eisenbarth GS (1993) Molecular aspects of the etiology of type I diabetes mellitus. *J Diabetes Complications* 7 (2): 142–150

5 Julier C, Hyer RN, Davies J, Merlin F, Soularue P, Briant L et al (1991) Insulin-IGF2 region on chromosome 11p encodes a gene implicated in HLA-DR4-dependent diabetes susceptibility. *Nature* 354 (6349): 155–159

6 Concannon P, Gogolin-Ewens KJ, Hinds DA, Wapelhorst B, Morrison VA, Stirling B et al (1998) A second-generation screen of the human genome for susceptibility to insulin-dependent diabetes mellitus. *Nat Genet* 19 (3): 292–296

7 Bennett ST, Wilson AJ, Esposito L, Bouzekri N, Undlien DE, Cucca F et al (1997) Insulin VNTR allele-specific effect in type 1 diabetes depends on identity of untransmitted paternal allele. The IMDIAB Group. *Nat Genet* 17 (3): 350–352

8 Davies JL, Kawaguchi Y, Bennett ST, Copeman JB, Cordell HJ, Pritchard LE et al (1994) A genome-wide search for human type 1 diabetes susceptibility genes. *Nature* 371 (6493): 130–136

9 Karges W, Hammond-McKibben D, Cheung RK, Visconti M, Shibuya N, Kemp D et al (1997) Immunological aspects of nutritional diabetes prevention in NOD mice: a pilot study for the cow's milk-based IDDM prevention trial. *Diabetes* 46 (4): 557–564

10 Oldstone MB (1998) Molecular mimicry and immune-mediated diseases. *Faseb J* 12 (13): 1255–1265

11 von Herrath MG, Holz A, Homann D, Oldstone MB (1998) Role of viruses in type I diabetes. *Semin Immunol* 10 (1): 87–100

12 Horwitz MS, Bradley LM, Harbertson J, Krahl T, Lee J, Sarvetnick N (1998) Diabetes

induced by Coxsackie virus: initiation by bystander damage and not molecular mimicry. *Nat Med* 4 (7): 781–785

13 Bach JF (1994) Insulin-dependent diabetes mellitus as an autoimmune disease. *Endocr Rev* 15 (4): 516–542

14 Dayer-Metroz MD, Wollheim CB, Seckinger P, Dayer JM (1989) A natural interleukin 1 (IL-1) inhibitor counteracts the inhibitory effect of IL-1 on insulin production in cultured rat pancreatic islets. *J Autoimmun* 2 (2): 163–171

15 Hanenberg H, Kolb-Bachofen V, Kantwerk-Funke G, Kolb H (1989) Macrophage infiltration precedes and is a prerequisite for lymphocytic insulitis in pancreatic islets of prediabetic BB rats. *Diabetologia* 32 (2): 126–134

16 Heitmeier MR, Scarim AL, Corbett JA (1997) Interferon-gamma increases the sensitivity of islets of Langerhans for inducible nitric-oxide synthase expression induced by interleukin 1. *J Biol Chem* 272 (21): 13697–13704

17 Kessler L, Jesser C, Lombard Y, Karsten V, Belcourt A, Pinget M et al (1996) Cytotoxicity of peritoneal murine macrophages against encapsulated pancreatic rat islets: *in vivo* and *in vitro* studies. *J Leukoc Biol* 60 (6): 729–736

18 Gepts W (1965) Pathologic anatomy of the pancreas in juvenile diabetes mellitus. *Diabetes* 14 (10): 619–633

19 Roep BO, De Vries RR (1992) T-lymphocytes and the pathogenesis of type 1 (insulin-dependent) diabetes mellitus. *Eur J Clin Invest* 22 (11): 697–711

20 Roep BO, Kallan AA, De Vries RR (1992) Beta-cell antigen-specific lysis of macrophages by CD4 T-cell clones from newly diagnosed IDDM patient. A putative mechanism of T-cell-mediated autoimmune islet cell destruction. *Diabetes* 41 (11): 1380–1384

21 Huang GC, Tremble J, Bailyes E, Arden SD, Kaye T, McGregor AM et al (1995) HLA-DR-restricted T cell lines from newly diagnosed type 1 diabetic patients specific for insulinoma and normal islet beta cell proteins: lack of reactivity to glutamic acid decarboxylase. *Clin Exp Immunol* 102 (1): 152–158

22 Stiller CR, Dupre J, Gent M, Jenner MR, Keown PA, Laupacis A et al (1984) Effects of cyclosporine immunosuppression in insulin-dependent diabetes mellitus of recent onset. *Science* 223 (4643): 1362–1367

23 Bougneres PF, Carel JC, Castano L, Boitard C, Gardin JP, Landais P et al (1988) Factors associated with early remission of type I diabetes in children treated with cyclosporine. *N Engl J Med* 318 (11): 663–670

24 Sibley RK, Sutherland DE, Goetz F, Michael AF (1985) Recurrent diabetes mellitus in the pancreas iso-and allograft. A light and electron microscopic and immunohistochemical analysis of four cases. *Lab Invest* 53 (2): 132–144

25 Lampeter EF, Homberg M, Quabeck K, Schaefer UW, Wernet P, Bertrams J et al (1993) Transfer of insulin-dependent diabetes between HLA-identical siblings by bone marrow transplantation. *Lancet* 341 (8855): 1243–1244

26 Wicker LS, Miller BJ, Mullen Y (1986) Transfer of autoimmune diabetes mellitus with splenocytes from nonobese diabetic (NOD) mice. *Diabetes* 35 (8): 855–860

27 Bendelac A, Carnaud C, Boitard C, Bach JF (1987) Syngeneic transfer of autoimmune diabetes from diabetic NOD mice to healthy neonates. Requirement for both L3T4⁺ and Lyt-2⁺ T cells. *J Exp Med* 166 (4): 823–832

28 Harrison LC, De Aizpurua H, Loudovaris T, Campbell IL, Cebon JS, Tait BD et al (1991) Reactivity to human islets and fetal pig proislets by peripheral blood mononuclear cells from subjects with preclinical and clinical insulin-dependent diabetes. *Diabetes* 40 (9): 1128–1133

29 Roep BO, Kallan AA, Duinkerken G, Arden SD, Hutton JC, Bruining GJ et al (1995) T-cell reactivity to beta-cell membrane antigens associated with beta-cell destruction in IDDM. *Diabetes* 44 (3): 278–283

30 Chang JC, Linarelli LG, Laxer JA, Froning KJ, Caralli LL, Brostoff SW et al (1995) Insulin-secretory-granule specific T cell clones in human IDDM. *J Autoimmun* 8 (2): 221–234

31 Foulis AK, McGill M, Farquharson MA (1991) Insulitis in type 1 (insulin-dependent) diabetes mellitus in man – macrophages, lymphocytes, and interferon-gamma containing cells. *J Pathol* 165 (2): 97–103

32 Kallan AA, Roep BO, Arden SD, Hutton JC, de Vries RR (1995) Beta-cell reactive T-cell clones from type I diabetes patients are not beta cell specific and recognize multiple antigens. *J Autoimmun* 8 (6): 887–899

33 Giorda R, Peakman M, Tan KC, Vergani D, Trucco M (1991) Glutamic acid decarboxylase expression in islets and brain. *Lancet* 338 (8780): 1469–1470

34 Kaufman DL, Erlander MG, Clare-Salzler M, Atkinson MA, Maclaren NK, Tobin AJ (1992) Autoimmunity to two forms of glutamate decarboxylase in insulin-dependent diabetes mellitus. *J Clin Invest* 89 (1): 283–292

35 Santamaria P, Nakhleh RE, Sutherland DE, Barbosa JJ (1992) Characterization of T lymphocytes infiltrating human pancreas allograft affected by isletitis and recurrent diabetes. *Diabetes* 41 (1): 53–61

36 Santamaria P, Lewis C, Jessurun J, Sutherland DE, Barbosa JJ (1994) Skewed T-cell receptor usage and junctional heterogeneity among isletitis alpha beta and gamma delta T-cells in human IDDM. *Diabetes* 43 (4): 599–606

37 Kontiainen S, Toomath R, Lowder J, Feldmann M (1991) Selective activation of T cells in newly diagnosed insulin-dependent diabetic patients: evidence for heterogeneity of T cell receptor usage. *Clin Exp Immunol* 83 (3): 347–351

38 Kontiainen S, James RL, Feldman M (1991) Human islet cell induced T cell lines and clones from diabetic children. *Autoimmunity* 8 (3): 193–197

39 Conrad B, Trucco M (1994) Superantigens as etiopathogenetic factors in the development of insulin-dependent diabetes mellitus. *Diabetes Metab Rev* 10 (4): 309–338

40 Conrad B, Weidmann E, Trucco G, Rudert WA, Behboo R, Ricordi C et al (1994) Evidence for superantigen involvement in insulin-dependent diabetes mellitus aetiology. *Nature* 371 (6495): 351–355

41 Lampeter EF, Seifert I, Lohmann D, Heise JW, Bertrams J, Christie MR et al (1994)

Inflammatory islet damage in patients bearing HLA-DR 3 and/or DR 4 haplotypes does not lead to islet autoimmunity. *Diabetologia* 37 (5): 471–475
42 Bottazzo GF, Dean BM, McNally JM, MacKay EH, Swift PG, Gamble DR (1985) *In situ* characterization of autoimmune phenomena and expression of HLA molecules in the pancreas in diabetic insulitis. *N Engl J Med* 313 (6): 353–360
43 Bottazzo GF, al-Sakkaf L, Dean BM, Schwarz G, Pujol-Borrell R (1985) Hypotheses on the etiology of insulin–dependent diabetes: published and recent ideas. *Journ Annu Diabetol Hotel Dieu* 135–147
44 Somoza N, Vargas F, Roura-Mir C, Vives-Pi M, Fernandez-Figueras MT, Ariza A et al (1994) Pancreas in recent onset insulin-dependent diabetes mellitus. Changes in HLA, adhesion molecules and autoantigens, restricted T cell receptor V beta usage, and cytokine profile. *J Immunol* 153 (3): 1360–1377
45 Daniel D, Gill RG, Schloot N, Wegmann D (1995) Epitope specificity, cytokine production profile and diabetogenic activity of insulin-specific T cell clones isolated from NOD mice. *Eur J Immunol* 25 (4): 1056–1062
46 Christianson SW, Shultz LD, Leiter EH (1993) Adoptive transfer of diabetes into immunodeficient NOD-scid/scid mice. Relative contributions of $CD4^+$ and $CD8^+$ T-cells from diabetic versus prediabetic NOD.NON-Thy-1a donors. *Diabetes* 42 (1): 44–55
47 Koike T, Itoh Y, Ishii T, Ito I, Takabayashi K, Maruyama N et al (1987) Preventive effect of monoclonal anti-L3T4 antibody on development of diabetes in NOD mice. *Diabetes* 36 (4): 539–541
48 Ilonen J, Surcel HM, Kaar ML (1991) Abnormalities within CD4 and CD8 T lymphocytes subsets in type 1 (insulin-dependent) diabetes. *Clin Exp Immunol* 85 (2): 278–281
49 Buschard K, Ropke C, Madsbad S, Mehlsen J, Sorensen TB, Rygaard J (1983) Alterations of peripheral T-lymphocyte subpopulations in patients with insulin-dependent (type 1) diabetes mellitus. *J Clin Lab Immunol* 10 (3): 127–131
50 Buschard K, Ropke C, Madsbad S, Mehlsen J, Rygaard J (1983) T lymphocyte subsets in patients with newly diagnosed type 1 (insulin-dependent) diabetes: a prospective study. *Diabetologia* 25 (3): 247–251
51 Al-Sakkaf L, Pozzilli P, Tarn AC, Schwarz G, Gale EA, Bottazzo GF (1989) Persistent reduction of CD4/CD8 lymphocyte ratio and cell activation before the onset of type 1 (insulin-dependent) diabetes. *Diabetologia* 32 (5): 322–325
52 Harrison LC, Honeyman MC, DeAizpurua HJ, Schmidli RS, Colman PG, Tait BD et al (1993) Inverse relation between humoral and cellular immunity to glutamic acid decarboxylase in subjects at risk of insulin-dependent diabetes. *Lancet* 341 (8857): 1365–1369
53 Ellis TM, Atkinson MA (1996) The clinical significance of an autoimmune response against glutamic acid decarboxylase. *Nat Med* 2 (2): 148–153
54 Campbell IL, Kay TW, Oxbrow L, Harrison LC (1991) Essential role for interferon-gamma and interleukin-6 in autoimmune insulin-dependent diabetes in NOD/Wehi mice. *J Clin Invest* 87 (2): 739–742
55 Debray-Sachs M, Carnaud C, Boitard C, Cohen H, Gresser I, Bedossa P et al (1991) Pre-

vention of diabetes in NOD mice treated with antibody to murine IFN gamma. *J Autoimmun* 4 (2): 237–48
56 Tisch R, Yang XD, Singer SM, Liblau RS, Fugger L, McDevitt HO (1993) Immune response to glutamic acid decarboxylase correlates with insulitis in non-obese diabetic mice. *Nature* 366 (6450): 72–75
57 Tisch R, McDevitt H (1996) Insulin-dependent diabetes mellitus. *Cell* 85 (3): 291–297
58 Han HS, Jun HS, Utsugi T, Yoon JW (1996) A new type of CD4⁺ suppressor T cell completely prevents spontaneous autoimmune diabetes and recurrent diabetes in syngeneic islet-transplanted NOD mice. *J Autoimmun* 9 (3): 331–339
59 Moore KW, O'Garra A, de Waal Malefyt R, Vieira P, Mosmann TR (1993) Interleukin-10. *Annu Rev Immunol* 11: 165–190
60 Moritani M, Yoshimoto K, Ii S, Kondo M, Iwahana H, Yamaoka T et al (1996) Prevention of adoptively transferred diabetes in nonobese diabetic mice with IL-10-transduced islet-specific Th1 lymphocytes. A gene therapy model for autoimmune diabetes. *J Clin Invest* 98 (8): 1851–1859
61 Pennline KJ, Roque-Gaffney E, Monahan M (1994) Recombinant human IL-10 prevents the onset of diabetes in the nonobese diabetic mouse. *Clin Immunol Immunopathol* 71 (2): 169–175
62 Zheng XX, Steele AW, Hancock WW, Stevens AC, Nickerson PW, Roy-Chaudhury P et al (1997) A noncytolytic IL-10/Fc fusion protein prevents diabetes, blocks autoimmunity, and promotes suppressor phenomena in NOD mice. *J Immunol* 158 (9): 4507–4513
63 Mueller R, Lee MS, Sawyer SP, Sarvetnick N (1996) Transgenic expression of interleukin 10 in the pancreas renders resistant mice susceptible to low dose streptozotocin-induced diabetes. *J Autoimmun* 9 (2): 151–158
64 Balasa B, Sarvetnick N (1996) The paradoxical effects of interleukin 10 in the immunoregulation of autoimmune diabetes. *J Autoimmun* 9 (2): 283–286
65 Vafiadis P, Bennett ST, Todd JA, Nadeau J, Grabs R, Goodyer CG et al (1997) Insulin expression in human thymus is modulated by INS VNTR alleles at the IDDM2 locus. *Nat Genet* 15 (3): 289–292
66 Pugliese A, Zeller M, Fernandez A Jr, Zalcberg LJ, Bartlett RJ, Ricordi C et al (1997) The insulin gene is transcribed in the human thymus and transcription levels correlated with allelic variation at the INS VNTR-IDDM2 susceptibility locus for type 1 diabetes. *Nat Genet* 15 (3): 293–297
67 De Smedt T, Van Mechelen M, De Becker G, Urbain J, Leo O, Moser M (1997) Effect of interleukin-10 on dendritic cell maturation and function. *Eur J Immunol* 27 (5): 1229–1235
68 Schuler G, Thurner B, Romani N (1997) Dendritic cells: from ignored cells to major players in T-cell-mediated immunity. *Int Arch Allergy Immunol* 112 (4): 317–322
69 Banchereau J, Steinman RM (1998) Dendritic cells and the control of immunity. *Nature* 392 (6673): 245–252
70 Pfeiffer C, Stein J, Southwood S, Ketelaar H, Sette A, Bottomly K (1995) Altered pep-

tide ligands can control CD4 T lymphocyte differentiation *in vivo*. *J Exp Med* 181 (4): 1569–1574
71 Lenschow DJ, Zeng Y, Hathcock KS, Zuckerman LA, Freeman G, Thistlethwaite JR et al (1995) Inhibition of transplant rejection following treatment with anti-B7-2 and anti-B7-1 antibodies. *Transplantation* 60 (10): 1171–1178
72 Newgard CB, Clark S, BeltrandelRio H, Hohmeier HE, Quaade C, Normington K (1997) Engineered cell lines for insulin replacement in diabetes: current status and future prospects. *Diabetologia* 40 (2): S42–S47
73 Sutherland DER, Moudry KC (1989) Results of pancreas-transplant registry. *Diabetes* 38 (1): 46–54
74 Weir GC, Bonner-Weir S (1997) Scientific and political impediments to successful islet transplantation. *Diabetes* 46: 1247–1256
75 Ricordi C (1996) Human islet cell transplantation: New perspectives for an old challenge. *Diabetes Reviews* 4 (3): 356–369
76 Platt JL (1998) Current status of xenotransplantation: research and technology. *Transplant Proc* 30 (5): 1630–1633
77 Platt JL (1998) New directions for organ transplantation. *Nature* 392 (6679): 11–17
78 Platt JL (1997) Approaching the clinical application of xenotransplantation. *Am J Med Sci* 313 (5): 315–321
79 Platt JL (1996) Xenotransplantation: recent progress and current perspectives. *Curr Opin Immunol* 8 (5): 721–728
80 Braun K, Kauert C, Dunger A, Hahn HJ (1987) Allogeneic transplantation of microencapsulated islets. *Transplant Proc* 19 (1 Pt 2): 931–932
81 Sun AM, Goosen MF, O'Shea G (1987) Microencapsulated cells as hormone delivery systems. *Crit Rev Ther Drug Carrier Syst* 4 (1): 1–12
82 Lim F, Sun AM (1980) Microencapsulated islets as bioartificial endocrine pancreas. *Science* 210 (4472): 908–910
83 Ao Z, Suarez-Pinzon WL, Rajotte RV, Korbutt GS, Flashner M, Rabinovitch A (1998) Transplantation of microencapsulated syngeneic and xenogeneic (neonatal porcine) islets in nonobese diabetic mice. *Transplant Proc* 30 (2): 500
84 Kawakami Y, Inoue K, Hayashi H, Wang WJ, Setoyama H, Gu YJ et al (1997) Subcutaneous xenotransplantation of hybrid artificial pancreas encapsulating pancreatic B cell line (MIN6): functional and histological study. *Cell Transplant* 6 (5): 541–545
85 Sandler S, Andersson A, Eizirik DL, Hellerstrom C, Espevik T, Kulseng B et al (1997) Assessment of insulin secretion *in vitro* from microencapsulated fetal porcine islet-like cell clusters and rat, mouse, and human pancreatic islets. *Transplantation* 63 (12): 1712–1718
86 De Vos P, De Haan BJ, Wolters GH, Strubbe JH, Van Schilfgaarde R (1997) Improved biocompatibility but limited graft survival after purification of alginate for microencapsulation of pancreatic islets. *Diabetologia* 40 (3): 262–370
87 Sun Y, Ma X, Zhou D, Vacek I, Sun AM (1996) Normalization of diabetes in sponta-

neously diabetic cynomologus monkeys by xenografts of microencapsulated porcine islets without immunosuppression. *J Clin Invest* 98 (6): 1417–1422
88 Weber CJ, Hagler MK, Chryssochoos JT, Larsen CP, Pearson TC, Jensen P et al (1996) CTLA4-Ig prolongs survival of microencapsulated rabbit islet xenografts in spontaneously diabetic Nod mice. *Transplant Proc* 28 (2): 821–823
89 Inaba K, Zhou D, Yang B, Vacek I, Sun AM (1996) Normalization of diabetes by xenotransplantation of cryopreserved microencapsulated pancreatic islets. Application of a new strategy in islet banking. *Transplantation* 61 (2): 175–179
90 Rajotte RV, Ao Z, Korbutt GS, Lakey JR, Flashner M, Colby CB et al (1995) Cryopreservation of microencapsulated canine islets. *Transplant Proc* 27 (6): 3389
91 Korbutt GS, Ao Z, Warnock GL, Flashner M, Rajotte RV (1995) Successful reversal of diabetes in nude mice by transplantation of microencapsulated porcine neonatal islet cell aggregates. *Transplant Proc* 27 (6): 3212
92 Zhou D, Sun YL, Vacek I, Ma P, Sun AM (1994) Normalization of diabetes in cynomolgus monkeys by xenotransplantation of microencapsulated porcine islets. *Transplant Proc* 26 (3): 1091
93 Horcher A, Zekorn T, Siebers U, Klock G, Frank H, Houben R et al (1994) Transplantation of microencapsulated islets in rats: evidence for induction of fibrotic overgrowth by islet alloantigens released from microcapsules. *Transplant Proc* 26 (2): 784–786
94 Chen CF, Chern HT, Leu FJ, Chang TM, Shian LR, Sun AM (1994) Xenotransplantation of microencapsulated canine islets into diabetic rats. *Artif Organs* 18 (3): 193–197
95 Soon-Shiong P, Feldman E, Nelson R, Komtebedde J, Smidsrod O, Skjak-Braek G et al (1992) Successful reversal of spontaneous diabetes in dogs by intraperitoneal microencapsulated islets. *Transplantation* 54 (5): 769–774
96 Calafiore R (1992) Transplantation of microencapsulated pancreatic human islets for therapy of diabetes mellitus. A preliminary report. *Asaio J* 38 (1): 34–37
97 Brunetti P, Basta G, Faloerni A, Calcinaro F, Pietropaolo M, Calafiore R (1991) Immunoprotection of pancreatic islet grafts within artificial microcapsules. *Int J Artif Organs* 14 (12): 789–791
98 Bonner-Weir S (1991) Anatomy of the islet of Langerhans. In: E Samols (ed): *The endocrine pancreas*. Raven Press, New York, 15–27
99 Csete ME, Afra R, Mullen Y, Drazan KE, Benhamou PY, Shaked A (1994) Adenoviral-mediated gene transfer to pancreatic islets does not alter islet function. *Transplant Proc* 26 (2): 756–757
100 Csete ME, Benhamou PY, Drazan KE, Wu L, McIntee DF, Afra R et al (1995) Efficient gene transfer to pancreatic islets mediated by adenoviral vectors. *Transplantation* 59 (2): 263–268
101 Naldini L, Blomer U, Gage FH, Trono D, Verma IM (1996) Efficient transfer, integration, and sustained long-term expression of the transgene in adult rat brains injected with a lentiviral vector. *Proc Natl Acad Sci USA* 93 (21): 11382–11388
102 Zufferey R, Nagy D, Mandel RJ, Naldini L, Trono D (1997) Multiply attenuated lentiviral vector achieves efficient gene delivery *in vivo*. *Nat Biotechnol* 15 (9): 871–875

103 Ju Q, Edelstein D, Brendel MD, Brandhorst D, Brandhorst H, Bretzel RG et al (1998) Transduction of non-dividing adult human pancreatic beta cells by an integrating lentiviral vector. *Diabetologia* 41 (6): 736–739

104 Liu Y, Rabinovitch A, Suarez-Pinzon W, Muhkerjee B, Brownlee M, Edelstein D et al (1996) Expression of the bcl-2 gene from a defective HSV-1 amplicon vector protects pancreatic beta-cells from apoptosis. *Hum Gene Ther* 7 (14): 1719–1726

105 Weber M, Deng S, Kucher T, Shaked A, Ketchum RJ, Brayman KL (1997) Adenoviral transfection of isolated pancreatic islets: a study of programmed cell death (apoptosis) and islet function. *J Surg Res* 69 (1): 23–32

106 Marconi P, Krisky D, Oligino T, Poliani PL, Ramakrishnan R, Goins WF et al (1996) Replication-defective herpes simplex virus vectors for gene transfer *in vivo*. *Proc Natl Acad Sci USA* 93 (21): 11319–11320

107 Glorioso JC, Goins WF, Schmidt MC, Oligino T, Krisky DM, Marconi PC et al (1997) Engineering herpes simplex virus vectors for human gene therapy. *Adv Pharmacol* 40: 103–136

108 Goins WF, Krisky D, Marconi P, Oligino T, Ramakrishnan R, Poliani PL et al (1997) Herpes simplex virus vectors for gene transfer to the nervous system. *J Neurovirol* 3 (1): S80–S88

109 Goins WF, Lee KA, Cavalcoli JD, O'Malley ME, DeKosky ST, Fink DJ et al (1999) Herpes simplex virus type 1 vector-mediated expression of nerve growth factor protects dorsal root ganglion neurons from peroxide toxicity. *J Virol* 73 (1): 519–532

110 Kafri T, van Praag H, Ouyang L, Gage FH, Verma IM (1999) A packaging cell line for lentivirus-vectors. *J Virol* 73 (1): 576–584

111 Guo Z, Mital D, Mo YY, Tian Y, Shen J, Chong AS et al (1998) Effect of gene gun-mediated CTLA4IG and Fas ligand gene transfection on concordant xenogeneic islet graft rejection. *Transplant Proc* 30 (2): 589

112 Gainer AL, Suarez-Pinzon WL, Min WP, Swiston JR, Hancock-Friesen C, Korbutt GS et al (1998) Improved survival of biolistically transfected mouse islet allografts expressing CTLA4-Ig or soluble Fas ligand. *Transplantation* 66 (2): 194–199

113 Gainer AL, Korbutt GS, Rajotte RV, Warnock GL, Elliott JF (1997) Expression of CTLA4-Ig by biolistically transfected mouse islets promotes islet allograft survival. *Transplantation* 63 (7): 1017–1021

114 Welsh N, Oberg C, Hellerstrom C, Welsh M (1990) Liposome mediated *in vitro* transfection of pancreatic islet cells. *Biomed Biochim Acta* 49 (12): 1157–1164

115 McClane SJ, Chirmule N, Burke CV, Raper SE (1997) Characterization of the immune response after local delivery of recombinant adenovirus in murine pancreas and successful strategies for readministration. *Hum Gene Ther* 8 (18): 2207–2216

116 McClane SJ, Hamilton TE, DeMatteo RP, Burke C, Raper SE (1997) Effect of adenoviral early genes and the host immune system on *in vivo* pancreatic gene transfer in the mouse. *Pancreas* 15 (3): 236–245

117 Raper SE, DeMatteo RP (1996) Adenovirus-mediated *in vivo* gene transfer and expression in normal rat pancreas. *Pancreas* 12 (4): 401–410

118 Cameron MJ, Arreaza GA, Zucker P, Chensue SW, Strieter RM, Chakrabarti S et al (1997) IL-4 prevents insulitis and insulin-dependent diabetes mellitus in nonobese diabetic mice by potentiation of regulatory T helper-2 cell function. *J Immunol* 159 (10): 4686–4692

119 Cameron MJ, Arreaza GA, Delovitch TL (1997) Cytokine-and costimulation-mediated therapy of IDDM. *Crit Rev Immunol* 17 (5–6): 537–544

120 Nickerson P, Pacheco-Silva A, O'Connell PJ, Steurer W, Kelley VR, Strom TB (1993) Analysis of cytokine transcripts in pancreatic islet cell allografts during rejection and tolerance induction. *Transplant Proc* 25 (1 Pt 2): 984–985

121 Mueller R, Krahl T, Sarvetnick N (1996) Pancreatic expression of interleukin-4 abrogates insulitis and autoimmune diabetes in nonobese diabetic (NOD) mice. *J Exp Med* 184 (3): 1093–1099

122 Smith DK, Korbutt GS, Suarez-Pinzon WL, Kao D, Rajotte RV, Elliott JF (1997) Interleukin-4 or interleukin-10 expressed from adenovirus-transduced syngeneic islet grafts fails to prevent beta cell destruction in diabetic NOD mice. *Transplantation* 64 (7): 1040–1049

123 Gallichan WS, Kafri T, Krahl T, Verma IM, Sarvetnick N (1998) Lentivirus-mediated transduction of islet grafts with interleukin 4 results in sustained gene expression and protection from insulitis. *Hum Gene Ther* 9 (18): 2717–2726

124 Tripp CS, Wolf SF, Unanue ER (1993) Interleukin 12 and tumor necrosis factor alpha are costimulators of interferon gamma production by natural killer cells in severe combined immunodeficiency mice with listeriosis, and interleukin 10 is a physiologic antagonist. *Proc Natl Acad Sci USA* 90 (8): 3725–3729

125 Chen WF, Zlotnik A (1991) IL-10: a novel cytotoxic T cell differentiation factor. *J Immunol* 147 (2): 528–534

126 MacNeil IA, Suda T, Moore KW, Mosmann TR, Zlotnik A (1990) IL-10, a novel growth cofactor for mature and immature T cells. *J Immunol* 145 (12): 4167–4173

127 Qin L, Ding Y, Pahud DR, Robson ND, Shaked A, Bromberg JS (1997) Adenovirus-mediated gene transfer of viral interleukin-10 inhibits the immune response to both alloantigen and adenoviral antigen. *Hum Gene Ther* 8 (11): 1365–1374

128 Bromberg JS, Debruyne LA, Qin L (1998) Interactions between the immune system and gene therapy vectors: bidirectional regulation of response and expression. *Adv Immunol* 69: 353–409

129 Benhamou PY, Mullen Y, Shaked A, Bahmiller D, Csete ME (1996) Decreased alloreactivity to human islets secreting recombinant viral interleukin 10. *Transplantation* 62 (9): 1306–1312

130 Lee MS, Wogensen L, Shizuru J, Oldstone MB, Sarvetnick N (1994) Pancreatic islet production of murine interleukin-10 does not inhibit immune-mediated tissue destruction. *J Clin Invest* 93 (3): 1332–1338

131 Lee MS, Mueller R, Wicker LS, Peterson LB, Sarvetnick N (1996) IL-10 is necessary and sufficient for autoimmune diabetes in conjunction with NOD MHC homozygosity. *J Exp Med* 183 (6): 2663–2668

132 Lee MS, Wicker LS, Peterson LB, Sarvetnick N (1997) Pancreatic IL-10 induces diabetes in NOD.B6 Idd3 Idd10 mice. *Autoimmunity* 26 (4): 215–221
133 Nitta Y, Tashiro F, Tokui M, Shimada A, Takei I, Tabayashi K et al (1998) Systemic delivery of interleukin 10 by intramuscular injection of expression plasmid DNA prevents autoimmune diabetes in nonobese diabetic mice. *Hum Gene Ther* 9 (12): 1701–1707
134 Gray JD, Hirokawa M, Horwitz DA (1994) The role of transforming growth factor beta in the generation of suppression: an interaction between CD8+ T and NK cells. *J Exp Med* 180 (5): 1937–1942
135 Lee MS, Sawyer S, Arnush M, Krahl T, von Herrath M, Oldstone MA et al (1996) Transforming growth factor-beta fails to inhibit allograft rejection or virus-induced autoimmune diabetes in transgenic mice. *Transplantation* 61 (7): 1112–1115
136 Piccirillo CA, Chang Y, Prud'homme GJ (1998) TGF-beta1 somatic gene therapy prevents autoimmune disease in nonobese diabetic mice. *J Immunol* 161 (8): 3950–3956
137 Deng S, Ketchum RJ, Kucher T, Weber M, Shaked A, Naji A et al (1997) IL-10 and TGF-beta gene transfer for xenogeneic islet transplantation: comparison of effect in concordant vs discordant combination. *Transplant Proc* 29 (4): 2204–2205
138 Lenschow DJ, Zeng Y, Thistlethwaite JR, Montag A, Brady W, Gibson MG et al (1992) Long-term survival of xenogeneic pancreatic islet grafts induced by CTLA4lg [see comments]. *Science* 257 (5071): 789–792
139 Thomson AW, Lu L, Murase N, Demetris AJ, Rao AS, Starzl TE (1995) Microchimerism, dendritic cell progenitors and transplantation tolerance. *Stem Cells* (Dayt) 13 (6): 622–639
140 Steurer W, Nickerson PW, Steele AW, Steiger J, Zheng XX, Strom TB (1995) *Ex vivo* coating of islet cell allografts with murine CTLA4/Fc promotes graft tolerance. *J Immunol* 155 (3): 1165–1174
141 Weber CJ, Hagler MK, Chryssochoos JT, Kapp JA, Korbutt GS, Rajotte RV et al (1997) CTLA4-Ig prolongs survival of microencapsulated neonatal porcine islet xenografts in diabetic NOD mice. *Cell Transplant* 6 (5): 505–508
142 Levisetti MG, Padrid PA, Szot GL, Mittal N, Meehan SM, Wardrip CL et al (1997) Immunosuppressive effects of human CTLA4Ig in a non-human primate model of allogeneic pancreatic islet transplantation. *J Immunol* 159 (11): 5187–5191
143 Chahine AA, Yu M, McKernan MM, Stoeckert C, Lau HT (1995) Immunomodulation of pancreatic islet allografts in mice with CTLA4Ig secreting muscle cells. *Transplantation* 59 (9): 1313–1318
144 Nagata S, Suda T (1995) Fas and Fas ligand: lpr and gld mutations. *Immunol Today* 16 (1): 39–43
145 Nagata S, Golstein P (1995) The Fas death factor. *Science* 267 (5203): 1449–1456
146 Nagata S (1996) Apoptosis mediated by the Fas system. *Prog Mol Subcell Biol* 16: 87–103
147 Kabelitz D (1998) Apoptosis, graft rejection, and transplantation tolerance. *Transplantation* 65 (7): 869–75

148 Stuart PM, Griffith TS, Usui N, Pepose J, Yu X, Ferguson TA (1997) CD95 ligand (FasL)-induced apoptosis is necessary for corneal allograft survival. *J Clin Invest* 99 (3): 396–402

149 Lau HT, Yu M, Fontana A, Stoeckert CJ Jr (1996) Prevention of islet allograft rejection with engineered myoblasts expressing FasL in mice. *Science* 273 (5271): 109–112

150 Kang SM, Schneider DB, Lin Z, Hanahan D, Dichek DA, Stock PG et al (1997) Fas ligand expression in islets of Langerhans does not confer immune privilege and instead targets them for rapid destruction. *Nat Med* 3 (7): 738–743

151 Fandrich F, Lin X, Zhu X, Kloppel G, Parwaresch R, Kremer B (1998) CD95L confers immune priviledge to liver grafts which are spontaneously accepted. *Transplant Proc* 30 (4): 1057–1058

152 Swenson KM, Ke B, Wang T, Markowitz JS, Maggard MA, Spear GS et al (1998) Fas ligand gene transfer to renal allografts in rats: effects on allograft survival. *Transplantation* 65 (2): 155–160

153 Suda T, Hashimoto H, Tanaka M, Ochi T, Nagata S (1997) Membrane Fas ligand kills human peripheral blood T lymphocytes, and soluble Fas ligand blocks the killing. *J Exp Med* 186 (12): 2045–2050

154 Miwa K, Asano M, Horai R, Iwakura Y, Nagata S, Suda T (1998) Caspase 1-independent IL-1beta release and inflammation induced by the apoptosis inducer Fas ligand. *Nat Med* 4 (11): 1287–1292

155 Kurrer MO, Pakala SV, Hanson HL, Katz JD (1997) Beta cell apoptosis in T cell-mediated autoimmune diabetes. *Proc Natl Acad Sci USA* 94 (1): 213–218

156 Yamada K, Takane-Gyotoku N, Yuan X, Ichikawa F, Inada C, Nonaka K (1996) Mouse islet cell lysis mediated by interleukin-1-induced Fas. *Diabetologia* 39 (11): 1306–1312

157 Stassi G, Maria RD, Trucco G, Rudert W, Testi R, Galluzzo A et al (1997) Nitric oxide primes pancreatic beta cells for Fas-mediated destruction in insulin-dependent diabetes mellitus. *J Exp Med* 186 (8): 1193–200

158 Sandberg JO, Eizirik DL, Sandler S, Tracey DE, Andersson A (1993) Treatment with an interleukin-1 receptor antagonist protein prolongs mouse islet allograft survival. *Diabetes* 42 (12): 1845–1851

159 Sandberg JO, Andersson A, Eizirik DL, Sandler S (1994) Interleukin-1 receptor antagonist prevents low dose streptozotocin induced diabetes in mice. *Biochem Biophys Res Commun* 202 (1): 543–548

160 Sandberg JO, Eizirik DL, Sandler S (1997) IL-1 receptor antagonist inhibits recurrence of disease after syngeneic pancreatic islet transplantation to spontaneously diabetic non-obese diabetic (NOD) mice. *Clin Exp Immunol* 108 (2): 314–317

161 Arnush M, Heitmeier MR, Scarim AL, Marino MH, Manning PT, Corbett JA (1998) IL-1 produced and released endogenously within human islets inhibits beta cell function. *J Clin Invest* 102 (3): 516–526

162 Arnush M, Scarim AL, Heitmeier MR, Kelly CB, Corbett JA (1998) Potential role of resident islet macrophage activation in the initiation of autoimmune diabetes. *J Immunol* 160 (6): 2684–2691

163 Kawahara A, Kobayashi T, Nagata S (1998) Inhibition of Fas-induced apoptosis by Bcl-2. *Oncogene* 17 (20): 2549–2554
164 Benhamou PY, Moriscot C, Richard MJ, Kerr-Conte J, Pattou F, Chroboczek J et al (1998) Adenoviral-mediated catalase gene transfer protects porcine and human islets *in vitro* against oxidative stress. *Transplant Proc* 30 (2): 459
165 Utsugi T, Nagata M, Kawamura T, Yoon JW (1994) Prevention of recurrent diabetes in syngenic islet-transplanted NOD mice by transfusion of autoreactive T lymphocytes. *Transplantation* 57 (12): 1799–1804
166 Han HS, Jun HS, Utsugi T, Yoon JW (1997) Molecular role of TGF-beta, secreted from a new type of CD4$^+$ suppressor T cell, NY4.2, in the prevention of autoimmune IDDM in NOD mice. *J Autoimmun* 10 (3): 299–307
167 Posselt AM, Barker CF, Tomaszewski JE, Markmann JF, Choti MA, Naji A (1990) Induction of donor-specific unresponsiveness by intrathymic islet transplantation [see comments]. *Science* 249 (4974): 1293–1295
168 Posselt AM, Naji A, Roark JH, Markmann JF, Barker CF (1991) Intrathymic islet transplantation in the spontaneously diabetic BB rat. *Ann Surg* 214 (4): 363–371; discussion 371–373
169 Posselt AM, Barker CF, Friedman AL, Naji A (1992) Prevention of autoimmune diabetes in the BB rat by intrathymic islet transplantation at birth. *Science* 256 (5061): 1321–1324
170 Posselt AM, Barker CF, Markmann JF, Roark JH, Naji A (1992) Successful islet transplantation in the thymus of spontaneously diabetic BB rats. *Transplant Proc* 24 (3): 1023–1024
171 Koevary SB, Blomberg M (1992) Prevention of diabetes in BB/Wor rats by intrathymic islet injection. *J Clin Invest* 89 (2): 512–516
172 Charlton B, Taylor-Edwards C, Tisch R, Fathman CG (1994) Prevention of diabetes and insulitis by neonatal intrathymic islet administration in NOD mice. *J Autoimmun* 7 (5): 549–560
173 Battan R, Mordes JP, Abreau S, Greiner DL, Handler ES, Rossini AA (1994) Evidence that intrathymic islet transplantation does not prevent diabetes or subsequent islet graft destruction in RT6-depleted, diabetes-resistant BioBreeding/Worcester rats. *Transplantation* 57 (5): 731–736
174 Zeng Y, Bluestone JA, Ildstad ST, Torres MA, Montag AG, Thistlethwaite RJ, Jr. (1993) Long-term functional xenograft tolerance after intrathymic islet transplantation (Lewis rat —> B6 mouse). *Transplant Proc* 25 (1 Pt 1): 438–439
175 Goss JA, Nakafusa Y, Finke EH, Flye MW, Lacy PE (1994) Induction of tolerance to islet xenografts in a concordant rat-to-mouse model. *Diabetes* 43 (1): 16–23
176 James T, Jin MX, Chowdhury NC, Oluwole SF (1993) Tolerance induction to rat islet allografts by intrathymic inoculation of donor spleen cells. *Transplantation* 56 (5): 1148–1152
177 Oluwole SF, Jin MX, Chowdhury NC, James T, Fawwaz RA (1993) Induction of spe-

cific unresponsiveness to rat islet allografts by intrathymic UVB donor spleen cells. *Transplantation* 56 (5): 1142–1147

178 Oluwole SF, Chowdhury NC, Fawwaz RA (1993) Induction of donor-specific unresponsiveness to rat cardiac allografts by intrathymic injection of UV-B-irradiated donor spleen cells. *Transplantation* 55 (6): 1389–1395

179 Posselt AM, Odorico JS, Barker CF, Naji A (1992) Promotion of pancreatic islet allograft survival by intrathymic transplantation of bone marrow. *Diabetes* 41 (6): 771–775

180 Oluwole SF, Jin MX, Chowdhury NC, Ohajekwe OA (1994) Effectiveness of intrathymic inoculation of soluble antigens in the induction of specific unresponsiveness to rat islet allografts without transient recipient immunosuppression. *Transplantation* 58 (10): 1077–1081

181 Singer SM, Tisch R, Yang XD, Sytwu HK, Liblau R, McDevitt HO (1998) Prevention of diabetes in NOD mice by a mutated I-Ab transgene. *Diabetes* 47 (10): 1570–1577

182 Cetkovic-Cvrlje M, Gerling IC, Muir A, Atkinson MA, Elliot JF, Leiter EH (1997) Retardation or acceleration of diabetes in NOD/Lt mice mediated by intrathymic administration of candidate beta-cell antigens. *Diabetes* 46 (12): 1975–1982

183 DeMatteo RP, Raper SE, Ahn M, Fisher KJ, Burke C, Radu A et al (1995) Gene transfer to the thymus. A means of abrogating the immune response to recombinant adenovirus. *Ann Surg* 222 (3): 229–239

184 Steptoe RJ, Thomson AW (1996) Dendritic cells and tolerance induction. *Clin Exp Immunol* 105 (3): 397–402

185 Takayama T, Nishioka Y, Lu L, Lotze MT, Tahara H, Thomson AW (1998) Retroviral delivery of viral interleukin-10 into myeloid dendritic cells markedly inhibits their allostimulatory activity and promotes the induction of T-cell hyporesponsiveness. *Transplantation* 66 (12): 1567–1574

186 Lee WC, Zhong C, Qian S, Wan Y, Gauldie J, Mi Z, Robbins PD, Thomson AW, Lu L (1998) Phenotype, function and *in vivo* migration and survival of allogeneic dendritic cell progenitors genetically engineered to express TGFβ. *Transplantation* 66: 1810–1817

187 Lu L, Khoury S, Sayegh M, Thomson AW (1999) Dendritic cell tolerogenicity and prospects for therapy of allograft rejection and autoimmune disease. In: MT Lotze, AW Thomson (eds): *Dendritic cells: Biology and clinical applications*. Academic Press, San Diego, 487–511

188 Lu L et al (1999) Transduction of dendritic cells with adenoviral vectors encoding CTLA4-Ig markedly reduces their allostimulatory activity. *Transplant Proc* 31 (1–2): 797

189 Lin SS, Weidner BC, Byrne GW, Diamond LE, Lawson JH, Hoopes CW et al (1998) The role of antibodies in acute vascular rejection of pig-to-baboon cardiac transplants. *J Clin Invest* 101 (8): 1745–1756

190 Cotterell AH, Collins BH, Parker W, Harland RC, Platt JL (1995) The humoral immune response in humans following cross-perfusion of porcine organs. *Transplantation* 60 (8): 861–868

191 Leventhal JR, John R, Fryer JP, Witson JC, Derlich JM, Remiszewski J et al (1995)

Removal of baboon and human antiporcine IgG and IgM natural antibodies by immunoadsorption. Results of *in vitro* and *in vivo* studies. *Transplantation* 59 (2): 294–300
192 Sandrin MS, Vaughan HA, Dabkowski PL, McKenzie IF (1993) Anti-pig IgM antibodies in human serum react predominantly with Gal (alpha 1-3)Gal epitopes. *Proc Natl Acad Sci USA* 90 (23): 11391–11395
193 Sandrin MS, Osman N, McKenzie IF (1997) Transgenic approaches for the reduction of Galalpha (1,3)Gal for xenotransplantation. *Front Biosci* 2: e1–e11
194 Takahashi T, Saadi S, Platt JL (1997) Recent advances in the immunology of xenotransplantation. *Immunol Res* 16 (3): 273–297
195 Schmoeckel M, Bhatti FN, Zaidi A, Cozzi E, Waterworth PD, Tolan MJ et al (1998) Orthotopic heart transplantation in a transgenic pig-to-primate model. *Transplantation* 65 (12): 1570–1577
196 Byrne GW, McCurry KR, Martin MJ, McClellan SM, Platt JL, Logan JS (1997) Transgenic pigs expressing human CD59 and decay-accelerating factor produce an intrinsic barrier to complement-mediated damage. *Transplantation* 63 (1): 149–155
197 Pruitt SK, Baldwin WMd, Marsh HC, Jr., Lin SS, Yeh CG, Bollinger RR (1991) The effect of soluble complement receptor type 1 on hyperacute xenograft rejection. *Transplantation* 52 (5): 868–873
198 Sandrin MS, Fodor WL, Mouhtouris E, Osman N, Cohney S, Rollins SA et al (1995) Enzymatic remodelling of the carbohydrate surface of a xenogenic cell substantially reduces human antibody binding and complement-mediated cytolysis [see comments]. *Nat Med* 1 (12): 1261–1267
199 McKenzie IF, Osman N, Cohney S, Vaughan HA, Patton K, Mouhtouris E et al (1996) Strategies to overcome the anti-Gal alpha (1-3)Gal reaction in xenotransplantation. *Transplant Proc* 28 (2): 537
200 Osman N, McKenzie IF, Ostenried K, Ioannou YA, Desnick RJ, Sandrin MS (1997) Combined transgenic expression of alpha-galactosidase and alpha1,2-fucosyltransferase leads to optimal reduction in the major xenoepitope Galalpha (1,3)Gal. *Proc Natl Acad Sci USA* 94 (26): 14677–14682
201 Bracy JL, Sachs DH, Iacomini J (1998) Inhibition of xenoreactive natural antibody production by retroviral gene therapy. *Science* 281 (5384): 1845–1847
202 Zhang HG, Liu D, Heike Y, Yang P, Wang Z, Wang X et al (1998) Induction of specific T-cell tolerance by adenovirus-transfected, Fas ligand-producing antigen presenting cells. *Nat Biotechnol* 16 (11): 1045–1049

Gene transfer to facilitate transplantation

Jonathan S. Bromberg[1], Lisa A. DeBruyne[3], Randall S. Sung[4] and Lihui Qin[2]

Departments of Surgery and [1]Gene Therapy and Molecular Medicine and [2]Pathology, Mt. Sinai School of Medicine, One Gustave L. Levy Place, Box 1496, New York, NY 10029-6574, USA; [3]Parke-Davis Warner Lambert, Ann Arbor, MI 48109-0331, USA; [4]Departments of Surgery and Microbiology and Immunology, University of Michigan, Medical Center, Ann Arbor, MI 48109-0331, USA

Introduction

Other chapters in this volume have focused on gene transfer approaches for inhibition of immune responses against autoantigens. This chapter will discuss treatment of inflammatory responses directed against alloantigens, as a result of allogeneic transplantation of solid parenchymal organs or dispersed cells. From an immunological standpoint, autoimmunity and alloimmunity share many of the same basic mechanisms of lymphocyte activation and recruitment, reliance on clonal and nonclonal receptors to mediate cellular communication, participation of cytokines and adhesion receptors in diverse aspects of lymphocyte function, and effector mechanisms involving $CD4^+$ and $CD8^+$ T cells, B cells and macrophages [1]. The major difference between the two types of responses is that major histocompatibility complex (MHC) antigens are responsible for the vast majority of alloresponses, while autoimmunity for the most part involves responses to non-MHC antigens. Functional consequences of these differences are that MHC antigens can be presented directly to class I or class II allorestricted $CD8^+$ or $CD4^+$ T cells, respectively, or processed MHC-derived peptides can be represented indirectly to self-restricted, alloreactive T cells. In contrast, autoantigens are usually presented in the context of self MHC, often class II, to autoreactive $CD4^+$ T cells. While these differences are clearly protean in nature and have enormous significance for the understanding and control of autoreactive and alloreactive immune responses, they have not resulted in clinically applicable experimental approaches or practical molecular interventions that substantially differentiate or affect one type of immune response in preference to the other. As a result, many of the approaches and considerations that are germane for control of alloimmunity are equally applicable to autoimmunity.

Gene Therapy in Inflammatory Diseases, edited by C. H. Evans and P. D. Robbins

Unique advantages of gene therapy in transplantation

Since allografting requires the removal of tissues from one individual and transfer to another, allogeneic transplantation offers the possibility of treating cells or organs *ex vivo* with gene transfer vectors, prior to implantation of the cells or organs. In this respect transplantation presents several opportunities and possibilities for improving gene transfer that are not available in the consideration of treatment of other disorders, in which vectors must be directly applied to pathologically involved regions *in vivo*. Thus, higher concentrations, volumes and doses of vector can be administered to organs *ex vivo*, or cells *in vitro*, and excess vector washed away, decreasing chances for toxicity, immunogenicity, and systemic transduction or expression of the vector. A recent report even suggests that the decrease in immunogenicity as a result of *ex vivo* gene transduction may permit prolonged transgene expression [2]. While tissue or organ specificity of expression is desirable for most gene transfer vectors, this is difficult to achieve *in vivo*. The requirement for specificity has resulted in the development of specialized physical administration techniques, such as catheters, to direct localized vector placement, and the use of tissue restricted or regulatable promoters and enhancers to compartmentalize expression further. These maneuvers, which are inefficient and not fully developed technically, may not be necessary in the transplant setting since *ex vivo* transfection already results in highly specific organ and tissue transduction, without the possibility of affecting other organs or tissues. In essence, *ex vivo* perfusion allows one to achieve functional vector specificity, which is an elusive or imperfect goal with other approaches to gene transfer.

As has been pointed out in previous chapters, one of the major limitations to all of gene therapy is that gene expression and protein production are transient. Immune responses against vectors or transgenes, and promoter silencing and extinction, limit the time period over which therapeutically useful gene expression can be achieved. For treatment of inborn errors of metabolism, genetic deficiencies, or chronic diseases, this significantly limits the ability of gene transfer techniques to cure disease. In the setting of transplantation, however, the transient production of an immunosuppressive molecule may be sufficient to prevent lymphocyte priming and to alter immune regulation, so that a negative regulatory network, rather than a positive immune response, is produced. In fact, transient gene expression may be desirable since the potential toxicities and adverse effects of prolonged vector persistence, vector expression, or immunosuppressive molecule production could be avoided. In addition, the delivery of immunosuppressive molecules may further prolong transgene expression by impeding the anti-vector immune response [3]. The anti-transgene immune response, while of paramount concern in many gene transfer applications, is not currently as germane to the gene therapy of transplantation, since many of the immunosuppressive effector molecules that will be considered (see below) are self molecules. However, it can be anticipated that immunosuppressive molecules would impede the immune response to themselves or other co-transfected, non-self transgene products.

Local immunosuppression

A ubiquitous problem with current immunosuppression is that antigen nonspecific drugs are given systemically, resulting in global immunosuppression and drug associated toxicities. Antigen specific immunosuppression, through the use of donor derived cells, MHC peptides or receptor specific reagents, has so far not been successful outside of highly defined rodent models. Toxicity free pharmaceuticals are also unlikely ever to be developed. An alternative to systemic immunosuppression is local immunosuppression. In general, local immunosuppression can achieve equivalent or better immune modulation, compared to systemic administration, without exposing the recipient to the effect of systemic levels of the drugs [4]. This prevents both systemic immunosuppression, which may lead to infection and malignancy, and systemic drug-specific toxicities. Unfortunately, local immunosuppression with catheter delivery techniques or implanted devices is costly and associated with device related complications and failures [4]. Furthermore, local immunosuppression is not currently used clinically other than in highly specialized ophthalmologic applications, where drugs are easily administered to the eye, or some pulmonary conditions where inhaled drugs are partially effective. The alternative to local immunosuppression with gene transfer approaches obviates the problems with physical delivery techniques [5]. Local immunosuppression can also achieve functional antigen specificity with antigen nonspecific molecules since the immunosuppression is limited to the site of the graft, or the interface of the host immune system with donor alloantigen. Thus, a gene therapy approach to transplant immunosuppression could potentially achieve antigen specific immunosuppression without systemic immunosuppression, drug toxicities, or device related complications. A variety of *in vitro* and *in vivo* studies provide proof of concept for these notions, demonstrating local production and activity of biologically relevant molecules limited to the sites of cellular transduction [6–10].

Vectors

Vectors that have been considered for use in organ or cellular transplantation are essentially the same for other applications of gene transfer and gene therapy and include both plasmid and virus based vectors [11, 12]. A number of studies have successfully demonstrated gene transfer and expression with plasmid, adenoviral, adeno-associated viral, and retroviral vectors into heart, myocytes, liver, hepatocytes, and lung [13–24]. Vector specific advantages and disadvantages have been discussed in previous chapters and will not be repeated here. It is worthwhile to note that issues related to vector and transgene immunogenicity, kinetics of gene expression levels, persistence of gene expression, persistence of vector nucleic acids, and use of specific promoters are all as relevant for gene therapy in transplantation as for other applications [25–32]. In this context, the advantages of gene transfer applications in transplantation, as noted above, are that *ex vivo* perfusion of organs or cells permits one to achieve site specificity without resorting to manipulation of promoters and enhancers, or complicated physical delivery methods.

Whole organ transplantation

Several distinct strategies for the use of gene transfer and gene therapy techniques can be delineated. For the transplantation of vascularized grafts, *ex vivo* or "back table" perfusion of organs such as liver, heart, and kidney with vectors followed by incubation, wash out, and surgical implantation is a likely scenario that can be directly applied to current clinical transplantation. This technique has been successfully demonstrated in a number of experimental models [6, 8, 14, 16]. Such incubations will have to be performed in hypothermic (~4° C) conditions over a short time period (a few hours), to avoid ischemic damage to the organs. These physical conditions may be major limitations to transduction efficiency as a consequence of a vector's ability to efficiently bind to and internalize into cells at low temperatures and will require experimental optimization. Nonetheless, efficient transduction under such conditions has been demonstrated [33]. A corollary of this back table gene transfer approach is the use of organs derived from transgenic donors. Thus, if a gene therapy technique can successfully deliver a gene product and suppress specific immunity, the next logical step is to construct transgenic donors. Since transgenic humans are not an ethical possibility in clinical transplantation, such considerations are limited to transgenic xenogeneic donors, such as pigs. Further issues related to xenotransplantation and transgenic donors are beyond the scope of this chapter and will not be considered in the discussion that follows.

Cellular transplantation

Allotransplantation also includes cellular transplants such as pancreatic islet β-cells, bone marrow stem cells, hepatocytes, myoblasts, or specifically engineered cells secreting a therapeutic product (e.g. myoblasts secreting factor VIII to correct hemophilia). Each of these cellular transplants requires an individualized approach and strategy for the use of gene transfer techniques. Allogeneic bone marrow transplantation or allogeneic hematopoietic stem cell transfer at the time of parenchymal organ allograft transplantation have been considered as ways to induce alloantigen specific tolerance and improve graft survival without the need for long term maintenance immunosuppression [34–36]. While it is uncertain if bone marrow or stem cell transplantation will eventually fulfill the promise of inducing tolerance, from a methodologic standpoint they are relatively well developed and mature clinical techniques. They are, however, associated with a number of problems, especially graft failure and graft-versus-host disease (GVHD). A logical alternative that may both improve engraftment and decrease GVHD is autologous bone marrow transplantation or hematopoietic stem cell transfer with cells modified *in vitro* with gene transfer vectors. The most appropriate vectors for this use are retroviral derived vectors which will incorporate into the genomic DNA of proliferating precursor cells [37–41]. The feasibility of such an approach has been demonstrated in both animals [37–40] and humans [42]. In experimental animal transplant models MHC class I and II antigens have been transfected into bone marrow or stem cell grafts, transferred to recipients, and used to induce alloantigen specific tolerance in mice and pigs [43–49]. Thus, instead of transferring immunosuppressive molecule genes into an allogeneic graft to suppress the local immune response, alloantigen genes are transferred into syngeneic hematopoietic stem cell grafts, which are used systemically to reconstitute and tolerize the recipient for a concurrent or subsequent allograft.

A second strategy for cellular transplantation is to transplant allogeneic cells to correct metabolic disorders, such as pancreatic islet β-cells for type I diabetes or hepatocytes for various inborn errors of metabolism. Gene transfer approaches for these transplants are expected to be similar to those for parenchymal organ allografts. It is anticipated that the cells would be prepared *in vitro*, transduced with vectors encoding immunosuppressive molecules, and transferred to an appropriate site in the recipient [6, 15, 22, 23]. A variation of this approach is the co-transplantation of the allogeneic cells with other cells, syngeneic to the recipient, that have been transduced to secrete an immunosuppressive molecule [50]. This latter approach may be technically more feasible since the syngeneic cells could be transfected and selected separately ahead of time and stored in liquid nitrogen prior to the availability of cells from an allogeneic cadaver or living donor. Another variation is syngeneic cellular transplants with the syngeneic cells engineered by gene transfer techniques to correct a metabolic disorder [23]. In this case it may also be necessary to provide local (i.e. by gene transfer) or systemic immunosuppression to abrogate the immune response to the transgene product. Yet another variation is to protect immunologically the allogeneic and/or syngeneic transduced cells with immunoisolation devices comprised of alginate or physical chambers [50]. Thus, a variety of potential approaches to cell transplantation are possible with various schemes to provide therapeutic gene products and to suppress immune responses to transgene products, viral vector components, and major and minor histocompatibility antigens.

Thymic gene transfer

The immune response to transgenes and vectors is one of the major limitations to successful sustained vector expression after gene transfer [25–27]. Approaches relying on systemic immunosuppression with anti-CD40, CTLA4Ig, anti-CD4 or tacrolimus are effective in experimental models [28–31], but carry all the risks of systemic immunosuppression. While local immunosuppressive approaches have been outlined above; alternative means to abrogate these immune responses rely on permanent tolerizing methods, in particular oral [52] or intrathymic [53–56] presentation of viral vectors to induce long lasting, specific tolerance. These observations have been extended in studies in which the thymus was injected with syngeneic myocytes expressing allogeneic class I MHC or directly transfected with plasmid DNA encoding class I MHC [57–59]. In both cases alloantigen specific tolerance was induced. Thus, intrathymic gene transfer may solve the immunologic response to transgenes, vectors, and alloantigen. The technique remains problematic, however, since it is not certain if this approach is applicable to large animal or human transplantation because of thymic involution and extrathymic T cell maturation.

Candidate genes

A number of potential molecular gene candidates have been considered and tested in experimental systems for their ability to provide immunosuppression in allotransplantation settings. Because it is currently difficult, if not impossible, to transduce all the cells of a graft, most consideration has been given to transferring genes encoding soluble gene products, with the notion that even if only a few cells are transduced the gene product would "bathe" the graft in the immunosuppressive protein. Many studies have thus focused on the use of immunoregulatory cytokines to attenuate the immune response. The cytokine TGFβ can suppress T cell, B cell, antigen presenting cell, neutrophil, and inflammatory cytokine function; and TGFβ gene transfer can inhibit local immune responses in hepatic [60] and cardiac [61, 62] allografts. The TH2 cytokine IL-4 inhibits TH1 differentiation and therefore IFNγ production and CTL development; and IL-4 gene transfer can prolong cardiac allograft survival [63] and inhibit autoimmune diabetes [64, 65]. The TH2 cytokine IL-10 inhibits diverse aspects of TH1, B cell, macrophage, and antigen presenting cell function; and IL-10 gene transfer can inhibit alloreactivity to pancreatic islets [66] and cardiac grafts [62, 67]. Gene transfer of cytokine inhibitors such as soluble TNFα p55 receptor can suppress a variety of inflammatory responses [68, 69], although its efficacy in allografting is untested. Because TNFα may participate in complex regulatory pathways, it may not necessarily be beneficial, at least for islet transplantation [70]. The adenovirus E3 region encodes a number of proteins, among them the 14.7 kD protein, which inhibits TNFα cytotoxicity [71–73]. Gene transfer of E3-14.7K can prolong islet allograft survival [74] and prevent anti-adenoviral immune responses [75]. Soluble CTLA4Ig [76], IL-12 p40 homodimers (which inhibit IL-12 p35-p40 heterodimer activity) [77], and VCAM-1 ligand binding fragments [78] have also been used with some success in allograft or inflammatory rodent models. In sum, a number of soluble immunosuppressive cytokines or inhibitors of inflammatory cytokines demonstrate efficacy in their ability to negatively modulate alloreactivity or other similar inflammatory responses.

It was noted earlier that gene transfer of MHC antigens to the thymus or hematopoietic stem cells could serve as a strategy to induce antigen specific tolerance. An alternative consideration is to interfere with MHC function and therefore antigen presentation. The adenovirus E3 region also encodes a 19 kD glycoprotein which binds MHC class I chains in the endoplasmic reticulum and prevents export to the cell surface [74, 75]. Gene transfer of E3-19K can also help prolong islet allograft survival [74] and inhibit anti-vector immunity [75, 79].

There has been much interest in the use of FasL as an immunosuppressive moiety. Initial studies suggested the expression of FasL could create immunologically privileged sites by deleting antigen reactive lymphocytes that trafficked to that site [80–82]. However, recent experience [83–86] suggests that the use of FasL will not be successful in many settings, as it may provoke a more robust inflammatory response, especially with a granulocytic infiltrate. In addition, many tissues of interest (e.g. liver, myocardium) express Fas and are directly susceptible to the cytotoxic effects of FasL.

It is worthwhile to consider other mechanistic approaches to improve graft survival that have not yet been applied to the transplant setting. A major cause of allograft failure and patient morbidity and mortality is chronic rejection, especially in renal and cardiac allografts. Chronic rejection presents microscopically as rapidly advancing intimal hyperplasia, atherosclerotic lesions, and interstitial fibrosis. The exact involvement of the immune system in chronic rejection is not well understood and is currently the subject of intensive scrutiny. Likewise, the molecular and cellular relationship of chronic rejection to common atherosclerotic intimal lesions is also not well delineated. Nonetheless, a variety of gene transfer approaches for atherosclerosis have shown some success in experimental models [87–92] and ought to be considered for use in improving the long term function of vascularized allografts.

Immune responses

Gene transfer vectors induce inflammatory responses

The general idea of gene transfer for transplantation is to express immunosuppressive molecules within the allograft, which would prevent graft rejection by inhibiting the local immune response. While a variety of gene therapy vectors have been successfully used to introduce immunosuppressive molecules into grafts, many of them have been demonstrated to initiate local inflammatory responses. These inflammatory responses consist not only of conventional antigen specific lymphocyte responses, but also nonspecific and innate mechanisms inherent to lymphocytes, neutrophils, macrophages, NK cells, and even organ parenchymal cells. Such inflammatory responses may eliminate transgene expression, which make gene therapy less effective, or serve as adjuvants to enhance graft rejection, which is undesirable for the purpose of transplantation. These issues should be considered when choosing and evaluating a gene transfer vector for transplantation so that it can be designed to minimize immunostimulatory effects.

Adenoviral vectors are attractive for gene transfer because of their broad host range, capacity for large DNA inserts, and high titers. However, the *in vivo* application of first generation recombinant adenoviruses (with E1 deletion) is limited by host anti-viral immune responses [25, 93, 94]. Recombinant adenoviral vectors express low levels of viral genes which stimulate cellular responses, which involve $CD8^+$ CTL, $CD4^+$ TH1 cells, IFNγ and IL-2 [25, 93, 94], and lead to destructive inflammation and transient transgene expression. Instillation of E1 deleted adenovirus elicits MHC class I restricted, $CD8^+$, CTL responses, leading to loss of transgene expression by mechanisms that included destruction of virus infected cells [96, 97]. Adenoviral capsid proteins also activate $CD4^+$ T cells, which is necessary for full realization of effector function of $CD8^+$ T cells [98, 99]. $CD4^+$ T cells contribute to the maturation of $CD8^+$ CTL and secrete IFNγ, which sensitizes the virus infected cells to CTLs through upregulation of MHC class I [95]. $CD4^+$ cells alone are capable of destroying virus infected hepatocytes, and depletion of $CD4^+$ cells leads to prolonged transgene expression. Studies utilizing immune deficient animals [94, 100, 101] further proved that T cell dependent, adenoviral-antigen specific immunity is the principal factor limiting the duration of primary transgene expression. Thus, the same cell types and mechanisms responsible for graft rejection are also responsible for adenoviral clearance.

Adenoviral vectors may also boost viral or alloantigen immunity by enhancing costimulatory signals for lymphocyte or neutrophil activation, homing, or effector function. For example, adenoviral vectors increase ICAM-1 expression on bronchial epithelium [102, 103] and cause IL-8 expression by airway epithelial cells [104]. Adenoviral vectors may also initiate an innate, antigen nonspecific immune response. Experiments demonstrate that following intravenous administration, 90% of adenoviral vector is eliminated from the mouse within the first 24 h [105]. This loss is independent of dose and transgene expression, and is also seen in immunodeficient animals. Thus, it appears that innate immune mechanisms, particularly Kupfer cells, contribute to elimination of vector and loss of transgene expression. This is commensurate with studies documenting antigen nonspecific components to the anti-adenoviral immune response [106–108].

Retroviral vectors have been used in many gene therapy trials, primarily due to their ability to stably integrate into the host genome, ensuring sustained gene expression [109]. There is little concern about generating an immune response to the retroviral vector, since most current protocols use an *ex vivo* approach in which the cells to be transduced are isolated from a patient, genetically modified *in vitro*, and then reintroduced into the patient [109, 110]. However, direct injection of retroviral vectors *in vivo* results in very low transfection efficiency and causes extensive endomysial cellular infiltration [111].

Plasmid DNA which is not methylated, unlike eukaryotic DNA, can be antigenic and evoke both cellular and humoral immune responses. Experiments utilizing synthetic oligonucleotides bearing randomly selected DNA sequences from *Mycobacterium bovis* demonstrated that the activation was due to a series of CpG motifs that generally followed the sequence 5'-purine-purine-C-G-pyrimidine-pyrimidine-3' [112–114]. These sequences were frequently palindromic, although palindromes were not essential for activity [115]. CpG motifs elicit interferon production, NK cell activation, antibody production, and B cell proliferation in both human and murine lymphocytes [116–120]. Unmethylated CpG DNA motifs directly activate B cells to secrete IL-6 and IL-12 within several hours and, as a result of the IL-6 production, to secrete IgM. CpG acts on NK cells and to a lesser degree on $CD4^+$ T cells to induce IFNγ production. Thus, immune activation induced by CpG DNA includes both humoral immunity through the induction of IL-6 secretion and increased cellular immunity through IFNγ secretion [120]. Macrophages can ingest and are activated by bacterial DNA containing CpG motifs as evidenced by TNFα, IL-1, plasminogen activator inhibitor-2, and increased NF-κB binding activity [121]. A recent study by Sato et al. [122] demonstrated that plasmids bearing CpG motifs can dramatically enhance the immune response to DNA immunization and limit transgene expression.

These examples demonstrate that different vectors can activate multiple pathways and effector cell types to enhance immunity and inflammation. Since these effects are likely to impede efforts to treat inflammatory responses, such as in transplantation, several strategies have been considered to minimize or inhibit immune responses to improve transgene expression.

Viral products inhibit immune responses

Although viruses induce vigorous humoral and cellular immune responses, they also produce a variety of molecules that can directly or indirectly regulate immune responses. In particular, virally encoded proteins may serve to evade or counteract immune defenses [123–125]. For example, many viruses encode proteins that interfere with proinflammatory cytokines, such as IL-1, IL-6, TNFα, and IFNγ [123–125]. The *Nef* gene product of HIV-1 interferes with the T cell antigen receptor function by binding directly to the p56^{lck} and MAP kinases and inhibiting their kinase activity. Many viruses also encode cytokine or chemokine homologues. Viruses inhibit antigen processing or transport, and expression and function of major histocompatibility complex (MHC) molecules. Some of these proteins are likely to be expressed by currently available gene transfer vectors [125]. These proteins could contribute to decreased immunogenicity of vector and transgene components and result in prolonged transgene expression.

While a detailed review of the alterations of immune function by viral proteins is beyond the scope of this chapter, two viral derived proteins are particularly interesting and currently used in experimental protocols. The *BCRF1* open reading frame of Epstein-Barr virus encodes viral IL-10, a homologue of cellular IL-10 [126–129]. Gene transfer and expression of vIL-10 prolongs allograft survival and inhibits the immune response to adenoviral antigens, thereby improving the persistence of the vector and extending transgene expression [3]. Adenovirus E3 region products decrease cell surface expression of MHC class I [130–134] and TNF function [71–73] and reduce cytotoxic T cell responses [74, 135]. Overexpression of the immunomodulatory products of the E3 region inhibits anti-vector humoral and cellular immune responses and enhances vector gene expression [75, 135]. Expression of E3 in pancreatic islets prolonged survival of allografts [74]. Understanding the mechanisms by which viruses escape from host immune surveillance might be useful in designing gene therapy vectors specific for the treatment of transplantation or autoimmune diseases.

Strategies to inhibit immune responses to improve transgene expression

Several approaches can be taken to circumvent the immune response to gene therapy vectors. The first approach is to engineer less immunogenic vectors. Initial adenoviral studies used first generation vectors rendered replication defective by deletion of E1 region genes, which control viral replication and the expression of other early and late genes [136]. However, it is now known that E1 deleted adenoviral vectors can still express low levels of both early and late viral genes, which induce a significant immune response [25, 93–101, 105–108]. Thus, second generation adenoviral vectors have been constructed, which in addition to being E1 deleted, have a temperature sensitive mutation within the E2A-encoded DNA binding protein [137, 138]. This E2A mutation reduces late gene expression and further cripples replication. Studies have shown that *in vivo* administration of this second generation vector results in a decreased CTL response and increased duration of transgene expression compared to first generation adenoviral vectors [137, 138]. Combined E1/E4 deleted adenoviral vectors [139, 140] and an adenoviral vector that lacks all viral genes [141, 142] have also been constructed to eliminate viral proteins that stimulate host immune responses.

Plasmids bearing certain CpG motifs can dramatically enhance the immune response and limit transgene expression. Sato et al. [122] demonstrated that injection of a plasmid vector encoding β-galactosidase and containing the ampicillin resistance gene produced a strong CTL and antibody response against the β-galactosidase transgene. However, injection of a similar vector containing the kanamycin resistance gene did not generate a humoral or cellular response to β-galactosidase. Further analysis showed that the ampicillin resistance gene contained two CpG motifs (5'-AACGTT-3'), whereas the kanamycin resistance gene contained none. The addition of one or two hexanucleotide repeats to the noncoding region of the vector with the kanamycin resistance gene dramatically enhanced the immune response to β-galactosidase in a dose related fashion. It is expected that the deletion of CpG motifs may be more desirable for gene therapy for transplantation. A better understanding of the mechanisms of CpG stimulation is required since both the position and the precise sequence of the motif within the plasmid backbone are important determinants of the immunostimulatory effect. As an alternative approach to the same issue, methylation of plasmids prior to gene transfer might reduce immunogenicity, although methylation inactivates promoters [143].

The second approach is to suppress the immune system of the host by using immunosuppressive drugs such as cyclophosphamide [94] and cyclosporine A [94, 137, 144], FK506 [31, 108], CTLA4Ig [29], anti-CD40 ligand [145], or anti-CD4 [30]. Studies have shown that various immunosuppressive protocols can result in prolonged transgene expression and a marked decrease in the appearance of neutralizing antibody [30, 31, 98]. Such systemic global immunosuppression, which is not attractive for other clinical applications, may be suitable for transplant patients since they normally receive such treatment.

The third approach is to induce unresponsiveness to adenoviral antigens by intrathymic inoculation [53, 54, 56]. Intrathymic transplantation of syngeneic pancreatic islet cells infected with adenovirus impaired the normal antiviral cytotoxic T-lymphocyte response and prolonged hepatic transgene expression after an intravenous challenge with adenovirus. The involuted thymus of adult humans make this approach not feasible for human gene therapy.

The fourth approach is to generate local immunosuppression by using gene therapy vectors which express both a gene of interest and a gene encoding an immunosuppressive molecule, such as the 19K glycoprotein of the adenovirus E3 region [74, 75, 135], interleukin-1 (IL-1) receptor antagonist [146], or viral IL-10 [3]. These methods have met with limited success and can induce local but not systemic immunosuppression. We demonstrated that adenovirus-mediated gene transfer and expression of vIL-10 prolonged allograft survival and inhibited the immune response to adenoviral antigens, thereby improving the persistence of the vector and extending transgene expression [3]. Thus, the efficacy of adenoviral vectors can be improved by incorporating immunosuppressive genes into the vector.

Alloresponses alter transgene expression

While expression of immunosuppressive molecules by gene transfer vectors could regulate allograft rejection, the alloresponse could also affect vector persistence and transgene expression. It would be expected that at least three mechanisms are involved in the interaction of the alloimmune response and vector expression:

(1) Alloresponses kill transduced cells. Most current gene therapy approaches for transplantation include *ex vivo* perfusion of donor organs with gene transfer vectors prior to transplantation [14, 59, 60, 147], direct injection of gene transfer vectors into grafts [3, 14, 62, 67, 148], or transplantation of genetically modified cells [66, 74, 77, 149]. In all these situations, the transgene expressing cells are of donor origin and may serve as targets for allo-specific rejection. As alloresponses destroy donor cells in an antigen-specific fashion, it would be expected that transgene expression will decrease as a result of loss of transduced cells, which in turn would decrease local immunosuppression and make further allo-specific attack more effective.

(2) Alloresponses augment vector-specific immune responses. Alloreactions, including lymphocytic infiltration, cytokine production, APC activation, and accessory molecule up-regulation, may serve as adjuvants to enhance vector-specific immunity and elimination of transduced cells.

(3) Alloresponses provide a cytokine-rich environment that inactivates cytokine-sensitive promoters. Transgene expression can be eliminated even in the presence of substantial amounts of vector DNA in the transduced cells [150–152], which suggests that mechanisms other than antigen-specific cytolytic cell death may mediate non-cytodestructive events that determine the persistence of transgene expression [153, 154]. Harms and Splitter [155] reported that IFNγ treatment of transiently or stably transfected cell lines, representing various tissues and species, resulted in suppression of transgene expression driven by the SV40 or CMV viral promoters, while transgene expression driven by the mammalian MHC I promoter was enhanced. Our recent data [156] indicate that the cytokines IFNγ and TNFα inhibit transgene expression from certain widely used viral promoters (CMV, RSV, SV40, MMLV-LTR) delivered by adenoviral, retroviral or plasmid vectors *in vitro*. Inhibition is at the mRNA level and cytokines do not cause vector DNA degradation, inhibit total cellular protein synthesis, or kill infected/transfected cells. Administration of neutralizing anti-IFNγ mAb results in enhanced transgene expression *in vivo*. This suggests that these cytokines represent basic cellular defenses against viral nucleic acids and that cells can distinguish viral from cellular promoter sequences. Thus, cytokines generated by alloresponses will not only augment vector-specific immune responses to eliminate transduced cells, but also alter transgene expression by other mechanisms, including promoter attenuation or extinction. Standard gene therapy vectors in current use may be improved by altering cytokine responsive regulatory elements. Utilizing cytokine-insensitive promoters may prolong transgene expression and provide further immunosuppression for transplantation.

Transplanted organs and tissues

Heart

In contrast to other tissues, skeletal and cardiac muscle possess an enhanced ability to take up and express naked DNA injected *in vivo* [157, 158]. Therefore, initial studies explored the possibility of cardiac graft gene transfer by directly injecting plasmid vector into the apex of heterotopically transplanted hearts [13]. This method of graft transduction resulted in reporter gene expression throughout the heart, but was primarily localized directly to the site of injection [13]. Subsequent studies of adenoviral vector injection into cardiac grafts also found transgene expression throughout the heart, but with much higher levels of expression at the site of injection [14, 159]. The approach of directly injecting vectors into cardiac tissue is inferior to coronary artery perfusion, which gives a more even distribution of transgene expression [14, 160]. In addition, since it is the vascular endothelium which forms the initial interface between the donor graft and the recipient immune system, it may be more effective to introduce immunomodulatory genes into the coronary vasculature instead of myocardium.

The amount and location of transgene expression in perfused cardiac grafts varies depending on how the gene is introduced into the graft and whether a plasmid or viral vector is used. In the murine vascularized heterotopic cardiac transplant model, reporter gene studies have indicated that cationic lipid-mediated gene transfer with Lipofectin resulted in gene expression predominately localized to coronary vasculature, with little myocyte involvement [161]. Using a luciferase transgene, investigators reported that perfusion of DNA-Lipofectin complexes via the coronary arteries resulted in expression of the transgene primarily in the coronary capillaries, in perivascular areas surrounding coronary arteries and veins, and the endocardia of both ventricles [160].

Other studies using adenoviral vectors to perfuse cardiac allografts and isografts have shown similar results, except that adenoviral transgene expression was found not only in the coronary vasculature (including endothelial cells and smooth muscle cells of the vessels), but was also present in myocytes [16, 147, 162]. Viral vectors are more efficient at delivering genes into cardiac grafts *in vivo* than nonviral vectors, as demonstrated by a direct comparison in which luciferase transgene activity was shown to be 10-fold higher in rat cardiac allografts transduced with an adenoviral vector compared to a plasmid vector [14]. Nonetheless, viral vectors still do not result in efficient gene transfer in cardiac perfusion applications, with most studies reporting less than 1% of the cells expressing the transgene [147, 162]. Although appealing because they can transduce a variety of nonreplicative cell types efficiently, adenoviral vectors can also induce an exuberant immune response and may be problematic in human applications since many individuals have pre-existing immunity to adenovirus [125].

Plasmid vectors may be safer than viral vectors and more suitable for human transplantation applications. However, new approaches will be required to improve gene transfer and expression such as optimization of nucleic acid delivery, transcellular transport, nuclear localizing signals, and selective promoters [59, 62, 125, 163]. Recently, a new cationic liposome preparation, designated γAP-DLRIE/DOPE, was shown to increase *in vivo* vascular gene expression by greater than 15-fold compared to naked DNA or previously described cationic lipids [163]. This represents a significant improvement in nonviral vector *in vivo* transfection efficiency and approaches levels observed with clinically acceptable doses of adenoviral vectors.

There have been many studies documenting reporter gene expression in cardiac transplantation models, but cellular IL-10, viral IL-10, and TGFβ are the only biologically active genes introduced into cardiac allografts described to date [61, 62, 67, 164]. A variety of plasmid and viral (retrovirus, adenovirus) vectors have been shown to successfully transfer and express these cytokine genes in nonvascularized cardiac allografts [61, 62, 67, 164]. These cytokines were chosen due to their inherent immunosuppressive activities. IL-10 is an important regulatory molecule that was originally identified by its ability to inhibit cytokine synthesis of Th1 cells [165]. However, in addition to negatively regulating immune responses, IL-10 also has growth factor activity and promotes the proliferation and differentiation of B cells, mast cells, and thymocytes [166–168]. Viral IL-10, which is a homologue of cellular IL-10, shares many of the biologic activities of cellular IL-10 including inhibition of cytokine synthesis and accessory cell function [126, 127, 165, 169], but does not possess the T cell costimulatory activities of cellular IL-10 [129, 170]. In a direct comparison utilizing retroviral vectors encoding either vIL-10 or cellular IL-10, we demonstrated that treatment of cardiac allografts with a retrovirus encoding vIL-10 results in enhanced graft survival (27.6 days), whereas retroviral delivered cellular IL-10 has no effect on survival (12.0 days) compared to controls (12.1 days) [67]. We have shown that the transient, local expression of vIL-10 generates local immunosuppression by inhibiting donor-specific helper and cytotoxic lymphocytes, as well as $CD4^+$ and $CD8^+$ lymphocytic infiltration within the graft [67].

These investigations utilized the nonvascularized, neonatal heart, ear pinna model. Although informative, this model system is not directly clinically applicable. Thus, our laboratory has recently addressed the plausibility of utilizing vIL-10 gene transfer in a clinically relevant, vascularized cardiac allograft model to inhibit rejection. Murine cardiac allografts perfused with plasmid DNA encoding vIL-10 complexed with the cationic lipid γAP DLRIE/DOPE demonstrated enhanced graft survival (16.00 days) compared to both unmodified allografts (8.14 days) and vIL-10 antisense controls (8.28 days) (unpublished observations). Prolonged graft survival was found to be specific to vIL-10 expression since treatment with an anti-vIL-10 monoclonal antibody abrogated the effect. A decrease in the number of graft infiltrating donor-reactive helper and cytotoxic lymphocytes in the heart correlated with enhanced graft survival. Viral IL-10 gene transfer inhibited the accumulation of donor-specific helper lymphocytes and expansion of donor-reactive cytotoxic lymphocytes in the spleen, and was associated with a marked decrease in IgM alloantibody production with little to no IgG isotype switching. Thus, vIL-10 gene transfer inhibits both humoral and cellular components of the immune response in this clinically relevant, vascularized cardiac transplant model.

Prolonged survival of vascularized cardiac allografts transduced with vIL-10 was associated with a novel histology characterized by a mononuclear infiltrate composed of unactivated leukocytes, edema, and diffuse collagen deposition in the interstitium, yet myocytes remained viable and vessels were patent. These manifestations did not occur in syngeneic grafts perfused with vIL-10 DNA-liposome complexes, implying that the observed fibrosis was not a direct effect of the vIL-10 gene product, lipid associated toxicity, or an artifact of the perfusion protocol. There was also no evidence of fibrosis in allografts perfused with antisense vIL-10 DNA-liposome complexes. These findings suggest that both the vIL-10 transgene product and an alloantigenic component are required for the observed fibrosis.

Little is known about the role of IL-10 in fibrosis. At present, it is not clear what is inducing fibrosis in vIL-10 transduced allografts, but one possible candidate may be TGFβ. TGFβ plays a role in promoting Th2 helper cells by inhibiting Th1 development, and is a prominent inducer of fibrosis [171, 172]. Because TGFβ itself possesses many immunosuppressive properties, cardiac allografts have been transduced with viral and nonviral vectors encoding TGFβ in the nonvascularized ear-heart model [61, 62, 164]. In this system, we have shown that TGFβ gene transfer prolongs allograft survival (26.3 days versus 12.6 days for controls) but does not induce any apparent fibrosis [165]. Preliminary results with TGFβ lipid-mediated gene transfer in the vascularized heart model, however, did show marked fibrosis of TGFβ transduced grafts (unpublished observations).

Lung

Most gene transfer studies involving the lung have focused on correcting cystic fibrosis and have utilized airway administration of adenoviral vectors to the lung *in situ* [136]. Airway administration of adenoviral vector transduces ciliated, secretory, basal, and undifferentiated cells of the pulmonary epithelium [173]. However, this method of delivery results in gene transfer only to the epithelium. In contrast, perfusion of the pulmonary vasculature results in gene transfer to both the endothelium and epithelium [174]. Because pulmonary artery administration of vector transduces vascular endothelial cells, it may be more effective in the transplant setting since the endothelium is the interface with the recipient immune system. One of the first reports to look at the feasibility of gene transfer into the pulmonary vasculature introduced a β-galactosidase encoding adenoviral vector into the pulmonary circulation of sheep, since sheep have pulmonary and bronchial circulation similar to humans [174]. The pulmonary artery and vein were temporarily occluded and the adenoviral vector was injected into the lumen of the pulmonary artery. After 15 min the circulation was restored, and 1 to 4 days later the animals were sacrificed and the lungs studied. Gene transfer was successful in 13 of 17 sheep, with transgene expression detected in endothelial cells of the pulmonary circulation, as well as epithelial cells of the alveoli and the airways, and in the epithelium of submucosal glands. All types of epithelial cells including ciliated, secretory, basal and undifferentiated cells expressed the reporter transgene. These initial studies transduced native lungs *in situ* but suggested that gene transfer via the pulmonary circulation might be a reasonable approach to transduce donor lung grafts *ex vivo*.

Another set of studies proceeded to test the feasibility of *ex vivo* adenovirus-mediated gene transfer to lung allografts in pigs [175]. An adenoviral vector encoding the β-galactosidase reporter was injected into the lumen of the upper lobe pulmonary artery of donor lung grafts, incubated for 2 h at 10° C, and then placed into recipients. Animals were sacrificed 3 days post transplant and β-galactosidase expression was determined histologically, with the lower left lobe serving as a control. Reporter transgene expression was detected in endothelial cells of the upper lobe and was also observed in airway and alveoli epithelial cells. Again, all categories of cells including ciliated, undifferentiated, and basal cells expressed β-galactosidase. However, it should be noted that less than 1% of the total cells actually expressed the transgene. Low level expression was attributed to short exposure to the vector, low temperature, and the low susceptibility of porcine cells to human adenovirus. Interestingly, even though the donor pulmonary vasculature was flushed prior to anastomosis, investigators were still able to detect adenoviral vector and β-galactosidase expression in other organs. Adenoviral DNA was detected in all of the organs tested including heart, liver, muscle, right lung, spleen, kidney, testis/ovaries; and mRNA transcripts were also detected in these organs, including the gonads. This finding questions the safety of viral vector mediated gene transfer, especially in the transplant setting where organ recipients are immunosuppressed.

Chapelier et al. suggested that the cold preservation conditions required to prevent ischemic injury to the graft probably also inhibited transfection efficiency [175]. This issue was directly addressed using *ex vivo* adenoviral mediated gene transfer to rat lung isografts under different conditions of cold preservation [33]. In this study, left lung isografts were flushed with a first generation adenoviral vector encoding β-galactosidase and then stored at either 4° or 10° C for 8 h prior to implantation into recipients. Animals were sacrificed 5 days after transplantation and both the left and right lungs removed for histologic evaluation with the native right lung serving as a control. Storage of lungs at 10° C showed significant transgene expression in all lung isografts, whereas storage at 4° C resulted in successful transgene expression in only half the grafts. Morphologically, transduced cells were primarily vascular endothelial cells with gene expression detected in pulmonary arterioles, capillaries and venules. Again, only approximately 1% of the total cells were transduced. Thus, it appears that adenoviral *ex vivo* gene transfer to lung grafts is feasible under cold preservation conditions, but not optimal. The authors did attribute other factors to the poor gene transfer efficiency including low viral load (given the large area of the pulmonary vasculature) and low viral viability in their adenovirus preparation.

Gene transfer to the pulmonary vasculature is still in the early stages of development and investigators are just now beginning to introduce biologically relevant molecules into lung allografts. However, early reports are providing results similar to those seen in cardiac allografts models. Mora et al. recently reported that rat lung allografts transduced with TGFβ improved gas exchange [176]. At present, the mechanism of how TGFβ improved lung function is unknown.

Kidney

Research on gene transfer into the kidney has been limited to studies of reporter gene expression. The most frequently employed vectors have been retrovirus and adenovirus; the advantages and limitations of these two vectors with respect to gene expression in the kidney are similar to those noted in other organ systems. However, several features of gene transfer specific to the kidney deserve mention. Gene transfer may be selectively targeted to particular renal cell types by altering the vector or route of administration. Glomerular cell targeting has been achieved utilizing retrovirus or liposomes, albeit with low efficiency [177]. Bosch et al. achieved selective distal tubular β-galactosidase expression using a retroviral vector injected directly into the kidney [178]; however, a nephrotoxic agent was required to induce tubular damage and regeneration, and expression was limited to the site of injection. For selective tubular expression, injection or perfusion of vector via the renal artery is limited to those vectors which can pass through the glomerular basement membrane [177]. While liposome or retroviral vectors are generally too large for this approach, adenoviral vectors have been successfully used to achieve selective β-galactosidase expression in the proximal tubules for 2 weeks [179]. Successful adenovirus-mediated gene transfer into the renal papilla and medulla has also been achieved by retrograde infusion into the urinary tract [177].

Several novel *ex vivo* systems have been developed to facilitate gene transfer in the kidney. Kitamura et al. have transfected cultured rat mesangial cells with the LacZ gene and subsequently transferred them via renal artery injection to the rat kidney [180]. The transferred mesangial cells, which are entrapped by the glomeruli, produced site-specific expression for 4 weeks; the duration of expression was doubled if transient mesangiolysis was induced by administration of an anti-mesangial cell monoclonal antibody. Two studies have used embryonic renal tissue as vehicles for gene transfer. Woolf et al. transplanted retrovirus-transduced mouse metanephros into the renal cortex of neonatal mouse kidneys, and demonstrated expression in glomerular epithelial cells and interstitial cells [181]. In contrast, Koseki et al., using a similar approach in a rat model, demonstrated expression primarily in tubular cells [182]. These findings further illustrate that species-specific, as well as organ-specific, differences may influence the efficacy of gene transfer approaches.

Ex vivo gene transfer has also been demonstrated in adult human kidneys. Ziegler et al. delivered an adenovirus-polylysine-DNA complex with a lacZ expression vector via the renal artery into three discarded cadaveric human kidneys [183]. After a 1-h cold incubation period, pulsatile perfusion using current clinical techniques allowed preservation of these kidneys for 60 h. Gene expression as demonstrated by X-gal staining, PCR, RT-PCR and *in situ* hybridization showed expression limited to the proximal tubular epithelium throughout the 60-h time period. These findings demonstrate that short-term gene transfer may be successful in procured human kidneys under standard preservation conditions.

Pancreatic islets

The limited success of clinical human islet allotransplantation in the treatment of type I diabetes is partly due to the fact that islets are subject both to allorejection and autoimmune destruction. Pancreatic islet and β-cell grafts, being a cellular transplant, are very appropriate targets for *ex vivo* gene therapy. The ideal β-cell replacement is both glucose responsive and able to elude allo- and autoimmune responses. Significant attention has been focused on the engineering of cells with low immunogenicity to replace β-cell function, and a number of gene therapy strategies have evolved to this end [184]. While immortalized pancreatic β-cell lines are less immunogenic than fresh intact islets, they lose glucose responsiveness with long-term culture; this problem has been circumvented by transfection of β-cell lines with the gene encoding the glucose transporter GLUT-2 [185]. Other transgene constructs have incorporated the use of a genetic switch to control growth of transplanted transformed β-cells [186, 187], and still others have utilized the transfection of genes encoding β-cell transcription factors into islet stem cells or pancreatic α-like cells in order to induce growth and differentiation into a β-cell phenotype [188, 189]. This raises the possibility of autotransplantation of engineered α- or islet stem cells to recreate β-cell function.

However, some investigators have focused on utilizing gene therapy techniques with the ultimate goal of rendering whole islet allografts less immunogenic. Reporter gene expression has been achieved in the islets of a number of species, including human, pig, and mouse [66, 190, 191]. Csete et al. established that adenoviral-mediated transfer of the lacZ gene to syngeneic murine islet grafts resulted in efficient short-term gene expression without impairing insulin secretion *in vitro* and without affecting the capacity of the graft to reverse diabetes *in vivo* [7]. These findings were subsequently duplicated and evidence of transgene expression at 38 days demonstrated [192]. Muruve et al., using a 10-fold higher multiplicity of infection, achieved β-galactosidase expression for 20 weeks, and demonstrated reduced neutralizing antibody activity in sera from islet recipients compared with mice injected intravenously with the same vector [2]. These findings provide further evidence that adenoviral vector administered *ex vivo* into a cellular transplant may induce less of an adenovirus-specific immune response than vector administered systemically. In a similar experiment, DeMatteo et al. showed that adenovirus-infected syngeneic islets placed into the rat thymus abrogated the adenovirus-specific immune response, while direct intrathymic injection of adenovirus did not [53].

A number of investigators have utilized gene transfer methods to induce local immunosuppression of pancreatic islet allografts. Gainer et al. used a "gene gun" approach to directly transfect murine islets with a cDNA encoding CTLA4Ig. Recipients of these transduced grafts had a mean survival time of 67 days compared with 13 days for nontransduced grafts [76]. Chahine et al., using a direct plasmid-mediated gene transfer approach, transfected murine myoblasts with the gene encoding CTLA4Ig, reasoning that the more frequently dividing myoblasts would achieve greater gene expression than islets [50]. They then co-transplanted the transduced myoblasts with the islet allografts. Serum CTLA4Ig was demonstrated in half of these animals up to 60 days after transplantation. The addition of CTLA4Ig transduced myoblasts prolonged mean survival time from 11.0 to 31.7 days provided that the myoblasts were syngeneic with the recipient; CTLA4Ig-secreting myoblasts of the same strain as the islet donor conferred no survival benefit.

This same group cotransplanted syngeneic myoblasts expressing Fas ligand [CD95L] with pancreatic islet allografts under the kidney capsule and also achieved prolongation of graft survival [82]. Myoblasts transplanted into the contralateral kidney from the islet allograft did not confer similar protection, demonstrating that local immunosuppression is a critical feature of this model. Interestingly, both islet allografts transduced with the gene encoding FasL via an adenovirus-mediated approach and fetal murine pancreas allografts from CD95L-expressing transgenic donors have been shown to undergo either normal or even accelerated rejection [83, 85]. Furthermore, CD95L expression induces a granulocytic infiltration of both pancreas grafts and transgenic pancreata. The mechanism of CD95L-mediated immunosuppression by myoblast expression versus immunostimulation by pancreas expression remains to be established.

Human islets have also been successfully transduced with genes encoding immunosuppressive molecules. Benhamou et al. used an adenoviral vector to transduce the vIL-10 gene into human islets and demonstrated significant protein production that was proportional to the viral dose [66]. An *in vitro* alloreactivity assay showed normal allogeneic lymphocyte proliferation with low viral dose and low vIL-10 production, but diminished alloreactivity when viral dose was increased and vIL-10 production was higher. However, at these higher transduction and protein expression levels, glucose-stimulated insulin secretion was blunted.

Liver-directed gene therapy

A number of approaches for liver-directed gene therapy have been developed. The three major approaches are (1) *in vivo* administration of vectors with affinity for the liver; (2) *ex vivo* gene transfer to isolated hepatocytes, with subsequent hepatocyte transplantation; (3) *in situ* or *ex vivo* administration of gene transfer vector to a whole organ liver graft. Direct administration of adenoviral vector to the liver either intravenously or via the biliary tract results in high efficiency transduction and expression of reporter genes by hepatocytes [25, 29, 30]. While attractive as a clinical model because of its simplicity and minimal morbidity, this model is limited by the transient nature of gene expression, as previously discussed. Retroviral vectors require hepatocyte division, a condition only satisfied by partial liver resection or administration of hepatotoxins. However, newer methods of gene transduction being developed may circumvent this requirement and thus may eliminate the need for hepatocyte transplantation in hepatic single-gene-defect metabolic deficiencies. Bosch et al. pretreated mice with keratinocyte growth factor prior to retroviral-mediated LacZ gene transfer and achieved a 40-fold increase in hepatocyte proliferation compared with nontreated animals [193]. This stimulation of proliferation resulted in a 600-fold increase in β-galactosidase expression, with 2% of hepatocytes transduced.

Hepatocytes

Theoretical advantages of allogeneic hepatocyte transplantation in liver-directed gene therapy compared with whole organ transplantation include lower surgical morbidity, the ability for *ex vivo* gene transfer at high efficiency with positive selection of transduced cells, and the potential for easy replenishment of hepatocyte function through the use of multiple donors or cryopreserved cells from the same donor. Disadvantages include a limit to the number of cells which may be transplanted into the portal system (the preferred site), the limited functional lifespan of isolated hepatocytes, and the limited survival of transplanted allogeneic hepatocytes due to rejection [23, 194].

For the latter reason, gene therapy in hepatocyte transplantation has been focused on autotransplantation for treatment of single-gene-defect metabolic deficiencies such as hemophilia B, ornithine transcarbamylase deficiency, Crigler-Najjar syndrome, and hereditary tyrosinemia [195-199]. However, a number of observations relevant to the development of gene therapy in allogeneic hepatocyte transplantation have been made. In the Watanabe heritable hyperlipidemic (WHHL) rabbit, an authentic model of human familial hypercholesterolemia, retrovirus-mediated transfer of the gene encoding the LDL receptor into hepatocytes transplanted intrasplenically resulted in a significant decrease in serum cholesterol [200]. This was short-lived in allogeneic hepatocytes but persisted for over 4 months in recipients of autologous hepatocytes. Preliminary results in human patients with FH show similar potential [201].

Few investigators have attempted to transduce genes encoding immunosuppressive molecules into allogeneic hepatocytes for the purposes of prolonging graft survival. Fabrega et al. used cationic lipid-mediated gene transfer to express hIL-10 in cultured Brown Norway rat hepatocytes for 14 days [202]. They then allotransplanted these hepatocytes into Nagasa analbuminemic rats and achieved a significant increase in serum albumin levels compared with nontransduced hepatocytes. Allograft survival as determined by albumin expression above baseline persisted for 40 days compared with 10 days in control animals. Although direct levels of hIL-10 production were not assayed, serum hIL-10 levels were undetectable, suggesting that local expression of hIL-10 was responsible for the prolonged graft survival.

Liver

Gene transfer techniques may also be applied to whole-organ liver grafts prior to recipient implantation. Shiraishi et al. perfused syngeneic rat liver grafts *in situ* with replication-defective adenoviral vectors encoding the LacZ gene driven by the human CMV promoter [203]. Viral DNA was demonstrated by PCR of graft DNA up to postoperative day 14, and β-galactosidase protein production was noted up to 7 days postoperatively whether the vectors were perfused into the hepatic artery or portal vein. Increased reporter expression was present when vectors were perfused into the hepatic artery compared with portal vein infusion.

Shaked and coworkers demonstrated efficient adenovirus-mediated transfer of LacZ in both cold-preserved rat hepatocytes and in syngeneic liver grafts following *ex vivo* portal vein infusion under hypothermic preservation conditions [15, 18]. Gene expression; as demonstrated by X-Gal staining, PCR, and RT-PCR; persisted for greater than 2 weeks. Drazan et al. utilized a similar model to transfer the genes encoding TGFβ1 and vIL-10 into ACI-to-Lewis rat liver allografts [8, 60]. Although graft survival was not assessed, transgene DNA, mRNA and protein were demonstrated throughout the 5–7 days of the experiment, and a decrease in intragraft cytokine levels of TNFα and IFNγ provided further evidence of TGFβ1 expression. This same group also achieved prolonged survival > 80 days in 5 of 6 ACI-to-Lewis liver allografts by adenovirus-mediated transfer of the gene encoding CTLA4Ig into the grafts [204]. Immunosuppression was not strictly local since systemic levels of CTLA4Ig were achieved. In this model, intragraft cytokine levels of TNFα and IFNγ diminished over time relative to controls, and the mononuclear graft infiltrate was delayed, less intense and associated with less parenchymal damage. The persistence of this infiltrate beyond 40 days despite graft function was suggestive of T-cell anergy.

A second method to diminish alloreactivity to liver grafts is that of tolerance induction by transduction of donor-specific genes to the thymus. Knechtle et al. have successfully transduced ACI donor MHC Class I antigen cDNA both directly into recipient thymus and into Lewis recipient myoblasts and myotubules which were then injected into recipient thymus [57, 58]. In both models the presence of the transduced DNA and/or the expression of MHC alloantigen gene product was demonstrated. Long-term survival of ACI-to-Lewis hepatic allografts was achieved in both models and donor-specific tolerance was demonstrated in the myoblast model. This tolerance appears to involve a combination of clonal deletion and suppressor type T-cell generation, which is consistent with other models of intrathymic tolerance.

Bone marrow

Hematopoietic progenitor cells are logical targets for gene transfer in that they are cellular transplants that are readily obtained and returnable to the host following manipulation. Transfer to a pluripotent stem cell could in principle allow indefinite repopulation of an individual, with a wide array of modified cells distributed throughout the body [205]. Vectors which integrate into genomic DNA, i.e. retroviral vectors, currently are required to take advantage of this longevity.

Gene marking permits the identification of the origin of cells following autologous bone marrow transplantation [41, 42, 205–208]. Both bone marrow and stem cell preparations have been marked by retroviral-mediated transfer of the *neo* gene at efficiencies sufficient to allow their use as a clinical graft. This allows for both the selection of transduced cells and for subsequent identification of graft-derived cells. Such information is critical for the evaluation of marrow purging techniques, and for analysis of engraftment and subsequent marrow regeneration [41, 205–207, 209–211]. Other investigators have achieved local production of TNFα for anti-leukemic effects and GM-CSF for neutrophil recovery following chemotherapy, thereby avoiding the systemic effects of these cytokines [211, 212]. Genes conferring resistance to methotrexate and trimetrexate have also been successfully transferred into bone marrow, providing the potential for *in vivo* selection of donor cells and more effective chemotherapeutic options following allogeneic or autologous bone marrow transplantation [213, 214].

A novel approach to the control of the allogeneic graft-versus-leukemia response has been developed utilizing gene transfer. Bonini et al. treated eight patients with relapse or EBV-induced lymphoma after T-cell depleted bone marrow transplantation with immunocompetent, nondepleted donor lymphocytes retrovirally transduced with the Herpes simplex thymidine kinase suicide gene [215]. Such therapy produced antitumor activity in five patients, with lymphocyte survival of up to 12 months. Three patients developed significant graft-versus-host disease as a result of the treatment, which was abrogated by ganciclovir-induced elimination of the transduced cells in all cases. Such an approach may be an attractive alternative to T-cell depletion in allogeneic bone marrow transplantation by restoration of the graft-versus-leukemia effect while providing an effective treatment for potential graft-versus-host disease.

Another strategy utilizes the infusion of autologous bone marrow transfected with genes encoding donor-type MHC molecules prior to organ transplantation. Sykes et al. used retroviral transduction of allogeneic class I MHC into syngeneic murine bone marrow cells to demonstrate prolonged survival of skin grafts expressing the introduced MHC antigen [44]. Gene transfer was demonstrated in 29 of 30 spleen colonies at day 14 following bone marrow transplantation, and was detectable in bone marrow cells and/or thymocytes in 3 of 6 animals tested at 12 to 24 weeks post-transplantation. Skin graft survival was prolonged from 28 to 131 days, and was specific for the transduced MHC antigen. Specific cytolytic T cell precursors persisted in these animals despite a hyporesponsive state. This finding, combined with the observation that skin grafts bearing the transduced MHC antigen were rejected if a fully disparate third-party skin graft was placed simultaneously, suggested that the hyporesponsive state may be a result of deficient T cell help [216].

Emery et al. transferred allogeneic MHC class II DRβ cDNA into swine bone marrow and demonstrated expression of the transgene in both long-term cultures and in the peripheral blood of irradiated swine up to 5 months after transplantation [45–47]. In transplanted animals, the transgene was expressed in several lineages including T lymphocytes and monocytes, and allogeneic RNA transcripts were detected at 5–10% of the level of endogenous DRβ message in peripheral blood. This same group used retroviral-transduced MHC class II DRβ cDNA into umbilical cord blood, with similar *in vitro* transgene expression [47]. This approach was utilized in a miniature swine renal allograft model [217]. Although the donor-recipient pair was fully mismatched at the class I locus, treatment with syngeneic bone marrow transduced with donor class II cDNA conferred long-term allograft survival. Swine MHC class II genes have also been transduced into $CD34^+$ cynomolgus monkey cells, with subsequent expression of the transgene 12 weeks after transplantation [218, 219]. This approach may be effective for tolerance induction toward xenogeneic organ transplants.

Myoblast

Myoblast-mediated gene therapy or transplantation of cultured, genetically engineered myoblasts into mature skeletal muscle, provides a therapeutic entry for correcting diseases of skeletal muscle and other tissues. Primary skeletal myoblasts can be stably infected or transfected with retroviral or plasmid vectors *in vitro*. Implanted myoblasts can fuse with existing myofibers of the host and form hybrid myofibers that contribute to the syncytium a normal gene product missing from the host [220–222]. This principle has been successfully applied to muscular dystrophies in mice [220, 223–224] and human [226]. Implanted myoblasts can also persist as muscle precursor or myogenic reserve cells that contribute to host muscle regeneration when myofibers are damaged, providing a mechanism to maintain persistent expression of transgenes [223].

Experiments on the mdx mouse, which is the genetic homologue of Duchenne muscular dystrophy, have suggested two possible therapeutic approaches for these myopathies. In one, implantation of normal muscle precursor cells into mdx skeletal muscle leads to the conversion of dystrophin-negative fibres to dystrophin-positive, with consequent improvement in muscle histology. However, implanted muscle precursor cells were rapidly rejected by non-tolerant hosts, even when the host and donor are compatible for major but not minor histocompatibility antigens [223, 224]. The alternative approach is direct injection of dystrophin cDNA into skeletal or cardiac muscle which also gives rise to dystrophin-positive fibers, although the efficiency of this gene transfer is extremely low [223, 224]. One way to circumvent this problem is to implant mpc of host origin, containing multiple copies of the dystrophin gene [220, 223, 224]. Although such myoblast-mediated gene therapy appears promising, there are a number of questions to be answered and refinements to be made before the technique could be considered as possible treatment for myopathies in man.

In addition to the treatment of intrinsic muscle diseases, genetically modified myoblast transplantation has been used for the treatment of non-muscle diseases in murine models. Primary myoblast-mediated gene transfer achieves long-term expression of human factor IX at therapeutic levels to correct hemophilia B [149, 226–229]; production of growth hormone in growth hormone-deficient Snell dwarf mice [17, 230, 231]; and sustained delivery of functionally active erythropoietin to correct anemia associated with end-stage renal failure in mice [233, 234]. In terms of transplantation applications, CTLA4Ig secreted by a myoblast cell line can prolong pancreatic islet allograft survival in a cotransplantation model [50]. Genetically modified myoblast transplantation has also found potential application in diabetes mellitus [235], lysosomal enzyme deficiency [236, 237], and Parkinson's disease [238].

Most of the current myoblast-mediated gene therapy models used genetic modification of autologous cells or transplantation into SCID recipients to circumvent alloimmunity. An alternate approach is the implantation of a genetically modified "universal" cell line to deliver desired gene products to nonautologous recipients [149, 232]. Hortelano et al. implanted mouse myoblasts secreting human factor IX into allogeneic mice and demonstrated long-term expression of human factor IX

[149]. Al-Hendy et al. implanted allogeneic myoblasts engineered to secrete mouse growth hormone into the growth hormone-deficient Snell dwarf mice; the treatment enhanced growth of these dwarf mice by a variety of physiological parameters [232]. The same cell line could be used to treat different patients with the same gene deficiency regardless of the recipient's histocompatibility tissue type. To avoid allograft rejection, the implanted cells were enclosed in alginate-polylysine-alginate microcapsules that function as an immunologic barrier permeable to low molecular weight transgene products (< 150 kD), but impermeable to high molecular weight immune mediators [51, 149, 232]. The encapsulated cells remained functional for at least 6 months. This simple method of delivery of recombinant gene products *in vivo* could have wide application to therapies requiring a continuous systemic supply of recombinant gene products.

Summary

Although the application of gene therapy to transplantation is a relatively recent development, a substantial body of knowledge has accrued defining optimal conditions for gene transfer and expression in specific organs and cell types with respect to type of vehicle, dosing, route of vector administration, toxicity, promoter specificity etc. In addition, the development of methods of efficient gene transfer into either whole organ or cellular transplants has been achieved utilizing protocols that closely mimic current clinical practice. Thus the scenario of organ-specific, local immunosuppression directed by gene therapy vectors has become a reasonable and attractive possibility for clinical transplantation. The current major limitations of gene therapy approaches in transplantation, as in other applications, continue to be the lack of transgene persistence and immune responses to both vector and transgene product. While strategies to circumvent these problems are being developed as actively in transplant research as in other fields, tolerance induction, which may only require short-term immunosuppression, may not be adversely affected by these limitations. Hence, approaches not well suited for gene therapy elsewhere may be perfectly appropriate or even advantageous for transplantation. Gene therapy in transplantation is currently targeted toward modulating the expression and function of cytokines, adhesion molecules, and effector cells, as in other inflammatory conditions, or it may be targeted directly at MHC disparities between donor and recipient. However, as new biologically important molecules in the alloimmune response are identified and characterized, many are potentially immunomodulatory transgene products, and gene transfer approaches utilizing these molecules can be anticipated. Rapid advances in gene therapy methodology are occurring in parallel with an increased understanding of transplant immunology and the rejection response. The convergence of these two areas holds considerable potential for therapies of benefit to the clinical transplant patient.

References

1 Bromberg JS (1997) Transplant immunology. In: *Surgery scientific principles and practice*. 2nd ed. Lippincott-Raven, Philadelphia, PA, 527–555

2 Muruve DA, Manfro RC, Strom TB, Libermann TA (1997) *Ex vivo* adenovirus-mediated gene delivery leads to long-term expression in pancreatic islet transplants. *Transplantation* 64: 542–546

3 Qin L, Ding Y, Pahud DR, Robson ND, Shaked A, Bromberg JS (1997) Adenovirus-mediated gene transfer of viral interleukin-10 inhibits the immune response to both alloantigen and adenoviral antigen. *Hum Gene Ther* 8: 1365–1374

4 Gruber SA (1996) *Local immunosuppression of organ transplants*. RG Landes Company and Chapman & Hall, Austin, TX

5 Bromberg JS, Qin L (1996) Gene transfer to the transplanted organ. In: *Local immunosuppression of organ transplants*. RG Landes Company and Chapman & Hall, Austin, TX, 169–180

6 Shaked A, Csete ME, Shiraishi M, Miller AR, Moen RM, Busuttil RW, Economou JS (1994). Retroviral-mediated gene transfer into rat experimental liver transplant. *Transplantation* 57: 32–34

7 Csete ME, Benhamou PY, Drazan KE, Wu L, McIntee DF, Afra R, Mullen Y, Busuttil RW, Shaked A (1995) Efficient gene transfer to pancreatic islets mediated by adenoviral vectors. *Transplantation* 59: 263–268

8 Drazan KE, Wu L, Olthoff KM, Jurim O, Busuttil RW, Shaked A (1995) Transduction of hepatic allografts achieves local levels of viral IL-10 which suppress alloreactivity *in vitro*. *J Surg Res* 59: 219–223

9 Nabel EG, Plautz G, Nabel GJ (1990) Site-specific gene expression *in vivo* by direct gene transfer into the arterial wall. *Science* 249: 1285–1288

10 Mehra MR, Stapleton DD, Cook JL, Zhang T, Ventura HO, Huang C, Maldonado B, Smart FW, Ré RN, Murgo JP, Barbee RW (1996) Adenovirus-mediated *in vivo* gene transfer in a rabbit model of allograft vasculopathy. *J Heart Lung Transplant* 15: 51–57

11 Hullett DA (1996) Gene therapy in transplantation. *J Heart Lung Transplant* 15: 857–862

12 Knechtle SJ (1996) Gene therapy and transplantation – A brief review. *Transplant Proc* 28: 19–23

13 Wang J, Jiao S, Wolff JA, Knechtle SJ (1992) Gene transfer and expression in rat cardiac transplants. *Transplantation* 53: 703–705

14 Wang J, Ma Y, Knechtle SJ (1996) Adenovirus-mediated gene transfer into rat allografts. *Transplantation* 61: 1726–1729

15 Csete ME, Drazan KE, Van Bree M, McIntee DF, McBride WH, Bett A, Graham FL, Busuttil RW, Berk AJ, Shakad A (1994) Adenovirus-mediated gene transfer in the transplant setting. *Transplantation* 57: 1502–1507

16 Donahue JK, Kikkawa K, Johns DC, Marban E, Lawrence JH (1997) Ultrarapid, highly efficient viral gene transfer to the heart. *Proc Natl Acad Sci USA* 94: 4664–4668

17 Barr E, Leiden JM (1991) Systemic delivery of recombinant proteins by genetically modified myoblasts. *Science* 254: 1507–1509

18 Shaked A, Csete ME, Drazan KE, Bullington D, Wu L, Busuttil RW, Berk AJ (1994) Adenovirus-mediated gene transfer in the transplant setting. *Transplantation* 57: 1508–1511

19 Drazan KE, Wu L, Shen X, Bullington D, Jurim O, Busuttil RW, Shaked A (1995) Adenovirus-mediated gene transfer in the transplant setting. *Transplantation* 59: 670–673

20 Lieber A, Vrancken Peeters MTFD, Meuse L, Fausto N, Perkins J, Kay MA (1995) Adenovirus-mediated urokinase gene transfer induces liver regeneration and allows for efficient retrovirus transduction of hepatocytes *in vivo*. *Proc Natl Acad Sci USA* 92: 6210–6214

21 Lieber A, Vrancken Peeters MTFD, Gown A, Perkins J, Kay MA (1995) A modified urokinase plasminogen activator induces liver regeneration without bleeding. *Hum Gene Ther* 6: 1029–1037

22 Bosch A, McCray Jr., Chang SMW, Ulich TR, Simonet WS, Jolly DJ, Davidson BL (1996) Proliferation induced by keratinocyte growth factor enhances *in vivo* retroviral-mediated gene transfer to mouse hepatocytes. *J Clin Invest* 98: 2683–2687

23 Raper SE (1995) Hepatocyte transplantation and gene therapy. *Clin Transplantation* 9: 249–254

24 Halbert CL, Standaert TA, Aitken ML, Alexander IE, Russell DW, Miller D (1997) Transduction by adeno-associated virus vectors in the rabbit airway: efficiency, persistence, and readministration. *J Virology* 71: 5932–5941

25 Yang Y, Nunes FA, Berencsi K, Furth EE, Gönczöl E, Wilson JM (1994) Cellular immunity to viral antigens limits E1-deleted adenoviruses for gene therapy. *Proc Natl Acad Sci USA* 91: 4407–4411

26 Riddell SR, Elliott M, Lewinsohn DA, Gilbert MJ, Wilson L, Manley SA, Lupton SD, Overell RW, Reynolds TC, Corey L, Greenberg P (1996) T-cell mediated rejection of gene-modified HIV-specific cytotoxic T lymphocytes in HIV-infected patients. *Nature Med* 2: 216–223

27 Tripathy SK, Black HB, Goldwasser E, Leiden JM (1996) Immune responses to transgene-encoded proteins limit the stability of gene expression after injection of replication-defective adenovirus vectors. *Nature Med* 2: 545–550

28 Kay MA, Meuse L, Gown AM, Linsley P, Hollenbaugh D, Aruffo A, Ochs HD, Wilson CB (1997) Transient immunomodulation with anti-CD40 ligand antibody and CTLA4Ig enhances persistence and secondary adenovirus-mediated gene transfer into mouse liver. *Proc Natl Acad Sci USA* 94: 4686–4691

29 Kay MA, Holterman A, Meuse L, Gown A, Ochs HD, Linsley PS, Wilson CB (1995) Long-term hepatic adenovirus-mediated gene expression in mice following CTLA4Ig administration. *Nature Genetics* 11: 191–197

30 DeMatteo RP, Markmann KF, Kozarsky KF, Barker CF, Raper SE (1996) Prolongation of adenoviral transgene expression in mouse liver by lymphocyte subset depletion. *Gene Therapy* 3: 4–12

31 Lochmüller H, Petrof BJ, Allen C, Prescott AS, Massie B, Karpati G (1995) Immuno-

suppression by FK506 markedly prolongs expression of adenovirus-delivered transgene in skeletal muscles of adult dystrophic [mdx] mice. *Biochem Biophys Res Comm* 213: 569–574

32 Vemuru RP, Davidson A, Aragona E, Chowdhury JR, Burk RD, Gupta S (1992) Immune tolerance to a defined heterologous antigen after intrasplenic hepatocyte transplantation: implications for gene therapy. *FASEB J* 6: 2836–2842

33 Boasquevisque CHR, Mora BN, Schmid RA, Lee TC, Nagahiro I, Cooper JD, Patterson GA (1997) *Ex vivo* adenoviral-mediated gene transfer to lung isografts during cold preservation. *Ann Thorac Surg* 63: 1556–1561

34 Colson YL, Lange J, Fowler K, Ildstad ST (1996) Mechanism for cotolerance in nonlethally conditioned mixed chimeras: negative selection of the V beta T-cell receptor repertoire by both host and donor bone marrow-derived cells. *Blood* 88: 4601–4610

35 Delaney CP, Murase N, Chen-Woan M, Fung JJ, Starzl TE, Demetris AJ (1996) Allogeneic hematolymphoid microchimerism and prevention of autoimmune disease in the rat. A relationship between allo- and autoimmunity. *J Clin Invest* 97: 217–225

36 Garcia-Morales R, Carreno M, Mathew J, Zucker K, Cirocco R, Ciancio G, Burke G, Roth D, Temple D, Rosen A et al (1997) The effects of chimeric cells following donor bone marrow infusions as detected by PCR-flow assays in kidney transplant recipients. *J Clin Invest* 99: 1118–1129

37 Eglitis MA, Kantoff P, Gilboa E, Anderson WF (1985) Gene expression in mice after high efficiency retroviral-mediated gene transfer. *Science* 230: 1395–1398

38 Keller G, Paige C, Gilboa E, Wagner EF (1985). Expression of a foreign gene in myeloid and lymphoid cells derived from multipotent haematopoietic precursors. *Nature* 318: 149–154

39 Snodgrass R, Keller G (1987) Clonal fluctuation within the haematopoietic system of mice reconstituted with retrovirus-infected stem cells. *EMBO J* 6: 3955–3960

40 Bowtell DDL, Johnson GR, Kelso A, Cory S (1987) Expression of genes transferred to hemopoietic stem cells by recombinant retroviruses. *Mol Biol Med* 4: 229–250

41 Chen BP, Fraser C, Reading C, Murray L, Uchida N, Galy A, Sasaki D, Tricot G, Jagannath S, Barlogie B et al (1995) Cytokine-mobilized peripheral blood $CD34^{+}Thy\text{-}1^{+}Lin^{-}$ human hematopoietic stem cells as target cells for transplantation-based gene therapy. *Leukemia* 9: S17–S25

42 Dunbar CE, Cottler-Fox M, O'Shaughnessy JA, Doren S, Carter C, Bereson R, Brown S, Moen RC, Greenblatt J, Stewart FM et al (1995) Retrovirally marked CD34-enriched peripheral blood and bone marrow cells contribute to long-term engraftment after autologous transplantation. *Blood* 85: 3048–3057

43 Madsen JC, Superina RA, Wood KJ, Morris PJ (1988) Immunological unresponsiveness induced by recipient cells transfected with donor MHC genes. *Nature* 332: 161–164

44 Sykes M, Sachs DH, Nienhuis AW, Pearson DA, Moulton AD, Bodine DM (1993) Specific prolongation of skin graft survival following retroviral transduction of bone marrow with an allogeneic major histocompatibility complex gene. *Transplantation* 55: 197–202

45 Emery DW, Smith CV, Shafer GE, Karson EM, Sachs DH, LeGuern C (1993) Expression of allogeneic class II cDNA in swine peripheral blood mononuclear cells following retroviral-mediated gene transfer into bone marrow. *Transplant Proc* 25: 140–141

46 Emery DW, Shafer GE, Karson EM, Sachs DH, LeGuern C (1993) Retrovirus-mediated transfer and expression of an allogeneic major histocompatibility complex class II DRB cDNA in swine bone marrow cultures. *Blood* 81: 2460–2465

47 Emery DW, Sablinski T, Arn JS, LeGuern C, Sachs DH (1994) Bone marrow culture and transduction of stem cells in a miniature swine model. *Blood Cells* 20: 498–503

48 LeGuern C, Shimada H, Emery DW, Germana S, Shafer GE, Sachs DH (1995) Retrovirus-mediated transfer of MHC class II cDNA into swine bone marrow cells. *J Mol Med* 73: 269–278

49 Fraser CC, Sykes M, Stanton Lee R, Sachs DH, LeGuern C (1995) Specific unresponsiveness to a retrovirally-transferred class I antigen is controlled through the helper pathway. *J Immunol* 154: 1587–1595

50 Chahine AA, Yu M, McKernan MM, Stoeckert C, Lau HT (1995) Immunomodulation of pancreatic islet allografts in mice with CTLA4Ig secreting muscle cells. *Transplantation* 59: 1313–1318

51 Carr-Brendel VE, Geller RL, Thomas TJ, Boggs DR, Young SK, Crudele J, Martinson LA, Maryanov DA, Johnson RC, Brauker JH (1997) Transplantation of cells in an immunoisolation device for gene therapy. *Methods Mol Biol* 63: 373–387

52 Ilan Y, Prakash R, Davidson A, Jona V, Droguett G, Horwitz MS, Chowdhury NR, Chowdhury JR (1997) Oral tolerization to adenoviral antigens permits long-term gene expression using recombinant adenoviral vectors. *J Clin Invest* 99: 1098–1106

53 DeMatteo RP, Raper SE, Ahn M, Fisher KJ, Burke C, Radu A, Wider G, Claytor BR, Barker CF, Markmann JF (1995) Gene transfer to the thymus a means of abrogating the immune response to recombinant adenovirus. *Annals Surgery* 222: 229–242

54 Ilan Y, Attavar P, Takahashi M, Davidson A, Horwitz MS, Guida J, Chowdhury NR, Chowdhury JR (1996) Induction of central tolerance by intrathymic inoculation of adenoviral antigens into the host thymus permits long-term gene therapy in Gunn rats. *J Clin Invest* 98: 2640–2647

55 Nakano N, Rooke R, Benoist C, Mathis D (1997) Positive selection of T cells induced by viral delivery of neopeptides to the thymus. *Science* 275: 678–683

56 DeMatteo RP, Chu G, Ahn M, Chang E, Barker CF, Markmann JF (1997) Long-lasting adenovirus transgene expression in mice through neonatal intrathymic tolerance induction without the use of immunosuppression. *J Virol* 71: 5330–5335

57 Knechtle SJ, Wang J, Jiao S, Geissler EK, Sumimoto R, Wolff J (1994) Induction of specific tolerance by intrathymic injection of recipient muscle cells transfected with donor class I major histocompatibility complex. *Transplantation* 57: 990–996

58 Knechtle SJ, Wang J, Graeb C, Zhai Y, Hong X, Fechner Jr. Geissler EK (1997) Direct MHC class I complementary DNA transfer to thymus induces donor-specific unresponsiveness, which involves multiple immunologic mechanisms. *J Immunol* 159: 152–158

59 Knechtle SJ, Zhai Y, Fechner J.(1996) Gene therapy in transplantation. *Transplant Immunology* 4: 257–264
60 Drazan KE, Olthoff KM, Wu L, Shen X, Gelman A, Shaked A (1996) Adenovirus-mediated gene transfer in the transplant setting. *Transplantation* 62: 1080–1084
61 Qin L, Ding Y, Bromberg JS (1996) Gene transfer of transforming growth factor-β1 prolongs murine cardiac allograft survival by inhibiting cell mediated immunity. *Hum Gene Ther* 7: 1981–1988
62 Qin L, Chavin KD, Ding Y, Favarro JP, Woodward JE, Lin J, Tahara H, Robbins P, Shaked A et al (1995) Multiple vectors effectively achieve gene transfer in a murine cardiac transplantation model: immunosuppression with TGF-β1 or vIL-10. *Transplantation* 59: 809–816
63 Levy AE, Alexander JW (1995) Administration of intragraft interleukin-4 prolongs cardiac allograft survival in rats treated with donor-specific transfusion/cyclosporine. *Transplantation* 60: 405–406
64 Mueller R, Krahl T, Sarvetnick N (1996) Pancreatic expression of interleukin-4 abrogates insulitis and autoimmune diabetes in nonobese diabetic (NOD) mice. *J Exp Med* 184: 1093–1099
65 Sarvetnick N (1996) Mechanisms of cytokine-mediated localized immunoprotection. *J Exp Med* 184: 1597–1600
66 Benhamou PY, Mullen Y, Shaked A, Bahmiller D, Csete ME (1996) Decreased alloreactivity to human islets secreting recombinant viral interleukin 10. *Transplantation* 62: 1306–1312
67 Qin L, Chavin KD, Tahara H, Ding Y, Favarro J, Woodward J, Lin J, Robbins PD, Lotze MT, Bromberg JS (1996) Retrovirus-mediated transfer of viral interleukin-10 gene prolongs murine cardiac allograft survival. *J Immunol* 156: 2316–2323
68 Kolls J, Peppel K, Silva M, Beutler B (1994) Prolonged and effective blockade of tumor necrosis factor activity through adenovirus-mediated gene transfer. *Proc Natl Acad Sci USA* 91: 215–219
69 Rogy MA, Auffenberg T, Espat NJ, Philip R, Remick D, Wollenberg GK, Copeland III EM, Moldawer L (1995) Human tumor necrosis factor receptor (p55) and interleukin 10 gene transfer in the mouse reduces mortality to lethal endotoxemia and also attenuates local inflammatory responses. *J Exp Med* 181: 2289–2293
70 Grewal IS, Grewal KD, Wong FS, Picarells DE, Janeway Jr, Flavell RA (1996) Local expression of transgene encoded TNFα in islets prevents autoimmune diabetes in nonobese diabetic (NOD) mice by preventing the development of auto-reactive islet-specific T cells. *J Exp Med* 184: 1963–1974
71 Tufariello J, Cho S, Horwitz MS (1994) The adenovirus E3 14.7-kilodalton protein which inhibits cytolysis by tumor necrosis factor increases the virulence of vaccinia virus in a murine pneumonia model. *J Virol* 68: 453–462
72 Tufariello J, Cho S, Horwitz MS (1994) Adenovirus E3 14.7-kilodalton protein, an antagonist of tumor necrosis factor cytolysis, increases the virulence of vaccinia virus in severe combined immunodeficient mice. *Proc Natl Acad Sci USA* 91: 10987–10991

73 Li Y, Kang J, Horwitz MS (1997) Interaction of an adenovirus 14.7-kilodalton protein inhibitor of tumor necrosis factor alpha cytolysis with a new member of the GTPase superfamily of signal transducers. *J Virol* 71: 1576–1582
74 Efrat S, Fejer G, Brownlee M, Horwitz MS (1995) Prolonged survival of pancreatic islet allografts mediated by adenovirus immunoregulatory transgenes. *Proc Natl Acad Sci USA* 92: 6947–6951
75 Ilan Y, Droguett G, Chowdhury NR, Li Y, Sengupta K, Thummala NR, Davidson A, Chowdhury JR, Horwitz MS (1997) Insertion of the adenoviral E3 region into a recombinant viral vector prevents antiviral humoral and cellular immune responses and permits long-term gene expression. *Proc Natl Acad Sci USA* 94: 2587–2592
76 Gainer AL, Korbutt GS, Rajotte RV, Warnock GL, Elliott JF (1994) Expression of CTLA4-Ig by biolistically transfected mouse islets promotes islet allograft survival. *Transplantation* 63: 1017–1044
77 Kato K, Shimozato O, Hoshi K, Wakimoto H, Hamada H, Yagita H, Okumura K (1996) Local production of the p40 subunit of interleukin 12 suppresses T-helper 1-mediated immune responses and prevents myoblast rejection. *Proc Natl Acad Sci USA* 93: 9085–9089
78 Chen S, Wilson JM, Vallance DK, Hartman JW, Davidson BL, Roessler BJ (1995) A recombinant adenoviral vector expressing a soluble form of VCAM-1 inhibits VCAM-1/VLA-4 adhesion in transduced synoviocytes. *Gene Therapy* 2: 469–480
79 Grunhaus A, Cho S, Horwitz MS (1994) Association of vaccinia virus-expressed adenovirus E3-19K glycoprotein with Class I MHC and its effects on virulence in a murine pneumonia model. *Virology* 200: 535–546
80 Bellgrau D (1995) A role for CD95 ligand in preventing graft rejection. *Nature* 377: 630–632
81 Griffith TS, Brunner T, Fletcher SM, Green DR, Ferguson TA (1995) Fas ligand-induced apoptosis as a mechanism of immune privilege. *Science* 270: 1189–1192
82 Lau HT, Yu M, Fontana A, Stoeckert CJ (1996) Prevention of islet allograft rejection with engineered myoblasts expressing FasL in mice. *Science* 273: 109–112
83 Kang S (1997) Fas ligand expression in islets of langerhans does not confer immune privilege and instead targets them for rapid destruction. *Nature Med* 3: 738–743
84 Chervonsky AV (1997) The role of Fas in autoimmune diabetes. *Cell* 89: 17–24
85 Allison J, Georgiou HM, Strasser A, Vaux DL (1997) Transgenic expression of CD95 ligand on islet beta cells induces a granulocytic infiltrate but does not confer immune privilege upon islet allograft. *Proc Natl Acad Sci USA* 94: 3943–3947
86 Seino K, Kayagaki N, Okumura K, Yagita H (1997) Antitumor effect of locally produced CD95 ligand. *Nature Med* 3: 165–170
87 Simons M, Edelman ER, DeKeyser J, Langer R, Rosenberg RD (1992) Antisense c-myb oligonucleotides inhibit intimal arterial smooth muscle cell accumulation *in vivo*. *Nature* 359: 67–70
88 Morishita R, Gibbons GH, Ellison KE, Nakajima M, Zhang L, Kaneda K, Ogihara T, Dzau V (1993) Single intraluminal delivery of antisense cdc2 kinase and proliferating-

cell nuclear antigen oligonucleotides results in chronic inhibition of neointimal hyperplasia. *Proc Natl Acad Sci USA* 90: 8474–8478
89 Ohno T, Gordon D, San H, Pompili VJ, Imperiale MJ, Nabel GJ, Nabel EG (1994) Gene therapy for vascular smooth muscle cell proliferation after arterial injury. *Science* 265: 781–784
90 Chang MW, Barr E, Seltzer J, Jiang Y, Nabel GJ, Nabel EG, Parmacek MS, Leiden JM (1995) Cytostatic gene therapy for vascular proliferative disorders with a constitutively active form of the retinoblastoma gene product. *Science* 267: 518–522
91 Von Der Leyen HE, Gibbons GH, Morishita R, Lewis NP, Zhang L, Nakajima M, Kaneda Y, Cooke JP, Dzau V (1995) Gene therapy inhibiting neointimal vascular lesion: *In vivo* transfer of endothelial cell nitric oxide synthase gene. *Proc Natl Acad Sci USA* 92: 1137–1141
92 Mann MJ, Gibbons GH, Tsao PS, Von Der Leyen HE, Cooke JP, Buitrago R, Kernoff R, Dzau VJ (1997) Cell cycle inhibition preserves endothelial function in genetically engineered rabbit vein grafts. *J Clin Invest* 99: 1295–1301
93 Yang Y, Ertl HCJ, Wilson JM (1994) MHC class I restricted cytotoxic T lymphocytes to viral antigens destroy hepatocytes in mice infected with E1 deleted recombinant adenoviruses. *Immunity* 1: 433–442
94 Dai Y, Schwarz EM, Gu D, Zhang WW, Sarvetnick N, Verma IM (1995) Cellular and humoral immune responses to adenoviral vectors containing factor IX gene: Tolerization of factor IX and vector antigens allows for long-term expression. *Proc Natl Acad Sci USA* 92: 1401–1405
95 Doherty PC, Allen W, Eichelberger M, Carding SR (1992) Roles of αβ and γδ T cell subsets in viral immunity. *Annu Rev Immunol* 10: 123–151
96 Yang Y, Li Q, Ertl HCJ, Wilson JM (1995) Cellular and humoral immune responses to viral antigens create barriers to lung-directed gene therapy with recombinant adenoviruses. *J Virol* 69: 2004–2015
97 Yang Y, Su Q, Wilson JM (1996) Role of viral antigens in destructive cellular immune responses to adenovirus vector-transduced cells in mouse lungs. *J Virol* 70: 7209–7212
98 Yang Y, Trinchieri G, Wilson JM (1995) Recombinant IL-12 prevents formation of blocking IgA antibodies to recombinant adenovirus and allows repeated gene therapy to mouse lung. *Nature Med* 1: 890–893
99 Yang Y, Xiang Z, Etrl HCJ, Wilson JM (1995) Upregulation of class I MHC antigens by interferon-γ is necessary for the T cell mediated elimination of recombinant adenovirus infected hepatocytes *in vivo*. *Proc Natl Acad Sci USA* 92: 7257–7261
100 Acsadi G, Lochmuller H, Jani A, Huard J, Massie B, Prescott S, Simoneau M, Petrof BJ, Karpati G (1996) Dystrophin expression in muscles of mdx mice after adenovirus-mediated *in vivo* gene transfer. *Hum Gene Ther* 7: 129–140
101 Zsengeller Z, Wert S, Hull W, Hu X, Yei S, Trapnell B, Whitsett J (1995) Persistence of replication-deficient adenovirus-mediated gene transfer in lungs of immune-deficient (nu/nu) mice. *Hum Gene Ther* 6: 457–467
102 Pilewski JM, Scott DJ, Wilson JM, Albelda SM (1995) ICAM-1 expression on bronchial

epithelium after recombinant adenovirus infection. *Am J Respir Cell Mol Biol* 12: 142–148

103 Stark JM, Amin RS, Trapnell BC (1996) Infection of A549 cells with a recombinant adenovirus vector induces ICAM-1 expression and increased CD-18-dependent adhesion of activated neutrophils. *Hum Gene Ther* 7: 1669–1681

104 Amin R, Wilmott R, Schwarz Y, Trapnell B, Stark J (1995) Replication-deficient adenovirus induces expression of interleukin-8 by airway epithelial cells *in vitro*. *Hum Gene Ther* 6: 145–153

105 Worgall S, Wolff G, Falck-Pedersen E, Crystal RG (1997) Innate immune mechanisms dominate elimination of adenoviral vectors following *in vivo* administration. *Hum Gene Ther* 8: 37–44

106 Yei S, Mittereder N, Wert S, Whitsett JA, Wilmott RW, Trapnell BC (1994) *In vivo* evaluation of the safety of adenovirus-mediated transfer of the human cystic fibrosis transmembrane conductance regulator DNA to lung. *Hum Gene Ther* 5: 733–746

107 Newman KD, Dunn PF, Owens JW, Schulick AH, Virmani R, Sukhova G, Libby P, Dichek DA (1995) Adenovirus-mediated gene transfer into normal rabbit arteries results in prolonged vascular cell activation, inflammation, and neointimal hyperplasia. *J Clin Invest* 96: 2955–2965

108 Vilquin JT, Guerette B, Kinoshita I, Roy B, Goulet M, Gravel C, Roy R, Tremblay JP (1995) FK506 immunosuppression to control the immune reactions triggered by first-generation adenovirus-mediated gene transfer. *Hum Gene Ther* 6: 1391–1401

109 Gordon EM, Anderson WF (1994) Gene therapy using retroviral vectors. *Curr Opin Biotech* 5: 611–616

110 Gunzburg WH, Salmons B (1996) Development of retroviral vectors as safe, targeted gene delivery systems. *J Mol Med* 74: 171–182

111 Schofield JP, and Caskey CT (1995) Non-viral approaches to gene therapy. *Br Med Bull* 51: 56–71

112 Yamamoto S, Yamamoto T, Kataoka T, Kuramoto E, Yano O, Tokunaga T (1992) Unique palindromic sequences in synthetic oligonucleotides are required to induce IFN and augment INF-mediated natural killer activity. *J Immunol* 148: 4072–4076

113 Yamamoto T, Yamamoto S, Kataoka T, Komuro K, Kohase M, Tokunaga T (1994) Synthetic oligonucleotides with certain palindromes stimulate interferon production of human peripheral blood lymphocytes *in vitro*. *Jpn J Cancer Res* 85: 775–779

114 Tokunaga T, Yano O, Kuramoto E, Kimura Y, Yamamoto T, Kataoka T, Yamamoto S (1992) Synthetic oligonucleotides with particular base sequences from the cDNA encoding proteins of mycobacterium bovis BCG induce interferons and activate natural killer cells. *Microbiol Immunol* 36: 55–66

115 Ballas ZK, Rasmussen WL, Krieg AM (1996) Induction of NK activity in murine and human cells by CpG motifs in oligodeoxynucleotides. *J Immunol* 157: 1840–1845

116 Yi AK, Klinman DM, Martin TL, Matson S, Krieg AM (1996) Rapid immune activation by CpG motifs in bacterial DNA. *J Immunol* 157: 5394–5402

117 Yi AK, Chace JH, Cowdery JS, Krieg AM (1996) IFN-g promotes IL-6 and IgM secre-

tion in response to CpG motifs in bacterial DNA oligodeoxynucleotides. *J Immunol* 156: 558–564
118 Yamamoto T, Yamamoto S, Kataoka T, Tokunaga T (1994) Lipofection of synthetic oligodeoxyribonucleotide having a palindromic sequence of AACGTT to murine splenocytes enhances interferon production and natural killer activity. *Microbiol Immunol* 38: 831–836
119 Kuramoto E, Yano O, Kimura Y, Baba M, Makino T, Yamamoto S, Yamamoto T, Kataoka, T, Tokunaga T (1992) Oligonucleotide sequences required for natural killer cell activation. *Jpn J Cancer Res* 83: 1128–1131
120 Klinman DM, Yi AK, Beaucage SL, Conover J, Krieg AM (1996) CpG motifs present in bacterial DNA rapidly induce lymphocytes to secrete interleukin 6, interleukin 12, and interferon-γ. *Proc Natl Acad Sci USA* 93: 2879–2883
121 Stacey KJ, Sweet MJ, Hume DA (1996) Macrophages ingest and are activated by bacterial DNA. *J Immunol* 157: 2116–2122
122 Sato Y, Roman M, Tighe H, Lee D, Corr M, Nguyen MD, Silverman GJ, Lotz M, Carson DA, Raz E (1996) Immunostimulatory DNA sequences necessary for effective intradermal gene immunization. *Science* 273: 352–354
123 Gooding LR (1992) Virus proteins that counteract host immune defenses. *Cell* 71: 5–7
124 Kotwal G (1996) The great escape: immune evasion by pathogens. *The Immunologist* 4/5: 157–164
125 Bromberg JS, DeBruyne LA, Qin L (1997) Interactions between the immune system and gene therapy vectors. Bidirectional regulation of response and expression. *Adv Immunol* 69: 353–409
126 Hsu DH, De Waal Malefyt R, Fiorentino DF, Dang MN, Vieira P, DeVries J, Spits H, Mosmann TR, Moore KW (1990) Expression of interleukin-10 activity by Epstein-Barr virus protein BCRF1. *Science* 250: 830–832
127 de Waal Malefyt R, Haanen J, Spits H, Roncarlol MG, te Velde A, Figdor C, Johnson C, Kastelein R, Yssel H, de Vries JE (1991) Interleukin 10 (IL-10) and viral IL-10 strongly reduce antigen-specific human T cell proliferation by diminishing the antigen-presenting capacity of monocytes via down-regulation of class II major histocompatibility complex expression. *J Exp Med* 174: 915–924
128 Vieira P, de Waal Malefyt R, Dang MN, Johnson KE, Kastelein R, Fiorentino DF, de Vries JE, Roncarolo MG, Mosmann TR, and Moore KW (1991) Isolation and expression of human cytokine synthesis inhibitory factor cDNA clones: homology to Epstein-Barr virus open reading frame BCRFI. *Proc Natl Acad Sci USA* 88: 1172–1176
129 Suzuki T, Tahara H, Narula S, Moore KW, Robbins PD, Lotze MT (1995) Viral interleukin 10 (IL-10), the human herpes virus 4 cellular IL-10 homologue, induces local anergy to allogeneic and syngeneic tumors. *J Exp Med* 182: 477–486
130 Routes JM, Metz BA, Cook JL (1993) Endogenous expression of E1A in human cells enhances the effect of adenovirus E3 on class I major histocompatibility complex antigen expression. *J Virol* 67: 3176–3181

131 Burgert HG, Kvist S (1985) An adenovirus type 2 glycoprotein blocks cell surface expression of human histocompatibility class I antigens. *Cell* 41: 987–997
132 Beier DC, Cox JH, Vining DR, Cresswell P, Engelhard VH (1994) Association of human class I MHC alleles with the adenovirus E3/19K protein. *J Immunol* 152: 3862–3872
133 Anderson M, Paäbo S, Nilsson T, Peterson A (1985) Impaired intracellular transport of class I MHC antigens as a possible means for adenoviruses to evade immune surveillance. *Cell* 43: 215–222
134 Feuerbach D, Etteldorf S, Ebenau-Jehle C, Abastado JP, Madden D, Burgert HG (1994) Identification of amino acids within the MHC module important for the interaction with the adenovirus protein E3/19k. *J Immunol* 153: 1626–1636
135 Lee MG, Abina MA, Haddada H, Perricaudet M (1995) The constitutive expression of the immunomodulatory gp 19k protein in E1-, E3- adenoviral vectors strongly reduces the host cytotoxic T cell response against the vector. *Gene Ther* 2: 256–262
136 Trapnell BC, Gorziglia M (1994) Gene therapy using adenoviral vectors. *Curr Opin Biotech* 5: 617–625
137 Engelhardt JF, Ye X, Doranz B, Wilson JM (1994) Ablation of E2A in recombinant adenoviruses improves transgene persistence and decreases inflammatory response in mouse liver. *Proc Natl Acad Sci USA* 91: 6196–6200
138 Yang Y, Nunes FA, Berencsi K, Gonczol E, Englehardt JF, Wilson JM (1994) Inactivation of E2a in recombinant adenoviruses improves the prospect for gene therapy in cystic fibrosis. *Nature Genetics* 7: 362–368
139 Dedieu JF, Vigne E, Torrent C, Jullien C, Mahfouz I, Caillaud JM, Aubailly N, Orsini C, Guillaume JM, Opolon P et al (1997) Long-term gene delivery into the livers of immunocompetent mice with E1/E4-defective adenoviruses. *J Virol* 71: 4626–4637
140 Armentano D, Zabner J, Sacks C, Sookdeo CC, Smith MP, St George JA, Wadsworth SC, Smith AE, Gregory RJ, St George JA (1997) Effect of the E4 region on the persistence of transgene expression from adenovirus vectors. *J Virol* 71: 2408–2416
141 Kochanek S, Clemens PR, Mitani K, Chen HH, Chan S, Caskey CT (1996) A new adenoviral vector: Replacement of all viral coding sequences with 28 kb of DNA independently expressing both full-length dystrophin and beta-galactosidase. *Proc Natl Acad Sci USA* 93: 5731–5736
142 Clemens PR, Kochanek S, Sunada Y, Chan S, Chen HH, Campbell KP, Caskey CT (1996) *In vivo* muscle gene transfer of full-length dystrophin with an adenoviral vector that lacks all viral genes. *Gene Ther* 3: 965–972
143 Challita PM, Kohn DB (1994) Lack of expression from a retroviral vector after transduction of murine hematopoietic stem cells is associated with methylation *in vivo*. *Proc Natl Acad Sci USA* 91: 2567–2571
144 Fang B, Eisensmith RC, Wang H, Kay MA, Cross RE, Landen CN, Gordon G, Bellinger DA, Read MS, Hu PC et al (1995) Gene therapy for hemophilia B: host immunosuppression prolongs the therapeutic effect of adenovirus-mediated factor IX expression. *Human Gene Ther* 6: 1039–1044
145 Yang Y, Su Q, Grewal IS, Schilz R, Flavell RA, Wilson JM (1996) Transient subversion

of CD40 ligand function diminishes immune responses to adenovirus vectors in mouse liver and lung tissues. *J Virol* 70: 6370–7377
146 McCoy RD, Davidson BL, Roessler BJ, Huffnagle GB, Simon RH (1995) Expression of human interleukin-1 receptor antagonist in mouse lungs using a recombinant adenovirus: effects on vector-induced inflammation. *Gene Therapy* 2: 437–442
147 Shiraishi M, Kusano T, Hara J, Hiroyasu S, Shao-Ping M, Makino Y, Muto Y (1996) Adenovirus-mediated gene transfer using *ex vivo* perfusion of the heart graft. *Surg Today* 26: 624–628
148 Ardehali A, Fyfe A, Laks H, Drinkwater DC Jr, Qiao JH, Lusis AJ (1995) Direct gene transfer into donor hearts at the time of harvest. *J Thoracic Cardiovas Surg* 109: 716–719
149 Hortelano G, Al-Hendy A, Ofosu FA, Chang PL (1996) Delivery of human factor IX in mice by encapsulated recombinant myoblasts: a novel approach towards allogeneic gene therapy of hemophilia B. *Blood* 87: 5095–5103
150 Dwarki VJ, Belloni P, Nijjar T, Smith J, Couto L, Rabier M, Clift S, Berns A, Cohen LK (1995) Gene therapy for hemophilia A: production of therapeutic levels of human factor VIII *in vivo* in mice. *Proc Natl Acad Sci USA* 92: 1023–1027
151 Rettinger SD, Kennedy SC, Wu X, Saylors RL, Hafenrichter DG, Flye MW, Ponder KP (1994) Liver-directed gene therapy: Quantitative evaluation of promoter elements by using *in vivo* retroviral transduction. *Proc Natl Acad Sci USA* 91: 1460–1464
152 Yao S, Farjo A, Roessler BJ, Davidson BL, Kurachi K (1996) Adenovirus-mediated transfer of human factor IX gene in immunodeficient and normal mice: evidence for prolonged stability and activity of the transgene in liver. *Viral Immunol* 9: 141–153
153 Guidotti LG, Ishikawa T, Hobbs MV, Matzke B, Schreiber R, Chisari FV (1996) Intracellular inactivation of the Hepatitis B virus by cytotoxic T lymphocytes. *Immunity* 4: 25–36
154 Tsui LV, Guidotti LG, Ishikawa T, Chisari FV (1995) Posttranscriptional clearance of hapatitis B virus RNA by cytotoxic T lymphocyte-activated hepatocytes. *Proc Natl Acad Sci USA* 92: 12398–12402
155 Harms JS, Splitter GA (1995) Interferon-g inhibits transgene expression driven by SV40 or CMV promoters but augments expression driven by the mammalian MHC I promoter. *Hum Gene Ther* 6: 1291–1297
156 Qin L, Ding Y, Pahud DR, Chang E, Imperiale MJ, Bromberg JS (1997) Promoter attenuation in gene therapy: IFNγ and TNFα inhibit transgene expression. *Hum Gene Ther* 8: 1851–1861
157 Lin H, Parmacek MS, Morle G, Bolling S, Leiden JM (1990) Expression of recombinant genes in myocardium *in vivo* after direct injection of DNA. *Circulation* 82: 2217–2221
158 Wolff JA, Malone RW, Williams P, Chang W, Ascadi G, Jani A, Felgner PL (1990) Direct gene transfer into mouse muscle *in vivo*. *Science* 247: 1456–1468
159 Guzman RJ, Lemarchand P, Crystal RG, Epstein SE, Finkel T (1993) Efficient gene transfer into myocardium by direct injection of adenovirus vectors. *Circ Res* 73: 1202–1207

160 Ardehali A, Fyfe A, Laks H, Drinkwater DC Jr, Qiao JH, Lusis AJ (1995) Direct gene transfer into donor hearts at the time of harvest. *J Thoracic Cardiovas Surg* 109: 716–719
161 Fyfe AI, Ardehali A, Laks H, Drinkwater DC, Lusis AJ (1995) Biologic modification of the immune response in mouse cardiac isografts using gene transfer. *J Heart Lung Transplant* 14: S165–170
162 Gojo S, Kitamur S, Niwaya K, Yoshida Y, Sakaguchi H, Kawachi K (1996) *Ex vivo* gene transfer to transplanted heart greats using adenoviral vector. *Transplant Proc* 28: 1818–1819
163 Stephan DJ,Yang Z-Y, San H, Simari RD, Wheeler CJ, Felgner PL, Gordon D, Nabel GJ, Nabel EG (1996) A new cationic liposome DNA complex enhances the efficiency of arterial gene transfer *in vivo*. *Hum Gene Ther* 7: 1803–1812
164 Qin L, Chavin KD, Ding Y, Woodward JE, Favaro JP, Lin J, Bromberg JS (1994) Gene transfer for transplantation: Prolongation of allograft survival with transforming growth factor-β1. *Annals Surg* 220: 508–519
165 Moore KW, Vieira P, Fiorentino DF, Trounstine ML, Khan TA, Mosmann TR (1990) Homology of cytokine synthesis inhibitory factor (IL-10) to the Epstein-Barr virus gene BCRFI. *Science* 248: 1230–1234.
166 Chen WF, Zlotnik A (1991) IL-10: a novel cytotoxic T cell differentiation factor. *J Immunol* 147: 528–534
167 Rousset F, Garcia E, Defrance T, Peronne C, Vezzio N, Hsu DH, Kastelein R, Moore KW, Banchereay J (1992) Interleukin 10 is a potent growth and differentiation factor for activated human B lymphocytes. *Proc Natl Acad Sci USA* 89: 1890–1893
168 Thompson-Snipes L, Dhar V, Bond MW, Mosmann TR, Moore KW, Rennick DM (1991) Interleukin 10: a novel stimulatory factor for mast cells and their progenitors. *J Exp Med* 173: 507–510
169 de Waal Malefyt R, Abrams J, Bennett B, Figdor CG, de Vries JE (1991) Interleukin 10 (IL-10) inhibits cytokine synthesis by human monocytes: an autoregulatory role of IL-10 produced by monocytes. *J Exp Med* 174: 1209–1220
170 Mosmann TR (1994) Properties and functions of interleukin-10. Adv Immunol 56: 1–26
171 Moses HL, Yang EY, Pietenpol JA (1990) TGF-β stimulation and inhibition of cell proliferation: New mechanistic insights. *Cell* 63: 245–247
172 Nilsen-Hamilton M (1990) Transforming growth factor-β and its actions on cellular growth and differentiation. *Curr Topics Develop Biol* 24: 95–136
173 Mastrangeli A, Danel C, Rosenfeld MA, Stratford-Perricaudet L, Perricaudet M, Pavirani A, Lecocq JP, Crystal RG (1993) Diversity of airway epithelial cell targets for *in vivo* recombinant adenovirus-mediated gene transfer. *J Clin Invest* 91: 225–234
174 Lemarchand P, Jones M, Danel C, Yamada I, Mastrangeli A, Crystal RG (1994) *In vivo* adenovirus-mediated gene transfer to lungs. *J Appl Physiol* 76: 2840–2845
175 Chapelier A, Danel C, Mazmanian M, Bacha EA, Sellak H, Gilbert MA, Herve P, Lemarchand P (1996) Gene therapy in lung transplantation: Feasibility of *ex vivo* adenovirus-mediated gene transfer to the lung. *Hum Gene Ther* 7: 1837–1845

176 Mora BN, Boasquevisque CHR, Boglione M Ritter JH, Scheule RK, Yew NS, Nietupski J, Qin L, DeBruyne L, Bromberg JS et al (1997) Improvement in lung allograft function following transfection with transforming growth factor β1. *The Society of Thoracic Surgeons*, meeting abstract
177 Kitamura, M (1994) Transfer of exogenous genes into the kidney. *Exp Nephrol* 2: 313–317
178 Bosch RJ, Woolf AS, Fine LG (1993) Gene transfer into the mammalian kidney: direct retrovirus transduction of regenerating tubular epithelial cells. *Exp Nephrol* 1: 49–54
179 Moullier P, Friedlander G, Calise D, Ronco P, Perricaudet M, Ferry N (1994) Adenoviral-mediated gene transfer to renal tubular cells *in vivo*. *Kidney International* 45: 1220–1225
180 Kitamura M, Taylor S, Unwin R, Burton S, Shimizu F, Fine LG (1994) Gene transfer into the rat glomerulus via a mesangial cell vector: Site-specific delivery, *in situ* amplification and sustained expression of an exogenous gene *in vivo*. *J Clin Invest* 94: 497–505
181 Woolf AS, Bosch RJ, Fine LG (1993) Gene transfer into the mammalian kidney: Microtransplantation of retrovirus-transduced metanephric tissue. Exp Nephrol 1: 41–48
182 Koseki C, Herzlinger D, Al-Aweqati Q (1991) Integration of embryonic nephrogenic cells carrying a reporter gene into functioning nephrons. *Am J Physiol* 261: C550–C554
183 Ziegler ST, Kerby JD, Curiel DT, Diethelm AG, Thompson JA (1996) Molecular conjugate-mediated gene transfer into isolated human kidneys. *Transplantation* 61: 812–817
184 Docherty K (1997) Gene therapy for diabetes mellitus. *Clin Science* 92: 321–330
185 Ferber S, Beltrande I, Rio H, Johnson JH, Noel RJ, Cassidy LE, Clark S, Becker TC, Hughes SD, Newgard CB (1994) GLUT-2 gene transfer into insulinoma cells confers both low and high affinity glucose-stimulated insulin release. *J Biol Chem* 269: 11523–11529
186 Deuschle U, Pepperkok R, Wang F, Giordano TJ, McAllister WT, Ansorge W, Bujard H (1989) Regulated expression of foreign genes in mammalian cells under the control of coliphage T3 RNA polymerase and lac repressor. *Proc Natl Acad Sci USA* 86: 5600–5604
187 Elfrat S, Fusco-Demane D, Lemberg H, Erman OA, Wang X (1995) Conditional transformation of a pancreatic β-cell line derived from transgenic mice expressing a tetracycline-regulated oncogene. *Proc Natl Acad Sci USA* 92: 3576–3580
188 Welsh M, Welsh N, Nilsson T, Arkhammar P, Pepinsky RB, Steiner DF, Berggren PO (1988) Stimulation of pancreatic islet beta-cell replication by oncogenes. *Proc Natl Acad Sci USA* 85: 116–120
189 Serup P, Jensen J, Andersen FG, Jaergensen MC, Blume N, Holst JJ, Madsen OD (1996) Induction of insulin and islet amyloid polypeptide production in pancreatic islet glucagonoma cells by insulin promoter factor I. *Proc Natl Acad Sci USA* 93: 9015–9020
190 Csete ME, Afra R, Mullen Y, Drazan KE, Benhamou PY, Shaked A (1994) Adenoviral-mediated gene transfer to pancreatic islets does not alter islet function. *Transplant Proc* 26: 756–757
191 Mirenda V, Charreau B, Sigalla J, Cassard A, Huvelin JM, David A, Soulilou JP, Le

Mauff B, Anegon I (1996) Xenoreactivity in the pig islet to human combination: Feasibility of adenovirus-mediated gene transfer into pig islets. *Transplant Proc* 28: 808–810

192 Korbutt GS, Smith DK, Rajotee RV, Elliott JF (1995) Expression of β-galactosidase in mouse pancreatic islets by adenoviral-mediated gene transfer. *Transplant Proc* 27: 3414

193 Bosch A, McCray PB Jr, Chang SM, Ulich TR, Simonet WS, Jolly DJ, Davidson BL (1996) Proliferation induced by keratinocyte growth factor enhances *in vivo* retroviral-mediated gene transfer to mouse hepatocytes. *J Clin Invest* 98: 2683–2687

194 Gupta S, Wilson JM, Chowdhury JR (1992) Hepatocyte transplantation: Development of new systems for liver repopulation and gene therapy. *Seminars in Liver Disease* 12: 321–331

195 Wolff JA, Yee JK, Skelly HF, Moores JC, Respess JG, Friedmann T, Leffert H (1987) Expression of retrovirally transduced genes in primary cultures of adult rat hepatocytes. *Proc Natl Acad Sci USA* 84: 3344–3348

196 Peng H, Armentano D, MacKenzie-Graham L, Shen RF, Darlington G, Ledley FD, Woo SL (1988) Retroviral-mediated gene transfer and expression of human phenylalanine hydroxylase in primary mouse hepatocytes. *Proc Natl Acad Sci USA* 85: 8146–8150

197 Hatzoglou M, Lamers W, Bosch F, Wynshaw-Boris A, Clapp DW, Hanson RW (1990) Hepatic gene transfer in animals using retroviruses containing the promoter from the gene for phosphoenolpyruvate carboxykinase *J Biol Chem* 265: 17285–17293

198 Armentano D, Thompson AR, Darlington G, Woo SL (1990) Expression of human factor IX in rabbit hepatocytes by retrovirus-mediated gene transfer: Potential for gene therapy of human hemophilia B. *Proc Natl Acad Sci USA* 87: 6141–6145

199 Kay MA, Baley P, Rothenberg S, Leland F, Fleming L, Parker Ponder K, Liu TJ, Finegold M, Darlington G, Pokorny W et al (1991) Expression of human α1-antitrypsin in dogs after autologous transplantation of retroviral transduced hepatocytes. *Proc Natl Acad Sci USA* 89: 89–93

200 Wilson JM, Johnston DE, Jefferson DM, Mulligan RC (1988) Correction of the genetic defect in hepatocytes from the Watanabe heritable hyperlipidemic rabbit. *Proc Natl Acad Sci USA* 85: 4421–4425

201 Grossman M, Raper SE, Kozarsky K, Stein EA, Engelhardt JF, Muller D, Lupien PJ, Wilson JM (1994) Successful *ex vivo* gene therapy directed to liver in a patient with familial hypercholesterolemia. *Nature Genetics* 6: 335–341

202 Fabrega AJ, Fasbender AJ, Struble S, Zabner J (1996) Cationic lipid-mediated transfer of the hIL-10 gene prolongs survival of allogeneic hepatocytes in Nagase analbuminemic rats. *Transplantation* 62: 1866–1871

203 Shirashi M, Kusano T, Hara J, Hiroyasu S, Shao-ping M, Makino Y, Muto Y (1997) Adenovirus-mediated gene transfer using in-situ perfusion of the liver graft. *Transplant International* 10: 202–206

204 Olthoff KM, Da Chen X, Gelman A, Turka L, Shaked A (1997) Adenovirus-mediated gene transfer of CTLA4Ig to liver allografts results in prolonged survival and local T-cell anergy. *Transplant Proc* 29: 1030–1031

205 Brenner MK, Heslop HE, Rill D, Li C, Nilson T, Roberts M, Smith C, Krance R, Rooney

C (1994) Gene transfer and bone marrow transplantation. *Cold Spring Harb Symp Quant Biol* 59: 691–697
206 Rill DR, Moen RC, Buschle M, Bartholomew C, Foreman NK, Mirro J Jr, Krance RA, Ihle JN, Brenner MK (1992) An approach for the analysis of relapse and marrow reconstitution after autologous marrow transplantation using retrovirus-mediated gene transfer. *Blood* 79: 2694–2700
207 Cornetta K, Srour EF, Moore A, Davidson A, Broun ER, Hromas R, Moen RC, Morgan RA, Rubin L, Anderson WF et al (1996) Retroviral gene transfer in autologous bone marrow transplantation for adult acute leukemia. *Hum Gene Ther* 7: 1323–1329
208 Fletcher FA, Moore KA, Williams DE, Anderson D, Maliszewski C, Belmont JW (1991) Effects of leukemia inhibitory factor (LIF) on gene transfer efficiency into murine hematolymphoid progenitors. *Adv Exp Med Biol* 292: 131–138
209 Luskey BD, Rosenblatt M, Zsebo K, Williams DA (1992) Stem cell factor, interleukin-3, and interleukin-6 promote retroviral-mediated gene transfer into murine hematopoietic stem cells. *Blood* 80: 396–402
210 Drize N, Chertov J, Sadovnikova E, Tiessen S, Zander A (1997) Long-term maintenance of hematopoiesis in irradiated mice by retrovirally transduced peripheral blood stem cells. *Blood* 89: 1811–1817
211 Yurasov S, Kollman TR, Kim A, Raker CA, Hachamovitch M, Wong-Staal F, Goldstein H (1997) Severe combined immunodeficiency mice engrafted with human T cells, B cells, and myeloid cells after transplantation with human fetal bone marrow or liver cells and implanted with human fetal thymus: A model for studying human gene therapy. *Blood* 89: 1800–1810
212 Kuhr T, Dougherty GJ, Klingermann H-G (1994) Transfer of the tumor necrosis factor a gene into hematopoietic progenitor cells as a model for site-specific cytokine delivery after marrow transplantation. *Blood* 84: 2966–2970
213 Rosenthal FM, Fruh R, Henschler R, Veelken H, Kulmburg P, Mackensen A, Gansbacher B, Mertelsmann R, Lindemannn A (1994) Cytokine therapy with gene-transfected cells: Single injection of irradiated granulocyte-macrophage colony-stimulating factor-transduced cells accelerates hematopoietic recovery after cytotoxic chemotherapy in mice. *Blood* 84: 2960–2965
214 Spencer HT, Sleep SE, Rehg JE, Blakley RL, Sorrentino BP (1996) A gene transfer strategy for making bone marrow cells resistant to trimetrexate. *Blood* 87: 2579–2587
215 Vinh DB, McIvor RS (1993) Selective expression of methotrexate-resistant dihydrofolate reductase (DHFR) activity in mice transduced with DHFR retrovirus and administered methotrexate. *J Pharmacol Exp Ther* 267: 989–996
216 Bonini C, Ferrari G, Verzeletti S, Servida P, Zappone E, Ruggieri L, Ponzoni M, Rossini S, Mavilio F, Traversari C et al (1997) HSV-TK gene transfer into donor lymphocytes for control of allogeneic graft-versus-leukemia. *Science* 276: 1719–1724
217 Fraser CC, Sykes M, Lee RS, Sachs DH, LeGuern C (1995) Specific unresponsiveness to a retrovirally-transferred class I antigen is controlled through the helper pathway. *J Immunol* 154: 1587–1595

218 Smith CV, Nakajima K, Mixon A, Guzetta PC, Rosengard BR, Fishbein JM, Sachs DH (1992) Successful induction of long-term specific tolerance to fully allogeneic renal allografts in miniature swine. *Transplantation* 53: 438–444

219 Banerjee PT, Ierino F, Kaynor GC, Giovino M, Sablinski T, Emery DW, Rosa MD, LeGuern C, Sachs DH, Monroy RL (1996) Retrovirus-mediated gene transfer and expression of swine MHC Class II genes in $CD34^+$ monkey stem cells. *Transplant Proc* 28: 747–748

220 Salminen A, Elson HF, Mickley LA, Fojo AT, Gottesman MM (1991) Implantation of recombinant rat myocytes into adult skeletal muscle: a potential gene therapy. *Hum Gene Ther* 2: 15–26

221 Rando TA, Blau HM (1994) Primary mouse myoblast purification, characterization, and transplantation for cell-mediated gene therapy. *J Cell Biol* 125: 1275–1287

222 Yao SN, Kurachi K (1993) Implanted myoblasts not only fuse with myofibers but also survive as muscle precursor cells. *J Cell Sci* 105: 957–963

223 Pagel CN, Morgan JE (1995) Myoblast transfer and gene therapy in muscular dystrophies. *Microscopy Research and Technique* 30: 469–479

224 Morgan, JE (1994) Cell and gene therapy in Duchenne muscular dystrophy. *Hum Gene Ther* 5:165–173

225 Law PK, Goodwin TG, Fang Q, Hall TL, Quinley T, Vastagh G, Duggirala V, Larkin C, Florendo JA, Li L et al (1997) First human myoblast transfer therapy continues to show dystrophin after 6 years. *Cell Transplant* 6: 95–100

226 Dai Y, Roman M, Naviaux RK, Verma IM (1992) Gene therapy via primary myoblasts: long-term expression of factor IX protein following transplantation *in vivo*. *Proc Natl Acad Sci USA* 89: 10892–10895

227 Yao SN, Smith KJ, Kurachi K (1994) Primary myoblast-mediated gene transfer: persistent expression of human factor IX in mice. *Gene Ther* 1: 99–107

228 Wang JM, Zheng H, Blaivas M, Kurachi K (1997) Persistent systemic production of human factor IX in mice by skeletal myoblast-mediated gene transfer: feasibility of repeat application to obtain therapeutic levels. *Blood* 90: 1075–1082

229 Baru M, Sha'anani J, Nur I (1995) Retroviral-mediated *in vivo* gene transfer into muscle cells and synthesis of human factor IX in mice. *Intervirology* 38: 356–360

230 Dhawan J, Pan LC, Pavlath GK, Travis MA, Lanctot AM, Blau HM (1991) Systemic delivery of human growth hormone by injection of genetically engineered myoblasts. *Science* 254: 1509–1512

231 Dahler A, Wade RP, Muscat GE, Waters MJ (1994) Expression vectors encoding human growth hormone (hGH) controlled by human muscle-specific promoters: prospects for regulated production of hGH delivered by myoblast transfer or intravenous injection. *Gene* 145: 305–310

232 Al-Hendy A, Hortelano G, Tannenbaum GS, Chang PL (1995) Correction of the growth defect in dwarf mice with nonautologous microencapsulated myoblasts—an alternate approach to somatic gene therapy. *Hum Gene Ther* 6: 165–175

233 Hamamori Y, Samal B, Tian J, Kedes L (1994) Persistent erythropoiesis by myoblast transfer of erythropoietin cDNA. *Hum Gene Ther* 5: 1349–1356
234 Hamamori Y, Samal B, Tian J, Kedes L (1995) Myoblast transfer of human erythropoietin gene in a mouse model of renal failure. *J Clin Invest* 95: 1808–1813
235 Simonson GD, Groskreutz DJ, Gorman CM, MacDonald MJ (1996) Synthesis and processing of genetically modified human proinsulin by rat myoblast primary cultures. *Hum Gene Ther* 7: 71–78
236 Shull RM, Lu X, McEntee MF, Bright RM, Pepper KA, Kohn DB (1996) Myoblast gene therapy in canine mucopolysaccharidosis. I: Abrogation by an immune response to alpha-L-iduronidase. *Hum Gene Ther* 7: 1595–1603
237 Naffakh N, Bohl D, Salvetti A, Moullier P, Danos O, Heard JM (1994) Gene therapy for lysosomal disorders. *Nouv Rev Fr Hematol* 36 (1): S11–S16
238 Jiao S, Gurevich V, Wolff JA (1993) Long-term correction of rat model of Parkinson's disease by gene therapy. *Nature* 362: 450–453

DNA vaccination as an anti-inflammatory strategy

Alexis Paul Godillot[1], Michael Madaio[2], David B. Weiner[3,4] and William V. Williams[1,4,5]

Department of Medicine, Divisions of [1]Rheumatology and [2]Nephrology, [3]Department of Pathology and Laboratory Medicine, [4]Institute for Biotechnology and Advanced Molecular Medicine, University of Pennsylvania School of Medicine, Philadelphia, PA 19104, USA: [5]Children's Hospital of Philadelphia, 913 Stellar-Chance Laboratories, 422 Curie Drive, Philadelphia, PA 19104-6100, USA

Introduction

Vaccination has become a paradigm of preventative medicine, as it is both efficacious and cost-effective. The ability of vaccines to elicit specific immune responses is the key to their efficacy. There are two methods by which vaccines elicit immune responses. The first vaccines developed consisted of live attenuated pathogens which infect the host and stimulate a protective immune response. This includes the smallpox vaccine and the Sabin polio vaccine. The second method of vaccination was the development of killed pathogens or subunits. This includes the Salk polio vaccine (killed polio virus) and the hepatitis vaccine (recombinant surface antigen glycoprotein). These killed and subunit preparations have been also of great utility.

These two methods of vaccination differ in the mechanism of antigen presentation to the immune system. Live attenuated viruses infect susceptible cells, and the viral proteins are produced by the host cells. This endogenous synthesis of viral proteins results in their being processed into antigenic peptides either in the cytosol or in the endoplasmic reticulum (ER). These peptides are transported to the ER where they associate with class I major histocompatibility (MHC molecules). This MHC class I-antigen (Ag) complex is then displayed on the cell surface, and recognized by T cell receptors (TCR) on $CD8^+$ T cells. Such $CD8^+$ T cells have several effector functions, including cytotoxicity (cytotoxic T cells or M) and secretion of certain cytokines (e.g. interferon γ (IFNγ)). Thus, this endogenous pathway of Ag presentation elicits $CD8^+$ mediated immunity.

Killed pathogens or subunit vaccines do not infect cells, but are endocytosed by specialized antigen presenting cells (APC). These exogenous Ag are processed into peptides in endocytic vesicles, and the peptides associate with class II MHC molecules. These MHC class II-Ag complexes are translocated to the cell surface, and are recognized by TCR on $CD4^+$ T cells. These T cells are then able to initiate cellular and humoral immunity. Two prototypical types of $CD4^+$ T cells have been recog-

Gene Therapy in Inflammatory Diseases, edited by C. H. Evans and P. D. Robbins

nized based on their ability to secrete specific cytokines. TH1 cells secrete IL-2 and IFNγ, inducing potent cellular immunity and antibody responses of the IgG2a isotype in mice. TH2 cells secrete IL-4 and IL-5, and induce predominately humoral responses (IgG1 and IgE responses in mice). Thus, this exogenous pathway of Ag presentation elicits $CD4^+$ mediated immunity.

These vaccination strategies have specific advantages and disadvantages. For example, killed or subunit vaccines fail to elicit strong $CD8^+$ T cell immunity. This includes CTL responses, which are felt to be critical in certain types of cellular immunity such as tumor immunity and in the regulation of autoreactivity. Attenuated viral vaccines suffer from other drawbacks, such as their potential pathogenicity (particularly in immunocompromised individuals), and the antigenic complexity of an intact virus. In addition, it is difficult to adapt attenuated viruses to cellular antigens, as in the case of tumor immunity and regulation of autoreactive cells.

Recently, studies have been performed assessing the utility of plasmid DNA as a vaccine directly. Theoretically, a DNA plasmid which encodes a gene under the control of an appropriate promoter, can be inoculated into an individual and taken up into the cells of that individual. These *in vivo* transfected cells would then synthesize the protein encoded by the gene just as if it had been infected with this gene as part of a viral infection. This is thus the genetic equivalent of a subunit or recombinant protein vaccine. The potential advantages of this strategy are many. There is no limit to the number of different protein antigens which can be delivered in this way, although it is only feasible to use protein antigens by this strategy. A single gene or many different genes can be targeted by this strategy, as can parts of genes (e.g. the nontoxic portion of toxins). The level of expression, the target cells transfected, and the intracellular localization of the antigen can all be manipulated with this technology.

These and many other considerations have made DNA vaccination a popular research tool in recent years. Here we will review the overall steps in developing DNA vaccines, and their potential applicability in the area of inflammatory diseases.

Development of DNA vaccines

Gene therapy, which involves the direct introduction of a normal, functional gene into a living animal, has great promise for replacing defective genetic information [1–3]. Similarly, direct immunization by DNA inoculation (DNA vaccination) appears to mimic some aspects of attenuated vaccines in that synthesis of specific foreign proteins would be accomplished in the host and be the subject of immune surveillance. DNA vaccination is accomplished by injection of a nucleic acid sequence directly into a host target tissue [1, 2]. While studies indicating the ability of genetic material to induce immune responses to the encoded genes date back to the 1970s [4], this technique was popularized more recently following investigations demonstrating gene expression following intramuscular injection of the human growth hormone and muscular dystrophy genes in mice [1, 2]. These gene products were antigenic in some circumstances and were shown to elicit antibody based immune responses [5].

These initial findings led to additional studies using DNA inoculation to induce immune responses to influenza virus [6, 7] and the human immunodeficiency virus [8]. The demonstration of elicitation of protective immunity by this technique has led to an explosion of interest in this topic, with hundreds of papers published since 1993. DNA vaccines have been demonstrated to elicit all arms of the immune system, and to induce protective immunity against both pathogens and pathogenic cells. In this section, we will discuss the essential components of DNA vaccines and their administration.

DNA vaccine design

DNA vaccines are typically designed with several considerations tailored to the system in which they are used. Vaccines which are targeted for human use must be developed with safety as the primary consideration. Bacterial plasmid DNA is used in all DNA vaccines developed to date, due to the ease of handling and low cost of producing these plasmids. Any potentially pathogenic genes encoded by such plasmids are not included. This includes genes for ampicillin resistance, which are typically incorporated into bacterial plasmids for growth selection purposes, as this may lead to increased ampicillin resistance by bacteria which may come in contact with the plasmid DNA. Many use kanamycin resistance instead, as this antibiotic is not used in humans. The plasmid also must have a bacterial origin of replication (preferably one which drives high copy number replication) to allow reproduction of the plasmid in the bacterial strains that are used to produce it. The remainder of the plasmid is involved in the antigenic gene to be expressed. A promoter sequence is introduced to drive expression of the gene in mammalian cells. The cytomegalovirus immediate early enhancer/promoter is typically used, as it has been shown to drive high levels of expression of genes in many different tissues [9]. Other enhancers may be added to boost expression, and other promoter systems can be employed if tissue-specific expression is desired. The antigenic gene is typically encoded as a complementary DNA (cDNA) to reduce the complexity of the constructs. Introns can be used, and have been by some investigators. Manipulation of the coding region of the gene will be discussed below. Finally, a polyadenylation signal is added to complete the transcript and the resultant mRNA to the correct intracellular compartment for translation.

This basic design (see Fig. 1) can be altered in many ways. Tissue-specific promoters can be introduced to limit expression of the genes to specific tissues

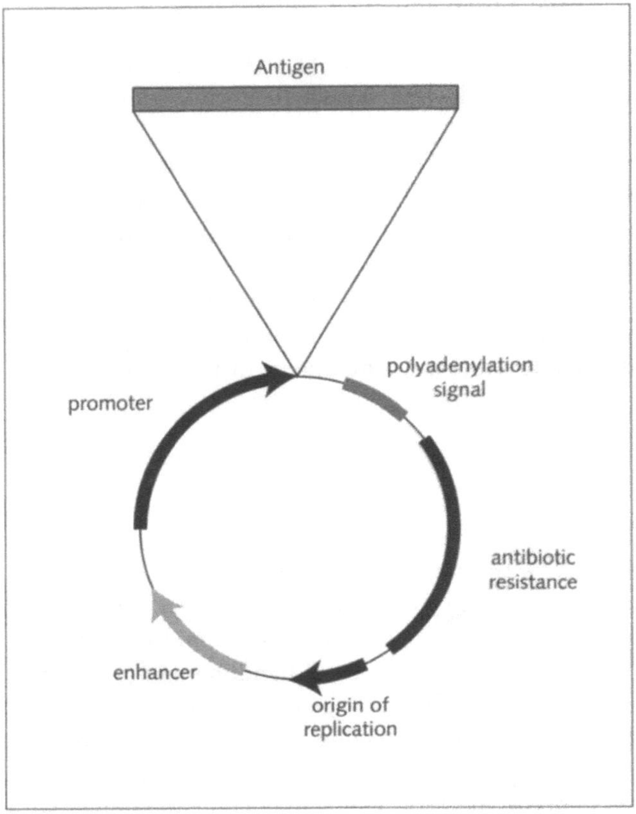

Figure 1
Structure of DNA vaccines.
A typical DNA vaccine backbone uses the CMV promoter with or without an enhancer to drive transcription of the inserted antigen gene. The inserts contain the coding region of the antigenic gene. The polyadenylation signal is needed for addition of polyA to the mRNA. The antibiotic resistance gene is needed to allow growth and selection of the plasmid in bacteria. As these resistance genes lack mammalian promoters, they are not produced in mammalian cells. The origin of replication is needed to drive replication of the plasmid.

(although leakiness is common for these "specific" promoters). More than one coding region can be introduced by the use of splice/donor sites or the use of internal ribosome entry sites. The coding region itself can be targeted to different intracellular compartments or targeted for secretion from the cell by using specific targeting sequences. The backbone structure of the plasmid is also important. Many recent studies indicate that bacterial DNA sequences which include specific motifs high in cytosine and guanosine (CpG motifs) are immunostimulatory [10–14]. Cytokine genes [15, 16], costimulatory molecules [17, 18], and other molecular adjuvants can also be added to DNA vaccine formulations to boost their immunogenicity. Many other modifications are possible.

DNA vaccine delivery

Delivery of DNA vaccines can be performed via many routes. The most prevalent currently used are intramuscular and intradermal. Intramuscular DNA inoculation (usually delivered by a needle) can be enhanced by facilitating agents which increase DNA uptake by muscle cells [19]. Intradermal inoculation has often used DNA-coated particles delivered via a "gene-gun" [20, 21]. Both of these routes are efficacious in eliciting immune responses to the inoculated genes. Other routes have also been shown to be efficacious in eliciting immune responses, including parenteral [61] and mucosal inoculation [22–25]. The route of inoculation has effects on the dose of vaccine needed to induce immunity (e.g. intradermal typically needs smaller doses than intramuscular) and may affect the character of the immune response (e.g. mucosal DNA may elicit higher IgA titers at mucosal surfaces compared with other routes of vaccination).

Immunity following DNA vaccination

Once delivered, DNA vaccines are capable of inducing both $CD4^+$ and $CD8^+$ T cell mediated immunity as well as humoral immunity (antibody responses). The mechanism for this is shown in Figure 2. The character of the immune response developed following DNA vaccination is dependent on several parameters. $CD8^+$ CTL responses are readily elicited by most DNA vaccines (Fig. 2A). This stems from the fact that the antigen is produced within the cell, thereby directly entering the endogenous pathway. In addition, multiple intracellular compartments are equipped, with the necessary proteases and transport proteins to ensure entry of antigenic peptides into the ER for loading onto class I MHC molecules. $CD4^+$ T cell responses are also readily elicited by DNA vaccines, and these can be thought of as a consequence of secretion of the gene product (Fig. 2B). In reality, the matter is more complex as intracellular antigens are also known to stimulate $CD4^+$ responses. However, the simple conceptual model of Ag secretion, uptake by a professional antigen presenting cell (APC), processing and presentation to $CD4^+$ T cells is shown here. Note that the Ag/MHC II complex developed by the professional APC (typically a macrophage or dendritic cell) is similarly developed by Ag-specific B cells which capture the secreted Ag using their surface immunoglobulin (Ig) mole-

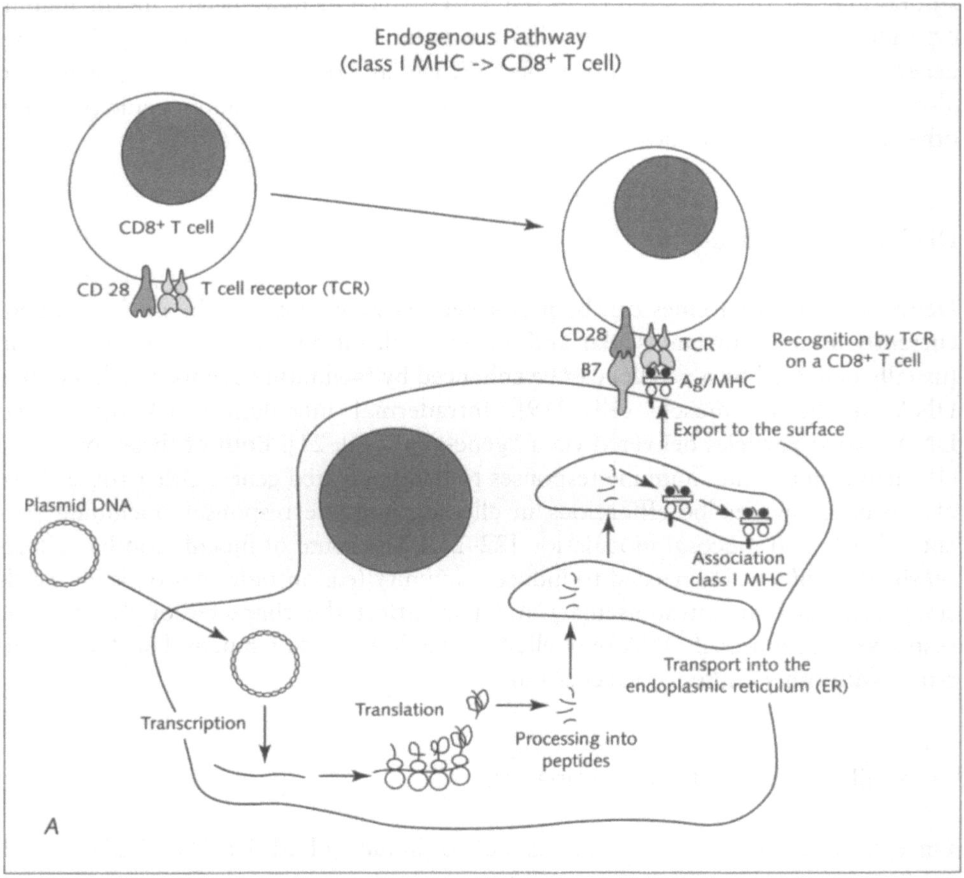

Figure 2
Antigen presentation following DNA vaccination
(A) Endogenous pathway antigen processing and presentation following DNA vaccination. The plasmid DNA is taken up and the gene transcribed to mRNA. The mRNA is translated and the protein (in this case shown as a cytosolic protein) is processed into peptides. The peptides are transported into the endoplasmic reticulum (ER) where they associate with a class I major histocompatibility complex (MHC) molecule. The Ag/MHC I is transported to the cell surface where it is recognized by an Ag/MHC I-specific CD8$^+$ T cell via the T cell antigen receptor (TCR). Co-stimulatory molecule interactions (B7$\rightarrow$CD28) are needed for stimulation of the T cell. This CD8$^+$ T cell can differentiate into a cytotoxic T cell (CTL) or secrete cytokines such as IFNγ.
(B) Exogenous pathway antigen processing and presentation following DNA vaccination. Step 1: The plasmid DNA is taken up and the gene transcribed to mRNA. The mRNA is translated in the endoplasmic reticulum (ER) and the protein is secreted from the cell. Step 2: The

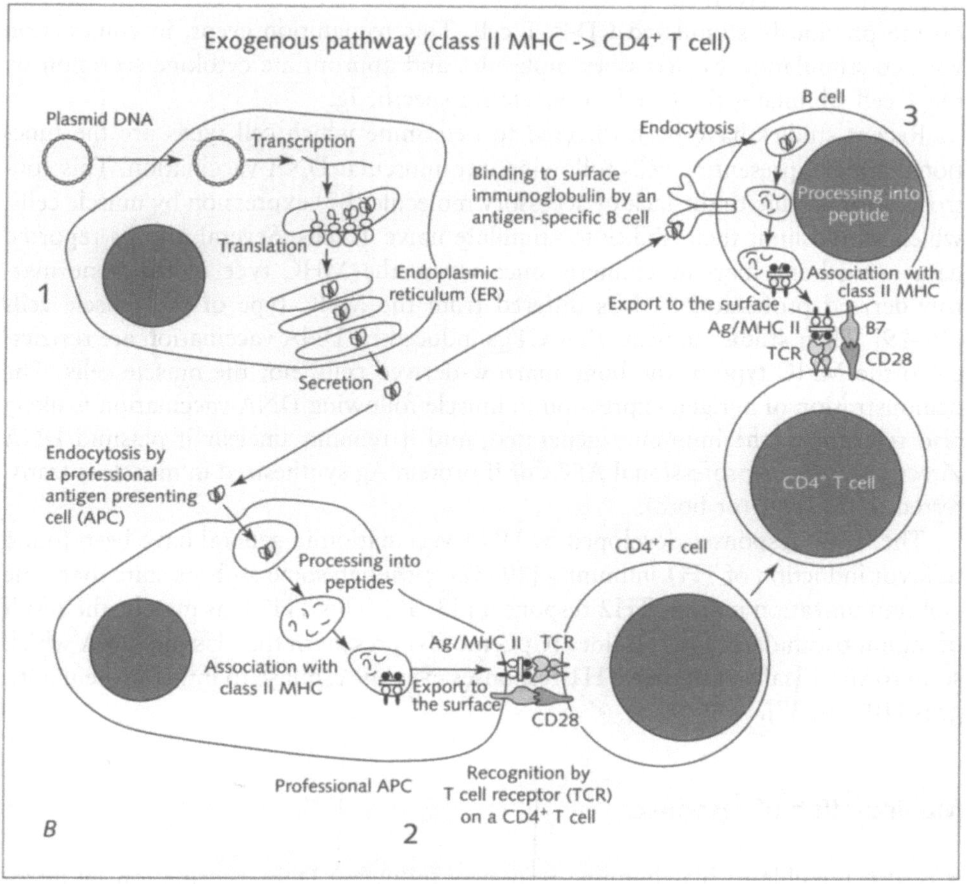

secreted protein endocytosed by a professional antigen presenting cell (APC) and processed into peptides. The peptides associate with class II MHC molecules in the endosomes, and the Ag/MHC II is transported to the cell surface where it is recognized by an Ag/MHC 11-specific CD4+ T cell via the TCR. Co-stimulatory molecule interactions (B7 -> CD28) are needed for stimulation of the T cell. The stimulated T cell then secretes cytokines which influence the character and extent of the immune response. Step 3: The secreted protein is bound by surface immunoglobulin (1 g) on an antigen-specific B cell. The Ig/Ag is endocytosed into endocytic vesicles where the Ag is processed into peptides which associate with class II MHC molecules. The Ag/MHC II is transported to the cell surface where it is recognized by an Ag/MHC II -specific CD4+ T cell via the TCR. This T cell (which is already activated in step 2) binds the Ag/MHC II via its TCR providing a specific signal to the B cell. This signal, along with the B7-CD28 interaction and local cytokine secretion by the T cell, stimulates the B cell to produce soluble Ig, with a resultant Ag-specific antibody response.

cules. This Ag/MHC II complex can then be recognized by the T cell receptor (TCR) on the previously stimulated $CD4^+$ T cell. This recognition event, in conjunction with co-stimulation by accessory molecules and appropriate cytokine secretion by the T cell stimulates the B cell to secrete Ag-specific Ig.

Recent studies have been directed to determine which cell types are the functional antigen presenting cells following intramuscular DNA vaccination. This controversy arose due to the lack of accessory molecule (B7) expression by muscle cells, which would limit their ability to stimulate naïve T cells. Several groups reported data using bone marrow chimeric mice where the MHC type of the bone marrow-derived professional APCs differed from the MHC type of the muscle cells [26–29]. Their studies indicate that CTLs induced by DNA vaccination are restricted to the MHC type of the bone marrow-derived cells, not the muscle cells. The demonstration of antigen expression in muscle following DNA vaccination is likely also relevant to the immunity generated, and it remains unclear if plasmid DNA directly transfects professional APCs or if protein Ag synthesized in muscle is transferred to the APC (or both).

The $CD4^+$ responses developed by DNA vaccination in general have been found to favor induction of TH1 immunity [30–32], although some authors state that gene gun immunization induces TH2 responses [33–35]. This TH1 bias may be the result of immunostimulatory nucleotides (CpG motifs) present in the plasmid DNA which seem to specifically stimulate TH1 responses even in response to intact protein antigens [10, 36, 37].

Manipulation of responses

It is also possible to bias immune responses following DNA vaccination by introducing cytokines or cytokine genes into the immunization process [15,16,38]. In general, TH1-inducing cytokines include IL-2, IFNγ, IL-12, IL-15 and IL-18. The TH2-inducing cytokines include IL-4, IL-5, and IL-10. Some of these, such as IL-12 [16, 38] and IL-4 [38], have already been shown to bias immune responses to DNA vaccines to TH1 and TH2 types respectively. These molecular adjuvants may be quite useful in biasing DNA vaccine responses toward desired pathways.

The efficacy of DNA vaccines can also be boosted by co-administration of accessory molecules, such as B7-1 (CD80) or B7-2 (CD86). Studies from two groups indicate that B7-2 co-administration with a plasmid DNA vaccine greatly boosts the immune response generated [17, 39]. This finding is somewhat surprising, as expression of B7-1 on tumor cells is more effective than expression of B7-2 in inducing protective anti-tumor immunity [18]. In addition, if DNA vaccines are expressed in professional APCs (which already express B7-1 and B7-2), it is unclear what role co-administered genes for B7-1 and B7-2 would play. Very recent studies suggest that these co-stimulatory molecule genes, when co-administered with a DNA vaccine, are both expressed on muscle cells and convert the muscle into an antigen-presenting cell (J.J. Kim et al., submitted). The ability to engineer somatic cells to become APCs has tremendous potential for altering tissue-specific immune responses.

Physiologic correlate to DNA vaccination

One question which arises with DNA vaccination is whether there is a physiological correlate in immunity. A potential correlate has recently been described by Klenerman et al. [40]. In this paper, they describe an RNA virus that infects mice. After the infection clears, they found evidence of DNA encoding the viral genes in the mouse spleens. The DNA was formed by endogenous reverse transcriptase (which many mammalian cells express). This viral DNA persisted in the mice and in mouse cell lines for some time. They postulated that this represents a naturally-occurring DNA vaccine against the virus. This implies a potentially general mechanism whereby DNA from infecting pathogens is taken up by cells. The genes encoded may be expressed to help boost immunity against the pathogen.

With this background in the basic aspects of DNA vaccination, we are now ready to address the potential applicability of this technique to inflammatory diseases.

DNA vaccination for inflammatory disease

There are several ways in which DNA vaccines can be employed to treat inflammatory diseases. As inflammatory diseases arise as a consequence of disordered immunity, one could intervene by altering the character of the immune response or inducing regulation of pathogenic cells. Both of these approaches have been tried with DNA vaccines with some success in experimental models.

Altering immune responses

As noted above, DNA vaccines in general seem to favor a TH1 type of immune response. This property can be used to advantage to alter aberrant TH2 immune responses, as TH1 and TH2 responses are often mutually antagonistic. One example of a disordered TH2 response is in the area of allergic disease and asthma. These diseases are linked to the production of IgE antibodies to specific antigens (allergens) which bind IgE receptors on mast cells. When the specific antigen cross-links the mast cell-bound IgE, histamine is released initiating an allergic response. IgE antibody production by B cells is stimulated by IL-4 and other TH2 cytokines. It stands to reason that encouraging a TH1 response to allergens would suppress IgE production and subsequent allergic responses.

At least two groups have reported that DNA immunization with an allergen suppresses IgE production. In the first, a model system was used with bacterial beta-galactosidase (β-gal) as the test antigen [31, 41]. This group used intradermal DNA vaccination with a construct encoding β-gal compared with recombinant protein immunization and monitored immune responses. They found that the β-gal gene immunization induced IgG2a subclass antibody responses and IFNγ production, both typical of TH1-mediated responses. In contrast, recombinant protein immunized animals developed IL-4 and IL-5 responses as well as IgE subclass antibodies indicating a TH2 responses. They then showed that β-gal gene inoculation prior to recombinant protein immunization prevented IgE antibody formation, and that this effect was antigen specific. Most significantly, this group demonstrated that β-gal DNA vaccination following recombinant protein vaccination (after an IgE response had already developed) down-modulated the IgE response by 66–75% [31]. Cell transfer experiments indicated that this result was mediated by both $CD4^+$ and $CD8^+$ T cells [41].

Similar results have been obtained using the gene for the house dust mite antigen [42, 43]. This group used intramuscular injection of rats with a plasmid DNA encoding a house dust mite allergen to explore the nature of the immune response, and its ability to block an IgE-mediated allergic response. They demonstrated that allergen DNA vaccination induced IgG production, prevented the induction of IgE synthesis, histamine release in bronchoalveolar fluids, and airway hyperresponsiveness in rats challenged with aerosolized allergen [42]. This effect was long-lasting, and was transferred by $CD8^+$ T cells. They also showed that rats previously immunized with the house dust mite allergen and with a pre-existing IgE response could be treated with DNA vaccination in an antigen-specific fashion with a subsequent 90% reduction in the IgE responses seen [43].

These results are not limited to allergic disorders. In the adjuvant arthritis model (AA), rats inoculated with Freund's adjuvant, which contains killed mycobacteria, develop arthritis in concert with development of immune responses to mycobacterial heat shock protein (hsp65). One group studied the effect of DNA vaccination with the hsp65 gene on the subsequent development of AA. They demonstrated significant protection from disease development in comparison with the control groups [44]. While the mechanism was not disclosed in this study, an immune response to hsp65 was clearly induced by the DNA vaccination.

These responses are postulated to involve development of certain cytokine profiles. Interestingly, direct inoculation of cytokine DNA is also capable of modulating autoimmune disease. In a murine model of systemic lupus erythematosus (SLE), Raz et al. investigated the effect of intramuscular inoculation of cytokine genes, TGFβ and IL-2 [45]. They found that TGFβ encoding plasmid treated animals had decreased anti-chromatin and rheumatoid factor antibody production, decreased total IgG production, and improved renal function. Survival was also improved to 70% at 26 weeks compared with 40% in the control group. In contrast, lupus mice that received the IL-2 gene had decreased survival (20% at 26 weeks), higher total IgG synthesis and increased autoantibody production. Thus, DNA inoculation may be useful in generalized autoimmunity as well as in antigen- specific autoimmune disease, by using cytokine genes to modulate disease. Clearly; the choice of cytokine is critical in this strategy.

Thus, it is clear that DNA vaccination shows great promise in developing genetic approaches to treating allergic and autoimmune diseases. However, these rodent models should be regarded as preliminary and will need significant additional experimentation before they are applicable to human allergic disorders.

Inducing anti-cellular immunity

Several human diseases are associated with the development of pathologic B and T cells. This includes malignancies such as lymphoma and leukemia, and autoimmune diseases, such as SLE where pathogenic autoantibodies mediate tissue injury, and autoimmune diabetes where autoreactive T cells mediate tissue destruction. Current therapy for these diseases is inadequate and treatment is associated with a high incidence of side-effects. A more logical approach to therapy for such diseases is to specifically eliminate the pathogenic B and/or T cells. This can be accomplished in a very specific fashion by targeting the antigen receptors expressed by these pathogenic cells. B cells bear surface Ig and T cells express TCR which are involved in immune recognition (see Fig. 2). These Ig and TCRs can themselves be the target of immune modulation. While many promising results have been obtained in experimental systems targeting clonotype-specific markers with a variety of immunotherapeutic approaches, these have not led to widespread clinical application. This stems at least in part from our lack of understanding of the basic immune mechanisms which lead to protective immunity. Thus, while it is clear that immunization with killed lymphoma cells [46, 47], and certain idiotype vaccines [48, 49] can induce protective anti-tumor immunity, these immunizations elicit multiple arms of the immune system (e.g.. both humoral and cellular immunity). This makes it difficult to dissect the responses responsible for protective immunity from other responses elicited which may not play a direct role.

DNA vaccines in tumor models

Targeting pathogenic cells is also a major goal in tumor-specific immunity. Several studies using DNA vaccination in tumor immunity are noted here, as they disclose principles which are useful in the development of approaches to eliminating autoreactive cells as well DNA-vaccination has been successfully used against a variety of model tumor antigens. Conry et al. [50] developed a polynucleotide vaccine against human carcinoembryonic antigen (CEA) using the CMV promoter. They used this vaccine to demonstrate that immunization of mice induced humoral and cellular immune responses [50]. Their study also demonstrated the induction of CEA-specific memory T cells by DNA vaccination. A later study by this group demonstrated that CEA DNA vaccination was capable of inducing protection from *in vivo* tumor challenge [51]. They noted that DNA vaccination was dose and schedule dependent. In their protection studies, they demonstrated that polynucleotide DNA vaccination was capable of eliciting protective responses against syngeneic CEA-transduced colon carcinoma cells as early as 3 weeks after the first vaccination.

We used a model system to investigate the utility of DNA vaccination in tumor immaturity. We employed a murine lymphoma cell which expressed human CD4 as a model tumor antigen [52]. Using human CD4 as the target antigen, we demonstrated that DNA vaccination against human CD4 elicited anti-CD4 antibodies, specific cellular proliferative responses against CD4, and CTL responses. Mice inoculated with the CD4 gene were protected from *in vivo* challenge with lymphoma cells expressing the human CD4 gene, and this protection was dependent on the timing of challenge and number of inoculations administered. Notably, the CTL response in mice which survived tagged-lymphoma challenge was markedly accentuated. These studies indicate the feasibility of using DNA inoculation to evoke protective immune responses against a model tumor antigen. They also suggest an important role for CTL responses in mediating protective immunity.

In a similar series of experiments, Irvine et al. [53] investigated the utility of DNA vaccination against a model tumor antigen using a pulmonary metastatic tumor which expressed the β-galactosidase gene. They demonstrated that epidermal DNA immunization against β-galactosidase (β-gal) induced specific antibody and cytolytic responses. They further demonstrated that DNA immunization against β-gal protected from pulmonary metastatic tumor, and that adoptive transfer of spleenocytes which were activated *in vitro* reduced the number of established pulmonary nodules. These authors found that while DNA immunization alone has no effect on established pulmonary metastases, significant reduction in the number of established metastases was observed if rIL-2, rIL-6, rIL-7, or particularly rIL-12 were given after DNA inoculation. This indicates the potential for DNA immunization to treat established tumors as well as to prevent tumor formation.

DNA immunization has also been shown to be effective in inducing CTL responses against a single epitope from a mutant form of the human p53 gene [54]. Using a minigene coding for a single epitope derived from mutant p53, these authors demonstrated that particle bombardment-mediated DNA transfer into the skin of mice induced CTL responses. This CTL response was enhanced if the DNA vaccine was fused in frame with the adenovirus E3 leader sequence, targeting the vaccine to the endoplasmic reticulum. This indicates that intracellular targeting can have a significant impact on the character of the immune responses elicited by DNA vaccines.

These studies establish the potential utility of DNA vaccination against model tumor antigens. However, all of the antigens used were in fact foreign proteins which typically are much more immunogenic than tumor antigens (which are self-antigens), which are the clinically relevant targets for cancer immunotherapy. A recent study by Syrengelas et al. [55] used the V_H and V_L regions of a murine lymphoma in an expression vector also encoding the human $C_\gamma l$ and C_κ with or without linked expression of human GM-CSF. Thus, their immunogen also had foreign antigenic determinants (human constant regions) linked to the self-V regions of interest. They demonstrated that intramuscular or intradermal DNA inoculation with these constructs resulted in an anti-idiotypic antibody response, as well as partial protection from tumor challenge *in vivo*. The linked expression of human GM-CSF markedly enhanced the responses elicited. They concluded that DNA immunization could induce immune responses against a weak, otherwise unrecognized tumor antigen, but that this was dependent on additional stimuli encoded by DNA (i.e. the human constant regions and GM-CSF).

A similar study has recently been published using a DNA vaccine against a lymphoma idiotype coupled to tetanus toxin fragment C [56]. These authors developed a DNA vaccine which fused the heavy and light chain variable regions (V_H and V_L respectively) to form a V_H-V_L heterodimer, also known as an F_V region. They compared a DNA vaccine encoding the F_V with one which fused the F_V region to tetanus toxin fragment C. They found a 50-fold enhancement in tumor-specific antibody responses, and these were largely directed against the Ig idiotype. A predominance of IgG2a antibodies was shown, consistent with a TH1 response.

These studies indicate the feasibility of developing anti-cellular immunity targeting lymphocyte variable regions with DNA vaccines.

DNA vaccines in autoimmune models

Idiotype-specific immunity can also modulate autoimmune disease when the pathogenic T cells are known by targeting their TCR. This approach was taken by Waisman et al. [57]. They used the model system of experimental allergic encephalomyelitis (EAE). EAE can be induced in susceptible mice by immunization with myelin basic protein (MBP), which is a protein found in the myelin sheath of neurons. These mice develop demyelination and a clinical picture similar to multiple sclerosis. Intact MBP and oligopeptides derived from the MBP sequence are both capable inducing EAE. MBP-reactive T cells in susceptible mice are dominated by T cells expressing TCRs encoded by the Vβ8 gene. Prior studies had shown that immunization of mice with peptides from Vβ8 is able to modulate the disease [58, 59]. Waisman et al. used the Vβ8 gene to immunize susceptible mice prior to the induction of EAE. They found that Vβ8 DNA vaccination completely protected mice from EAE-induced by MBP-peptide immunization, and partially protected

A Expression vector — Inserts and targeting strategy

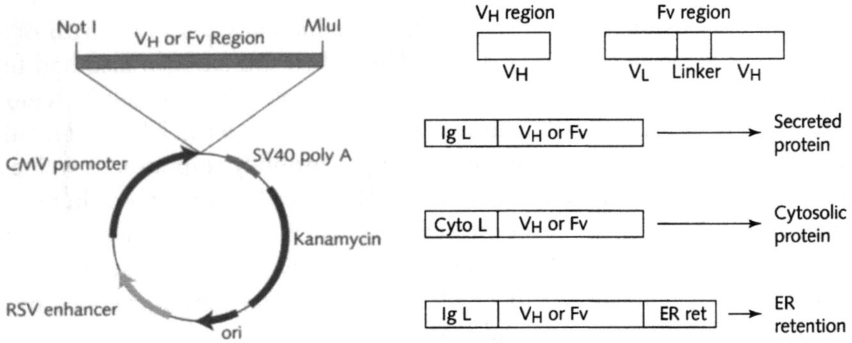

B Sequences of inserts

Immunoglobulin Leader (Ig L) for Secretion or ER Retention
Met asp met arg val pro ala gln leu leu gly leu leu leu leu trp leu pro gly ala lys cys ser arg

Cytosolic Leader (Cyto L)
Met gly trp ser cys lys arg arg ser ser glu glu thr ala thr ala gly val his ser arg

Anti-DNA IL/IM (H221) VL Region
asp ile val ile ser gln ser pro ser thr leu ala val ser ala gly glu lys val thr met asn cys lys ser ser gln ser leu phe asn ser arg thr arg lys asn tyr leu ala trp phe gln gln lys pro gly gln ser pro lys leu leu ile tyr trp ala ser thr arg glu ser gly val pro asp arg phe thr gly ser gly ser gly thr asp phe thr leu thr ile ser ser val gln ala glu asp leu ala val tyr tyr cys lys gln ser tyr tyr leu arg thr phe gly gly gly thr arg leu glu

Linker
arg ala asp ala ala glu gly lys ser ser gly ser gly ser glu ser lys ser tyr gln gly ser glu ser lys ser tyr gln

Anti-DNA IL/IM (H221) VH Region
glu val gln len gln gln ser gly ala glu leu val lys ser gly ala ser val lys leu ser cys lys ala ser gly phe thr phe thr ser tyr trp ile asn trp val lys gln arg ala gly gln gly leu glu trp ile gly asn ile tyr pro gly ser asn thr ile asn tyr ser glu asn phe lys lys lys ala thr leu thr val asp thr ser ser ser thr ala tyr met gln leu ser ser leu thr ser asp asp ser ala val tyr tyr cys ala arg glu arg leu leu gly phe val tyr trp gly gln gly thr leu val thr val ser thr ala lys thr thr ala

CD4 transmembrane and E19 cytoplasmie Domains (ER ret) for ER retention
met ala leu ile val leu gly gly val ala gly leu leu leu phe ile gly leu gly ile phe phe arg ser arg arg ser phe ile asp glu lys lys met pro

mice from EAE induced by intact MBP immunization. This effect was not due to depletion of Vβ8+ T cells from the mice, but rather due to an alteration in the character of the immune response elicited. Normally in the development of EAE and strong TH1 -type of response develops. DNA vaccination with the Vβ8 gene diminished IL-2, TNFα and IFNγ production in response to MBP while enhancing IL-4 and IL-10 production. Thus, Vβ8-gene immunization shifted the cytokine profiles and induced protective immunity against autoimmunity in this model.

We have performed preliminary studies to evaluate DNA vaccination against an autoantibody V region. The autoantibody-producing hybridoma anti-DNA IL/IM (also called H221) was selected from a large panel of hybridomas derived from MRL-1pr/lpr mice [60]; when anti-DNA IL/IM producing hybridoma cells are administered intraperitoneally to histocompatible mice, they produce glomerulonephritis, characterized by dense intramembranous and intraluminal deposits, associated with capillary wall thickening, mesangial interposition and expansion, aneurysmal dilatation and intraluminal occlusion of glomerular capillary loops, and heavy proteinuria. This provides an *in vivo* system in which we could evaluate the efficacy of DNA vaccination targeting a pathogenic autoantibody V region in eliciting protective immunity.

We cloned the heavy and light chain variable (V) regions of anti-DNA IL/IM into a standard DNA vaccine vector (Fig. 3). As noted above, antigen processing is handled differently in different intracellular compartments. To investigate the effect of targeting these DNA vaccines to distinct intracellular compartments, gene expression was targeted to specific intracellular versus extracellular compartments (cytosolic, endoplasmic reticulum (ER) for secretion, and ER for retention). Vaccination against a single V region (the V_H region) and against the entire F_V (V_H linked to V_L) fragment were employed. The gene constructs developed are shown in Figure 3. Ini-

Figure 3.
(A) Structure of DNA vaccines. The DNA vaccine backbone used was the pBBkan backbone [61]. This uses the CMV promoter and RSV enhancer to drive transcription. The inserts are shown below, with V_H or F_V (V_L linked to V_H) regions following a leader peptide (either a hydrophobic leader from murine IgG (Ig Leader), or a hydrophilic leader for cytosolic targeting [62] (Cyto Leader)), and an added transmembrane and cytosolic tail with an endoplasmic reticulum retention signal (CD4 TM and E19 Cyto).
(B) Sequences of the V regions and targeting sequences. A murine immunoglobulin leader sequence was used to target the gene product to the ER for secretion or ER retention. The cytosolic leader was a sequence previously reported for intracellular expression of antibodies [62]. The V_H and V_L sequences were determined following cloning of the PCR products. The linker peptide is one previously used by our group and others for functional expression of F_H regions [63]. The human CD4 transmembrane region was combined with the adenovirus E19 targeting sequence for ER retention [64].

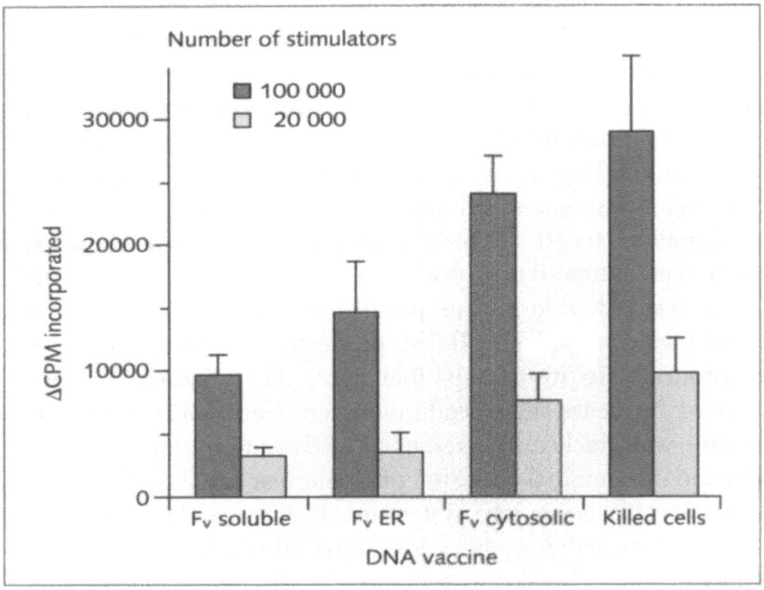

Figure 4
Proliferative response of spleenocytes following DNA inoculation.
Mice were inoculated once with 100 µg plasmid DNA in 0.25% bupivacaine. The vaccines were: F_V soluble (DNA vaccine using the F_V region targeted to the ER for secretion); F_V ER (DNA vaccine using the F_V region retained in the ER); and F_V cytosolic (DNA vaccine using the F_V region targeted to the cytosol). Killed cells refers to 5×10^6 irradiated (10 000 rads) H221 hybridoma cells. One week later, the splenocytes (5×10^5/well) were removed and incubated either in media alone or with killed H221 cells. Proliferation was evaluated by stimulating the immune splenocytes with killed anti-DNA IL/AM hybridoma cells (20 000 or 100 000/well). Following a 3-day culture, the cells were pulsed overnight with tritiated thymidine, and counts per minute (CPM) incorporated determined. The mean ΔCPM (experimental minus media only) ± the standard deviation of triplicate wells is shown for two concentrations of killed H221 cells.

tial studies indicated that the isolated V_H genes were poorly immunogenic, so we focused our studies on the FV constructs. Initially, we vaccinated histocompatible (but not syngeneic) AKR × DBA/2 mice with the constructs and monitored them for the development of anti-idiotypic antibody responses. No discernible antibody responses were elicited with these constructs even following several boosts.

However, we did see evidence of cellular immune responses even following a single vaccination. These studies employed fully syngeneic MRL-lpr/lpr x Balb/c mice. Groups of five MRL-lpr/lpr × Balb/c mice were immunized once with 100 µg plas-

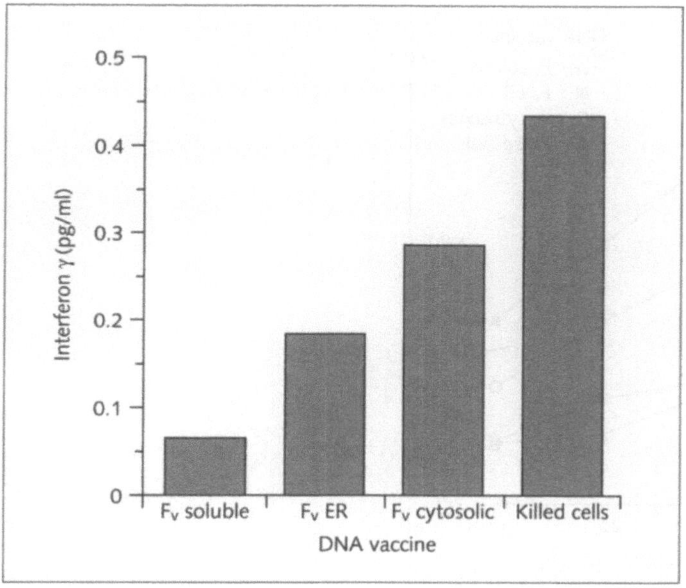

Figure 5
IFNγ production by spleenocytes following DNA inoculation.
Mice were inoculated with vaccines and splenocyte cultures set-up 1 week later as noted in Fig. 4. Following a 3-day culture, supernatants were removed and assayed for IFNγ using a commercially available kit (Genzyme, Cambridge, MA). Abbreviations are as in Fig. 4. The mean IFNγ produced for groups of five mice is shown for splenocytes stimulated with 100 000 killed H221 cells.

mid DNA in 0.25% bupivacaine simultaneously. One week later, they were sacrificed and evaluated for cytotoxic T cell and proliferative responses. Proliferation was evaluated by stimulating the immune splenocytes with 20 000 or 100 000 killed anti-DNA IL/IM hybridoma cells for 72 h, followed by a pulse with tritiated thymidine overnight. The results are shown in Figure 4. Clearly the weakest immunogen for stimulating proliferation was the secreted construct, while the ER-retained and cytosolic targeted constructs elicited higher proliferative responses. The cytosolic construct elicited responses nearly as high as inoculation with killed anti-DNA IL/IM cells (which was the positive control). A similar result was found for IFNγ production in these cultures (Fig. 5), with the cytosolic construct inducing production of levels of IFNγ close to those elicited by killed cell vaccination. In parallel with the proliferation result, the ER-retained construct was less potent, while the soluble construct elicited the weakest response. CTL activity was also assessed in

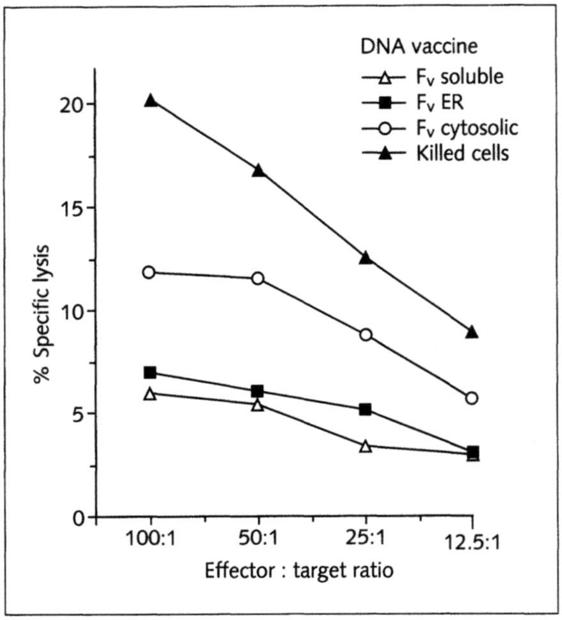

Figure 6
Cytotoxic T cell (CTL) response following a single DNA inoculation.
Mice were inoculated once with 100 μg plasmid DNA in 0.25% bupivacalne or with 5 × 10⁶ killed H221 cells. One week later, the splenocytes were removed and incubated with concanavalin A and killed H221 cells (20:1 effector:stimulator ratio). After 24–48 h the Con A was removed, the cells fed, and the culture continued for 5 days total. Following the 5-day culture, the effector cells were isolated by discontinuous gradient centrifugation, and used to lyse ^{51}Cr labeled H221 target cells at the various ratios shown. The % specific lysis was calculated, and the mean % specific lysis is shown for triplicate determinations.

these experiments, with the result shown in Figure 6. The target cells used here were the anti-DNA IL/IM hybridoma cells. While the levels of lysis seen were only modest in these experiments, it is clear that the killed cell immunization did elicit cytolytic activity, as did the cytosolic construct. The ER-retained and soluble constructs did not elicit significant CTL activity.

To evaluate the efficacy of these DNA vaccines in protecting from challenge with autoantibody-producing hybridoma cells *in vivo*, we used histocompatible AKR × DBA/2 mice (due to their commercial availability). Groups of six mice were immunized intramuscularly three times with 100 μg of the DNA vaccines in 0.25% bupivacaine or with 5×10^6 killed anti-DNA IL/IM hybridoma cells. The mice were challenged with anti-DNA IL/IM hybridoma cells intraperitoneally. Four weeks later, the mice were evaluated for tumor burden and mortality. The results are shown in Fig-

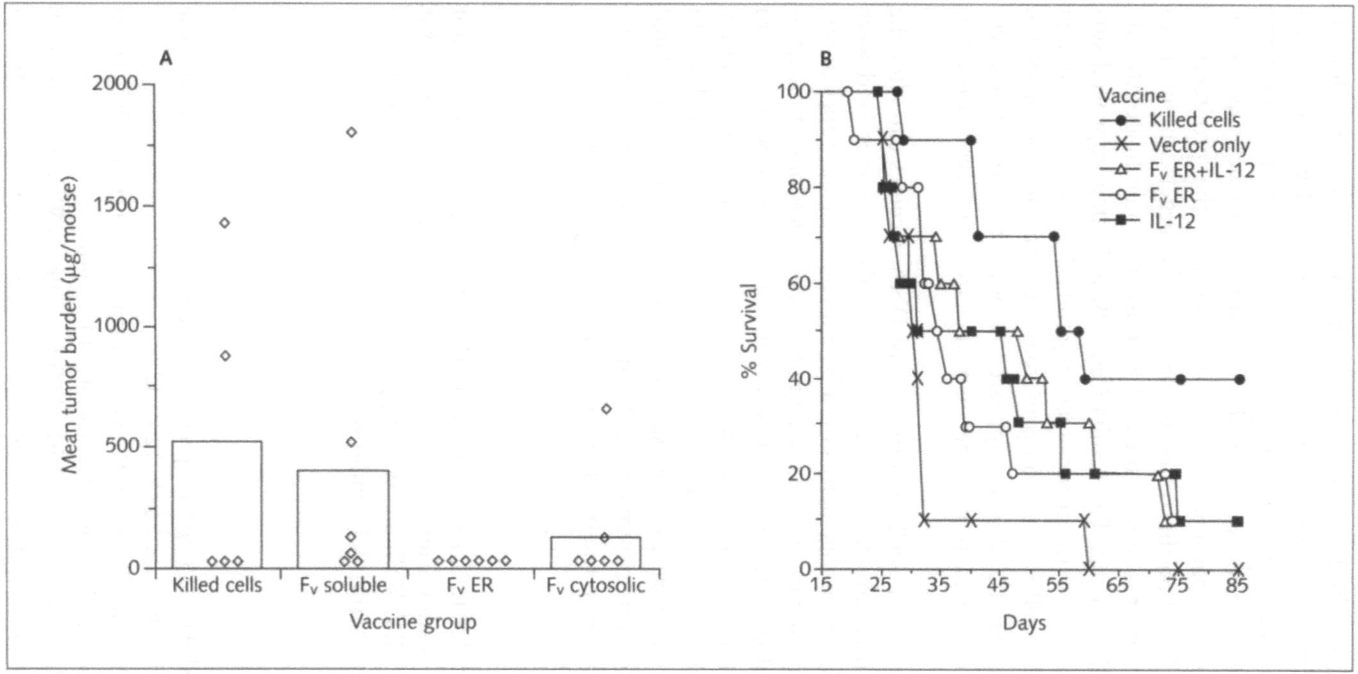

Figure 7.

Survival and tumor burden following DNA inoculation and challenge.

Groups of six mice were inoculated three times at biweekly intervals with 100 μg, of the various DNA vaccines in, bupivacalne, and challenged with 10^6 live H221 cells intraperitoneany one week later. Four weeks later all mice with tumors or ascites were sacrificed, tumors excised and tumor burden determined. (A) Tumor mass for each vaccinated group. The mean value is shown in a bar graph, with the values for individual mice superimposed. (B) In a similar experiment, groups of 10 mice were inoculated three times at biweekly intervals with 100 μg of the F_V ER DNA vaccines in bupivacaine with or without IL-12 encoding plasmids [16], or with IL-12 plasmid alone. One week later the mice were challenged with 1.5×10^6 live H221 cells intraperitoneally, and followed for mortality.

ure 7A. Several of the DNA vaccines showed specific effects, as evidenced by reduced mean tumor burden. The F_V ER-retained vaccine prevented tumor formation in 6/6 mice at this timepoint, compared with 3/6 immunized with the killed cells. The F_V cytosolic construct appeared to reduce tumor burden, but tumors were found in 4/6 of these mice on autopsy. Again, the F_V soluble construct was poorly protective in this experiment, paralleling the results seen in the proliferation, cytokine and CTL assays. Based on this result, we performed a larger experiment to determine if the protective effect seen with the F_V ER construct could be boosted by co-administration of the IL-12 gene. The results (Fig. 7B) indicated improved survival compared with vector only in the groups receiving the DNA vaccines, although in this experiment the killed cell vaccination protected a greater proportion of the mice. Co-administration of the IL-12 genes appeared to boost the protective effect seen, although IL-12 gene inoculation alone also appeared to have anti-tumor effects.

These results indicate that intracellular targeting of DNA vaccines can alter the immune responses elicited. Although the variable region DNA vaccines used were poorly immunogenic, their immunogenicity could be enhanced by appropriate targeting of the vaccines to specific intracellular compartments. This is one of the great advantages of this technology: the ease with which the antigen can be altered to probe the effects of a variety of manipulations on the immune responses elicited. The studies cited herein point out the tremendous potential of this technology. In human studies, these vaccines have appeared safe with over 100 patients inoculated to date. While this vaccine strategy remains in its infancy, there is a great potential for applying DNA vaccination to the treatment of inflammatory conditions.

Acknowledgments

We would like to acknowledge L.G. for inspiration. M.M. was supported by a grant from NIH. D.B. Weiner was supported by grants from the American Foundation for AIDS Research and NIH. W.V. Williams was supported by grants from the American Cancer Society and the Arthritis Foundation.

References

1 Nabel EG, Plautz G, Nabel GJ (1990) Site-specific gene expression *in vivo* by direct gene transfer into the arterial wall. *Science* 249: 1285–1288

2 Wolff JA, Malone RW, Williams P, Chong W, Acsadi G, Jani A, Feigner PL (1990) Direct gene transfer into mouse muscle *in vivo*. *Science* 247: 1465–1468

3 Acsadi G, Dickson G, Love DR, Jani A, Walsh FS, Gurusinghe A, Wolff JA, Davies KE (199 1) Human dystrophin expression in mdx mice after intramuscular injection of DNA constructs. *Nature* 352: 815–818

4 Israe' MA, Chan TW, Hourihan SL, Rowe WP, Martin MA (1979) Biological activity of polyma viral DNA in mice and hamsters. *J Virol* 29: 990–996

5 Tang DC, De Vit M, Johnston SA (1992) Genetic immunization is a simple method for eliciting an immune response. *Nature* 356: 152–154

6 Fynan EF, Robinson HL, Webster RG (1993) Use of DNA encoding influenza hemagglutin and avian influenza vaccine DNA. *DNA and Cell Biology* 12: 785–789

7 Ulmer JB, Donnelly JJ, Parker SE, Rhodes GH, Feigner PL, Dwarki VJ, Gromkowski SH, Deck RR, De Witt CM, Friedman A et al (1993) Heterologous protection against influenza by injection of DNA encoding a viral protein. *Science* 259: 1745–1749

8 Wang B, Ugen KE, Srikantan V, Agadjanyan MG, Dang K, Refaeli Y, Sato Al, Boyer J, Williams WV, Weiner DB (1993) Gene inoculation generates immune responses against human immunodeficiency virus type 1. *Proc Natl Acad Sci USA* 90: 4156–4160

9 Cheng L, Ziegelhoffer PR, Yang NS (1993) *In vivo* promoter activity and transgene expression in mammalian somatic tissues evaluated by using particle bombardment. *Proc Natl Acad Sci USA* 90: 4455–4459

10 Carson DA, Raz E (1997) Oligonucleotide adjuvants for T helper I (Th 1)-specific vaccination. *J Exp Med* 186: 1621–1622

11 Klinman DM, Yi AK, Beaucage SL, Conover J, Krieg AM (1996) CpG motifs present in bacteria DNA rapidly induce lymphocytes to secrete interleukin 6, interleukin 12, and interferon gamma. *Proc Natl Acad Sci USA* 93: 2879–2883

12 Krieg AM, Yi AK. Matson S, Waldschmidt TJ, Bishop GA, Teasdale R, Koretzky GA, Klinman DM (1995) CpG motifs in bacterial DNA trigger direct B-cell activation. *Nature* 374: 546–549

13 Sato Y, Roman M, Tighe H, Lee D, Corr M, Nguyen MD, Silverman GJ, Lotz M, Carson DA, Raz E (1996) immunostimulatory DNA sequences necessary for effective intradermal gene immunization. *Science* 273: 352–354

14 Yi AK, Chace JH, Cowdery JS, Krieg AM (1996) IFN-gamma promotes IL-6 and IgM secretion in response to CpG motifs in bacterial DNA and oligodeoxynucleotides. *J Immunol* 156: 558–564

15 Xiang Z, Ertl HC (1995) Manipulation of the immune response to a plasmid-encoded viral antigen by coinoculation with plasmids expressing cytokines. *Immunity* 2: 129–135

16 Kim JJ, Ayyavoo V, Bagarazzi ML, Chattergoon MA, Dang K, Wang B, Boyer JD, Weiner DB (1997) *In vivo* engineering of a cellular immune response by co-administration of IL-12 expression vector with a DNA immunogen. *J Immunol* 158: 816–826

17 Kim JJ, Bagarazzi ML, Trivedi N, Hu Y, Kazahaya K, Wilson DM, Ciccarelli R, Chattergoon MA, Dang K, Mahalingarn S, Chalian AA, Agadjanyan MG, Boyer JD, Wang B, Weiner DB (1997) Engineering of *in vivo* immune responses to DNA immunization via co-delivery of co-stimulator molecule genes. *Nat Biotechnol* 15: 641–646

18 Bueler H, Mulligan RC (1996) Induction of antigen- specific tumor immunity by genetic and cellular vaccines against MAGE: enhanced tumor protection by co-expression of granulocyte-macrophage colony-stimulating factor and B7-1. *Mol Med* 2: 545–555

19 Coney L, Wang B, Ugen KE, Boyer J, McCallus D, Srikantan V, Agadjanyan M, Pachuk CJ, Herold K, Merva M et al (1994) Facilitated DNA inoculation induces anti-HIV- I immunity *in vivo*. *Vaccine* 12: 1545–1550
20 Johnston SA, Tang DC (1993) The use of microparticle injection to introduce genes into animal cells *in vitro* and *in vivo*. *Genet Eng* 15: 225–236
21 Johnston SA, Tang DC (1994) Gene gun transfection of animal cells and genetic immunization. *Methods Cell Biol* 43: 353–365
22 Flynn EF, Webster RG, Fuller DH, Haynes JR, Santoro JC, Robinson HL (1993) DNA vaccines: protective immunizations by parenteral, mucosal, and gene-gun inoculations. *Proc Natl Acad Sci USA* 90: 11478–11482
23 Livingston JB, Lu S, Robinson HL, Anderson DJ (1995) The induction of mucosal immunity in the female genital tract using gene-gun technology. Part 1: Antigen expression. *Ann NY Acad Sci* 772: 265–257
24 Wang B, Dang K, Agadjanyan MG, Srikantan V, Li F, Ugen KE, Boyer J, Merva M, Williams WV, Weiner DB (1997) Mucosal immunization with a DNA vaccine induces immune responses against HIV-1 at a mucosal site. *Vaccine* 15: 821–825
25 Okada E, Sasaki S, Ishii N, Aoki I, Yasuda T, Nishioka K, Fukushima J, Miyazaki J, Wahren B, Okuda K (1997) Intranasal immunization of a DNA vaccine with IL-12- and granulocyte-macrophage colony-stimulating factor (GM-CSF)-expressing plasmids in liposomes induces strong mucosal and cell-mediated immune responses against HIV-1 antigens. *J Immunol* 159: 3638–3647
26 Corr M, Lee DJ, Carson DA, Tighe H (1996) Gene vaccination with naked plasmid DNA: mechanism of CTL priming. *J Exp Med* 184: 1555–1560
27 Fu TM, Ulmer JB, Caulfield MJ, Deck RR, Friedman A, Wang S, Liu X, Donnelly JJ, Liu MA (1997) Priming of cytotoxic T lymphocytes by DNA vaccines: requirement for professional antigen presenting cells and evidence for antigen transfer from myocytes. *Mol Med* 3: 362–371
28 Iwaski A, Torres CA, Ohashi PS, Robinson HL, Barber BH (1991) The dominant role of bone marrow-derived cells in CTL induction following plasmid DNA immunization at different sites. *J Immunol* 159: 11–14
29 Doe B, Selby M, Barnett S, Baenziger J, Walker CM (1996) Induction of cytotoxic T lymphocytes by intramuscular immunization with plasmid DNA is facilitated by bone marrow-derived cells. *Proc Natl Acad Sci USA* 93: 8578–8583
30 Martinez X, Brandt C, Saddallah F, Tougne C, Barrios C, Wild F, Dougan G, Lambert PH, Siegrist CA (1997) DNA immunization circumvents deficient induction of T helper type I and cytotoxic T lymphocyte responses in neonates and during early life. *Proc Natl Acad Sci USA* 94: 8726–8731
31 Raz E, Tighe H, Sato Y, Corr M, Dudler JA, Roman M, Swain SL, Spiegelberg HL, Carson DA (1996) Preferential induction of a Thl immune response and inhibition of specific IgE antibody formation by plasmid DNA immunization. *Proc Natl Acad Sci USA* 93: 5141–5145
32 Inchauspe G, Vitvitski L, Major ME, Jung G, Spengler U, Maisonnas M, Trepo C (1997)

Plasinid DNA expressing a secreted or a non-secreted form of hepatitis C virus nucleocapsid: comparative studies of antibody and T-helper responses following genetic immunization. *DNA and Cell Biology* 16: 185–195
33 Barry MA, Johnston SA (1997) Biological features of genetic immunization. *Vaccine* 15: 788–791
34 Feltquate DM, Heaney S, Webster RG, Robinson HL (1997) Different T helper cell types and antibody isotypes generated by saline and gene gun DNA immunization. *J Immunol* 158: 2278–2284
35 Pertmer TM, Roberts TR, Haynes JR (1996) Influenza virus nucleoprotein-specific immunoglobulin G subclass and cytokine responses elicited by DNA vaccination are dependent on the route of vector DNA delivery. *J Virol* 70: 6119–6125
36 Leclerc C, Deroaid E, Rojas M, Whalen RG (1997) The preferential induction of a Th 1 immune response by DNA-based immunization is mediated by the immunostimulatory effect of plasmid. *DNA and Cell Immunology* 179: 97–106
37 Halpern MD, Kurlander RJ, Pisetsky DS (1996) Bacterial DNA induces murine interferon-γ production by stimulation of interleukin-12 and tumor necrosis factor-α. *Cell Immunol* 1: 72–78
38 Maecker HT, Umetsu DT, DeKruyff RH, Levy S (1997) DNA vaccination with cytokine fusion constructs biases the immune response to ovalbumin Vaccine 15: 1687–1696
39 Iwasaki A, Stiernholm BJ, Chan AK, Berinstein NL, Barber BH (1997) Enhanced CTL responses mediated by plasmid DNA immunogens encoding costimulatory molecules and cytokines. *J Immunol* 158: 4591–601
40 Klenerman P, Hengartner H, Zinkernagel RM (1997) A non-retroviral RNA virus persists in DNA form. *Nature* 390: 298–301
41 Lee DJ, Tighe H, Corr M, Roman M, Carson DA, Spiegelberg HL, Raz E (1997) Inhibition of IgE antibody formation by plasmid DNA immunization is mediated by both $CD4^+$ and $CD8^+$ T cells Int. *Arch Allergy Immunol* 113: 227–230
42 Hsu CH, Chua KY, Tao MH, Lai YL, Wu HD, Huang SK, Hsieh KH (1996) Immunoprophylaxis of allergen-induced immunoglobulin E synthesis and airway hyperresponsiveness *in vivo* by genetic immunization. *Nat Med* 2: 540–544
43 Hsu CH, Chua KY, Tao MH, Huang SK, Hsieh KH (1996) Inhibition of specific IgE response *in vivo* by allergen-gene transfer. *Int Immunol* 8: 1405–1411
44 Ragno S, Colston MJ, Lowrie DB, Winrow VR, Blake DR, Tascon R (1997) Protection of rats from adjuvant arthritis by immunization with naked DNA encoding for mycobacterial heat shock protein 65. *Arthritis Rheum* 40: 277–283
45 Raz E.DudlerJ, Lotz M, Baird SM, Berry CC, Eisenberg RA, Carson DA (1995) Modulation of disease activity in murine systemic lupus erythematosus by cytokine gene delivery. *Lupus* 4: 286–292
46 Ghosh SK, Wong J, Banked RB (1987) Idiotype- specific T lymphocytes responsible for the selection 6T somatic variants of a B cell hybrid. *J Immunol* 145: 365–370
47 Ghosh SK, White LM, Ghosh R, Bankert RB (1990) Vaccination with membrane asso-

ciated idiotype provides greater and more prolonged protection of animals from tumor challenge than the soluble form of idiotype. *J Immunol* 145: 365–370

48 Campbell MJ, Esserman L, Byars NE, Allison AC, Levy R (1990) Idiotype vaccination against murine B cell lymphoma. Humoral and cellular requirements for the full expression of antitumor Immunity. *J Immunol* 145: 1029–1036

49 Tao M-H, Levy R (1993) Idiotype/granulocyte-macrophage colony-stimulating factor fusion protein as a vaccine for B-cell lymphoma. *Nature* 362: 755–758

50 Conry RM, Lo Buglio AF, Kantor J, Schlom J, Loechel F, Moore SE, Sumerel LA, Barlow DL, Abrams S, Curiel DT (1994) Immune response to a carcinoembryonic antigen polynucleotide vaccine. *Cancer Res* 54: 1164–1168

51 Conry RM, Lo Buglio AF, Loechel F, Moore SE, Sumerel LA, Barlow DL, Curiel DT (1995) A carcinoembryonic antigen polynucleotide vaccine has *in vivo* antitumor activity. *Gene Ther* 2: 59–65

52 Wang B, Merva M, Dang K, Ugen KE, Williams WV, Weiner DB (1995) Immunization by direct DNA inoculation induces rejection of tumor cell challenge. *Hum Gene Ther* 6: 407–418

53 Irvine KR, Rao JB, Rosenberg SA, Restifo NP (1996) Cytokine enhancement of DNA immunization leads to effective treatment of established pulmonary metastases. *J Immunol* 156: 238–245

54 Ciernik T, Berzofsky JA, Carbone DP (1996) Induction of cytotoxic T lymphocytes and antitumor immunity with DNA vaccines expressing single T cell epitopes. *J Immunol* 156: 2369–2375

55 Syrengelas AD, Chen TT, Levy R (1996) DNA immunization induces protective immunity against B-cell lymphoma. *Nat Med* 2: 1038–1041

56 Spellerberg MB, Zhu D, Thompsett A, King CA, Hamblin TJ, Stevenson FK (1997) DNA vaccines against lymphoma: promotion of anti-idiotypic antibody responses induced by single chain F_V genes by fusion to tetanus toxin fragment C. *J Immunol* 159: 1885–1892

57 Waisman A, Ruiz PJ, Hirschberg DL, Gelman A, Oksenberg JR, Brocke S, Mor F, Cohen IR, Steinman L (1996) Suppressive vaccination with DNA encoding a variable region gene of the T-cell receptor prevents autoirnmime encephalomyelitis and activates Th2 immunity. *Nat Med* 2: 899–905

58 Desquenne-Clark L, Esch TR, Otvos L, Heber-Katz E (1991) T-cell receptor peptide immunization leads to enhanced and chronic experimental allergic encephalomyelitis. *Proc Natl Acad Sci USA* 88: 7219–7223

59 Howell M, Winters S, Olee T, Powell H, Carlo D, Brostoff S (1989) Vaccination against experimental allergic encephalomyelitis with T cell receptor peptides.. *Science* 246: 668–670

60 Vlahakos DV. Foster MH, Adams S, Katz M, Uccl AA, Barrett KJ, Datta SK, Madaio MP (1992) Anti-DNA antibodies form immune deposits at distinct glomerular and vascular sites. *Kidney Int* 41: 1690–1700

61 Boyer JD, Wang B, Ugen K-E, Agadjanyan M, Javadian A, Frost P, Dang K, Carrano

RA, Ciccarelli R, Coney L, Williams WV, Weiner DB (1996) *In vivo* protective anti-HIV immune responses in non-human primates through DNA immunization. *J Med Primatol* 25: 242–250

62 Biocca S, Neuberger MS, Cattaneo A (1990) Expresssion and targeting of intracellular antibodies in mammalian cells. *EMBO J* 9: 101–108

63 Srikantan V, Wang B, Satre MA, Ugen KE, Dang K, Scales F, Godillot AP, Williams WV, Weiner DB (1994) Cloning and biological characterization of human single-chain F_v fragments that mediate neutralization of HIV-1. *Aids* 8: 1525–1532

64 Nilsson T, Jackson M, Peterson PA (1989) Short cytoplasmic sequences serve as retention signals for transmembrane proteins in the endoplasmic reticulum. *Cell* 58: 707–719

Naked DNA as a gene delivery vehicle in inflammatory diseases

Masayuki Miyata, Yukio Sato and Reiji Kasukawa

Department of Internal Medicine II, Fukushima University School of Medicine, Fukushima 960-1295, Japan

Introduction

The systemic injection of cytokines and related peptide is being used therapeutically with increasing success in animal models of inflammatory diseases. However, its applications are limited, because of the need for large amounts of purified proteins and the short-lived effects of these proteins. As described in the chapter by Evans and Robbins, this volume, gene transfer strategies offer novel possibilities for overcoming these limitations.

Gene transfer utilizing naked DNA is one strategy being evaluated in this regard. We describe here the therapeutic application of naked DNA for the synthesis of immunomodulatory molecules such as cytokines, in inflammatory diseases.

Manipulation of antibody production by naked DNA (plasmid DNA) encoding IL-2, IL-4 or TGFβ_1

Topical administration of plasmids encoding cytokines were first investigated by Raz et al. [1]. They injected plasmids encoding interleukin-2 (IL-2), IL-4 or transforming growth factor β_1 (TGFβ_1) (p-IL-2, p-IL-4 or p-TGFβ_1) directly into mouse skeletal muscle, to study the systemic immunological effects of the respective proteins.

They found intramuscular injection of p-IL-2 or p-IL-4 enhanced antibody production to the immunizing antigen (keyhole limpet hemocyanin: KLH) injected at the same site as that of plasmid. In contrast, p-TGFβ_1, whose product TGFβ_1 is known to antagonize the effects of IL-2 in *in vitro* experiments, suppressed the production of antibody as shown in Figure 1A. Intramuscular injection of p-IL-2 or p-TGFβ_1 influenced similarly the production of antibodies to transferrin injected at the different site from that of the plasmid, demonstrating that the cytokines influence immune responses not only locally but also systemically as shown in Figure 1B.

Gene Therapy in Inflammatory Diseases, edited by C. H. Evans and P. D. Robbins

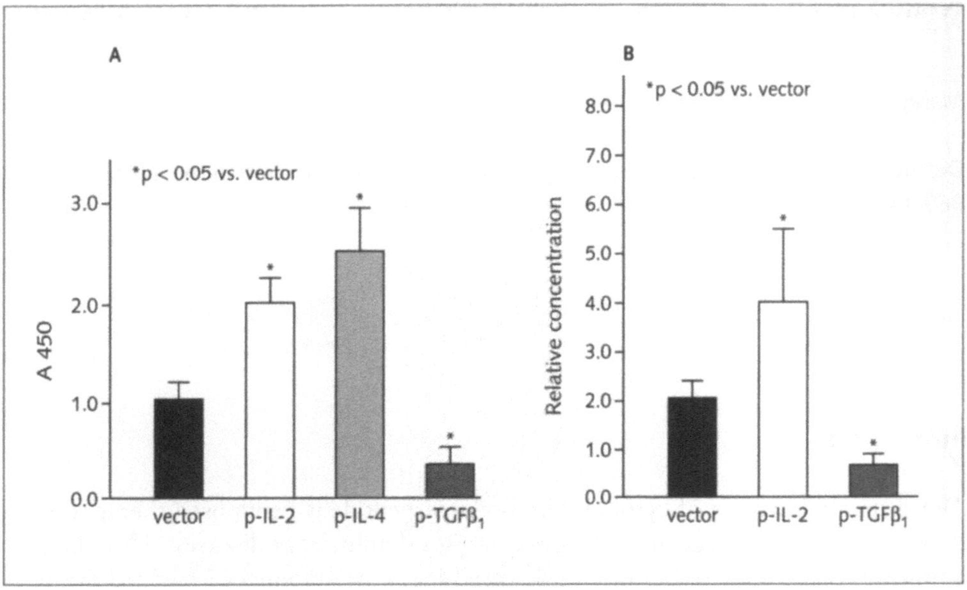

Figure 1
Effects of cytokine gene injections on antibody responses.
Groups of four BALB/c mice were injected i.m. on days 0, 7 and 14 with p-IL-2, p-IL-4 or p-TGFβ_1 (A). On day 3, 10, and 17, the animals were immunized at the same site with keyhole limpet hemocyanin; KLH. Following the same time schedule of injection, a group of eight mice were injected with expression vectors for IL-2 or TGFβ_1 (B). However, here the animals were immunized at a separate site, with human transferrin.
Antibody responses were measured by ELISA. Representative data observed week 10 were shown in A and B, respectively.
(From [1], reproduced by permission with modification.)

Their results demonstrate that the topical administration of plasmids encoding cytokines can regulate immune responses.

Subsequent to this report, several applications of this form of therapy on animal models of inflammatory diseases have been reported. Two experimental applications of p-TGFβ_1 in murine lupus nephritis by Raz et al. [2] and experimental rat colitis by Giladi et al. [3] will be presented, and then, two experimental applications of IL-10, which ameliorates the effects of proinflammatory cytokines and converts a T helper (Th)1-immune response to a Th2-immune response, on herpetic stromal keratitis in mice by Daheshia et al. [4] and murine collagen-induced arthritis by us [5] will be presented.

Murine lupus nephritis

Raz et al. [2] evaluated the effects of intramuscular injections of p-TGFβ_1 or p-IL-2 into MRL/lpr/lpr mice. TGFβ_1 was used since it is a potent suppressor of the proliferation of CD4$^+$ and CD8$^+$ T lymphocytes and thymocytes, and downregulates MHC class II expression [6]. By contrast, IL-2 stimulates immune responses.

In their experiment, p-TGFβ_1 exhibited beneficial effects on murine lupus leading to a prolongation of survival, up to 26 weeks in 80% of treated animals compared with 40% of animals in the control group. Decreases in the total IgG production and the antinuclear antibody titers, and a decrease in the severity of renal inflammation as estimated by histological scores were noted as shown in Figure 2A and B, respectively.

In contrast, intramuscular injection of p-IL-2 shortened the survival rate up to 26 weeks in 20% of treated animals, and increased total IgG production and antinuclear antibody titers.

Circulating levels of these cytokines were estimated and were demonstrated to be significantly elevated, confirming their previous report [1]. The specific immunological effects persisted for several weeks after the injection. Their results demonstrate that TGFβ_1 has therapeutically desirable effects while IL-2 amplifies the spontaneously occurring immunopathogenetic processes of murine lupus nephritis.

Experimental rat colitis

Giladi et al. [3] modulated experimental colitis induced with the intracolonic administration of trinitrobenzene sulfonic acid by the direct intramuscular injection of p-TGFβ_1.

In their experiment, the p-TGFβ_1 treated rats had less swelling of the colon, as estimated by measurement of the wet weight of a 10 cm long segment of the distal colon and a smaller lesional area in the colon, compared to controls. The amelioration of tissue injury was accompanied by a significant decrease in mucosal leukotriene C4 generation as shown in Figure 3A, B and C, respectively. However, plasma TGFβ_1 levels were similar in p-TGFβ_1-injected and control rats.

Their results confirm that intramuscular DNA injection may induce systemic effects, indicating a possibility of the therapeutic application of naked DNA inoculation in inflammatory bowel disease.

Herpetic stromal keratitis in mice

Most observations concur with the hypothesis that herpetic stromal keratitis (HSK) is caused by CD4$^+$ T cells that produce cytokines having a Th1 profile [7, 8]. The

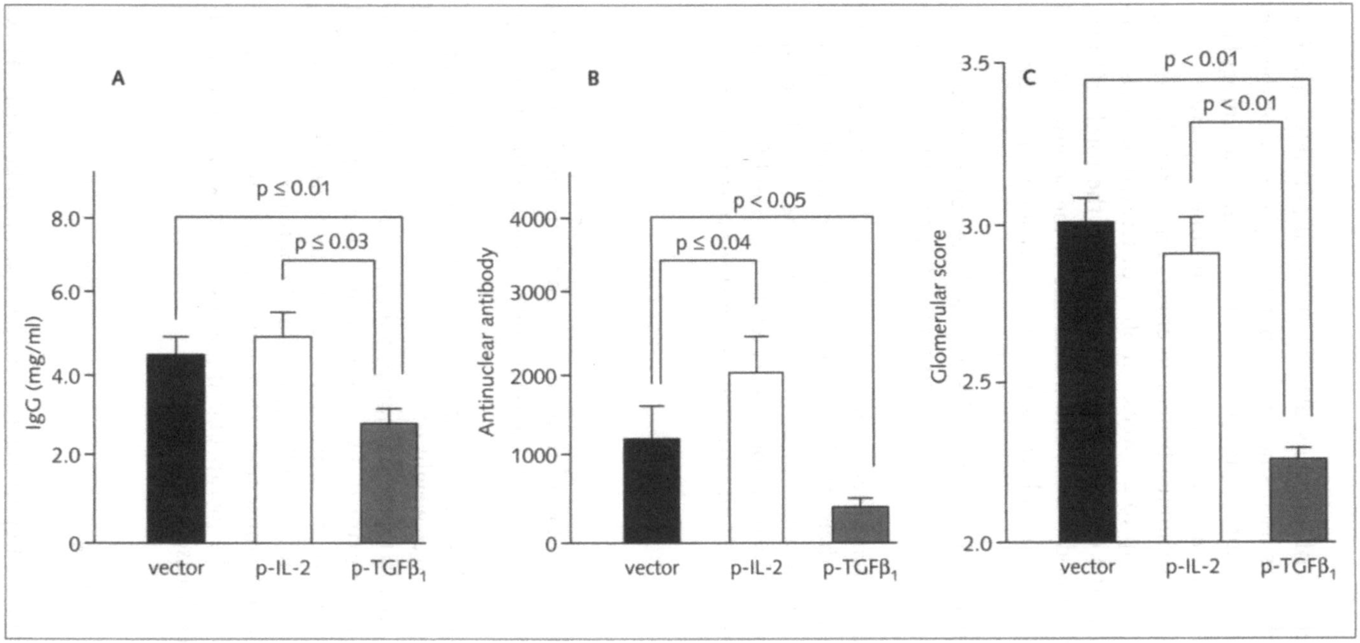

Figure 2
Effects of cytokine gene injections on murine lupus.
(A) Serum IgG levels. IgG levels in the p-TGFβ_1 *are significantly lower than in the vector control or the p-IL-2 groups (*$p \leq 0.01$ *and* $p \leq 0.03$*, respectively).*
(B) Titers of antinuclear antibodies. The titers in the p-IL-2 group are significantly higher than the vector control group ($p \leq 0.04$*). The titers in the p-TGF*β_1 *group are lower than in the vector control group, and the difference achieves statistical significance in week 18 (*$p < 0.05$*). Representative data observed week 18 were shown in A and B, respectively.*
(C) Mean glomerular score. The mean score obtained in the p-TGFβ_1 *group is significantly lower than in the vector control group or the p-IL-2 group (*$p \leq 0.01$ *in each case). (From [2], reproduced by permission with modification.)*

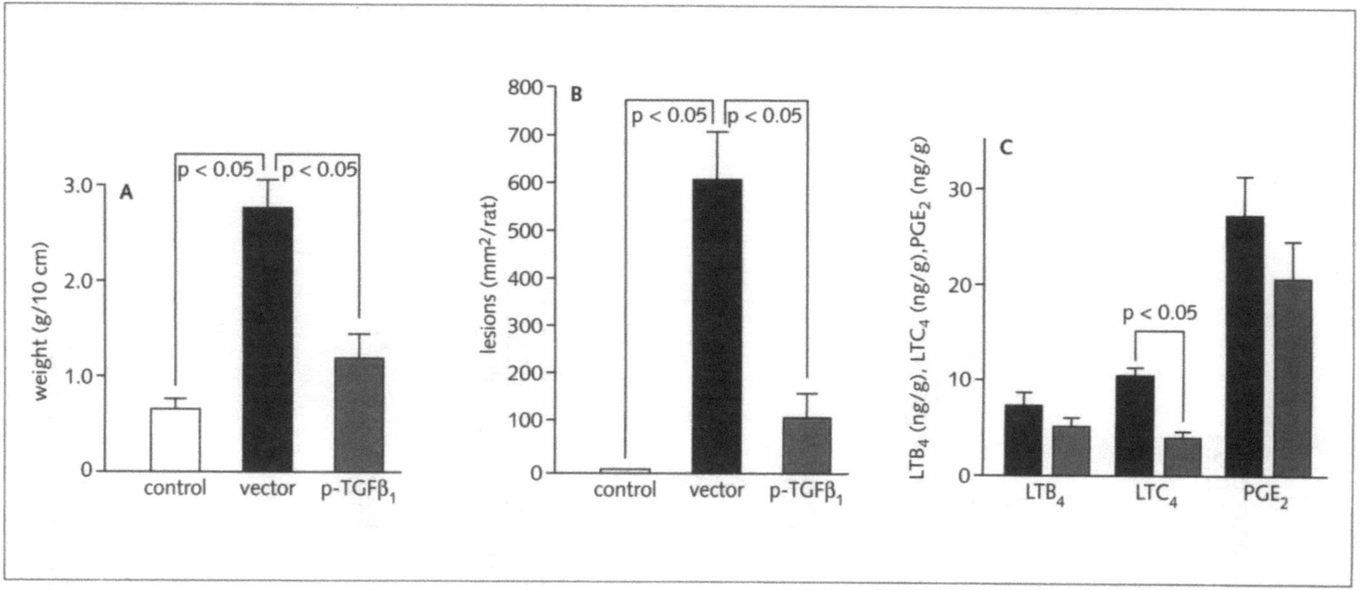

Figure 3

Effects of cytokine gene injections on colitis in rats

(A) Effect of intramuscular injection of p-TGFβ_1 on colonic weight (g/10 cm colon) in trinitrobenzene sulfonic acid (TNB)-treated rats. The wet weight of a 10 cm long distal colonic segment in the p-TGFβ_1 treated group was 52.5% of the wet weight of a similar segment isolated from the vector group ($p < 0.05$).

(B) Effect of intramuscular injection of p-TGFβ_1 on lesional area in TNB-treated rats. Lesional area was significantly smaller in the p-TGFβ_1 treated group than in the vector group ($p < 0.05$).

(C) Effect of intramuscular injection of p-TGFβ_1 on colonic prostaglandin E_2 (PGE_2), leukotriene (LT) B_4 and C_4 generation in TNB-treated rats. There was no significant difference in mucosal generation of PGE_2 and LTB_4 between the two groups of rats. In contrast, mucosal LTC_4 generation was significantly lower in the p-TGFβ_1 treated group than in the vector group ($p < 0.05$).

(From [3], reproduced by permission with modification.)

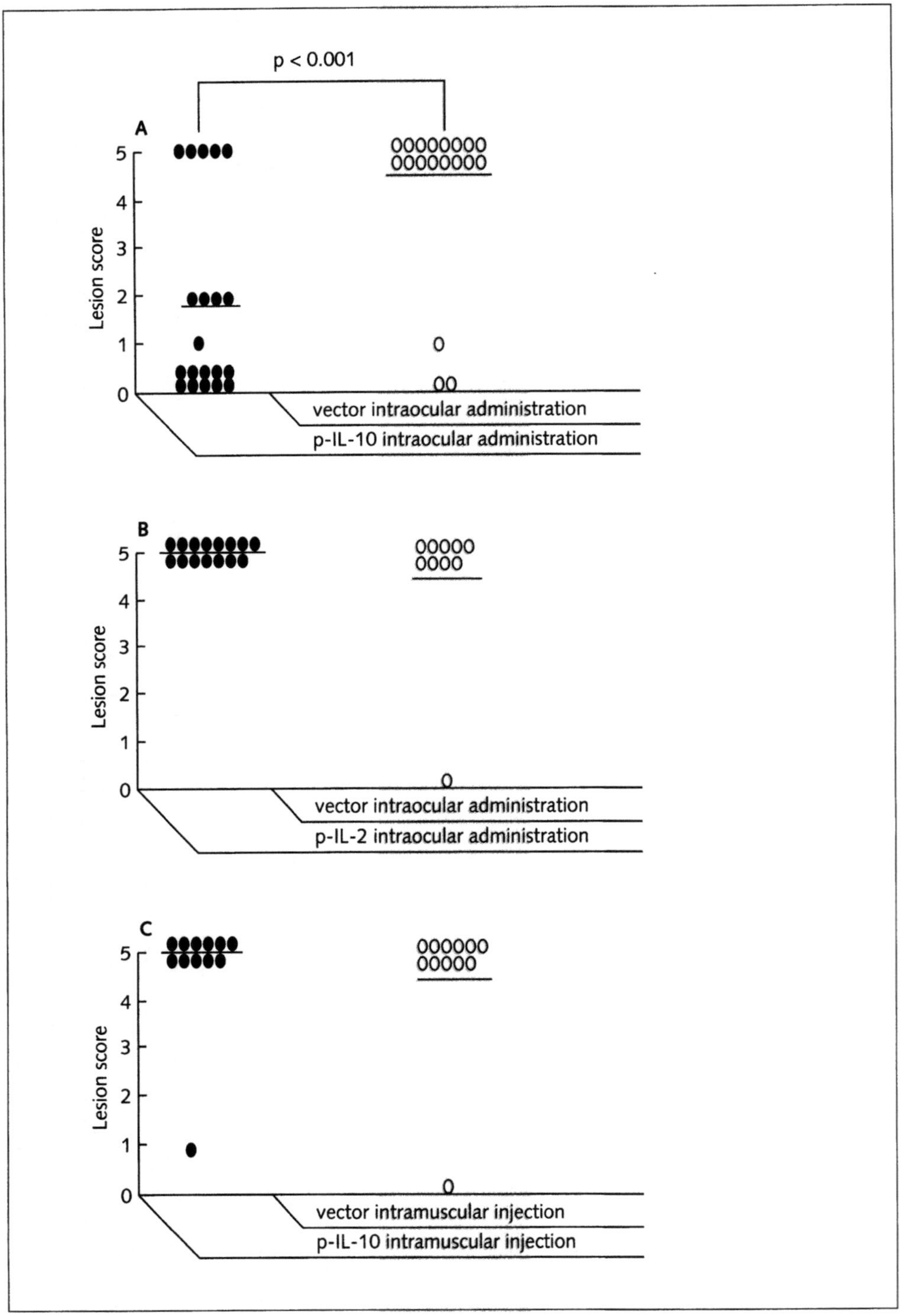
p < 0.001
A
Lesion score
5
4
3
2
1
0
vector intraocular administration
p-IL-10 intraocular administration
B
Lesion score
5
4
3
2
1
0
vector intraocular administration
p-IL-2 intraocular administration
C
Lesion score
5
4
3
2
1
0
vector intramuscular injection
p-IL-10 intramuscular injection

characteristics of a Th2 cytokine pattern are observed in animals which exhibit resolution of HSK. IL-10 was first identified as a product of Th2 clones, and can suppress cytokine synthesis by Th1 cells. HSK is minimized in severity or completely suppressed when the infected animals are treated by daily ocular and systemic administration of IL-10 [9].

Therefore, Daheshia et al. [4] examined the effects of a single topical administration of p-IL-10 on the herpetic stromal keratitis in mice. Plasmid DNA was applied on a single occasion to the sacrificed corneas, and the progress of clinical lesions was followed in individual mice over the subsequent 3-week observation period. In each experiment, animals received either cytokine DNA or control plasmid DNA. The majority of animals received topical p-IL-10 administration exhibited lesions of diminished severity in comparison with control as shown in Figure 4A. Topical p-IL-2 administration or a single intramuscular injection of p-IL-10 failed to improve HSK in mice as shown in Figure 4B and C, respectively.

These results indicate that the single topical administration of naked DNA, using an eyedropper, to the lesion would lead to improvement of HSK.

Murine collagen-induced arthritis

Murine type II collagen-induced arthritis (CIA) is a prototype model of rheumatoid arthritis and the cytokine pattern in CIA is considered to be consistent with a Th1 profile.

Therefore, we investigated whether inoculation of p-IL-10 inhibits murine CIA. p-IL-10 was inoculated intradermally into DBA/1 Lac/J mice (CIA-IL-10 group), followed by immunization with type II collagen (CII) in complete Freund's adjuvant (FA) after a week. CIA mice without inoculation of p-IL-10 (CIA group) and mice without any treatment (C group) were examined as controls. At the third and fifth week after immunization with CII in complete FA, booster injections of CII in

Figure 4
Effect of cytokine gene injection on the course of clinical lesions in murine keratitis. Groups of animals with a score of 2^+ clinical lesions were administered p-IL-10 or p-IL-2 or vector control, intraocularly or intramuscularly. Scores of individual eyes are shown on the graph
(A) Lesion score of animals administered with p-IL-10 intraocularly. Administration of p-IL-10 significantly suppressed the lesion score compared with vector control at day 32 ($p < 0.001$)
(B) Lesion score of animals administered with p-IL-2 intraocularly
(C) Lesion score of animals administered with p-IL-10 intramuscularly
(From [4], reproduced by permission with modification.)

Table 1

		CIA	CIA-IL-10	Control
Foot pad thickness (mm)	2nd week	2.81	2.67	2.45
	4th week	2.91	2.69	2.46
	6th week	2.91	2.62	2.48
	8th week	3.56	2.83	2.52
	10th week	3.4	2.69	2.52
IgG2a/IgG1 anti-type II collagen antibody	4th week	1.14	0.19	Not detectable
	6th week	4.32	0.32	Not detectable
	8th week	12.46	0.31	Not detectable
Histology	Arthritis	(+++)	(–) or (±)	(–)
	Synovial cell proliferation	(+++)	(–) or (±)	(–)
	Inflammatory cell infiltration	(+++)	(–) or (±)	(–)

PCM_V vector encoding IL-10 was inoculated intradermally into mice (CIA-IL-10) followed by induction of CIA. CIA-IL-10 mice exhibited a lower thickness of foot pads at the 8th and 10th weeks, a lower IgG2a/IgG1 antibody ratio and less severe inflammation of ankle joints than CIA mice.

incomplete FA were administered. Foot pad thickness, IgG1 (Th2 type) and IgG2a (Th1 type) isotype antibody titers to CII and histology of the ankle joints were examined at the tenth week.

The results are summarized in Table 1. CIA-IL-10 mice exhibited a lower thickness of foot pads at the eighth and tenth week, a lower IgG2a/IgG1 antibody ratio to CII and less severe inflammation of ankle joints than CIA mice. These results suggest that the p-IL-10 can suppress Th1 type immune response in CIA, resulting in complete suppression of CIA.

Conclusion

Treatment with naked DNA could be the cheapest and most feasible method of gene therapy. Delivery of plasmid leads to a unique immune response in animal models, although the clinical application of this method remains undetermined.

If it works in humans, this will prove to be a new and extremely effective strategy in the treatment of inflammatory diseases.

References

1 Raz E, Watanabe A, Baird SM, Eisenberg RA, Parr TB, Lotz M Kipps TJ, Carson DA (1993) Systemic immunological effects of cytokine genes injected into skeletal muscle. *Proc Natl Acad Sci USA* 90: 4523–4527

2 Raz E, Dudler J, Lotz M, Baird SM, Berry CC, Eisenberg RA, Carson DA (1995) Modulation of disease activity in murine systemic lupus erythematosus by cytokine gene delivery. *Lupus* 4: 286–292

3 Giladi E, Raz E, Karmeli F, Okon E, Rachmilewitz D (1995) Transforming growth factor-β gene therapy ameliorates experimental colitis in rats. *Eur J Gastro Hepatology* 7: 341–347

4 Daheshia M, Kuklin N, Kanangat S, Manickan E, Rouse BT (1997) Suppression of ongoing ocular inflammatory disease by topical administration of plasmid DNA encoding IL-10. *J Immunol* 159: 1945–1952

5 Miyata M, Sato Y, Sato H, Saito A, Irisawa A, Nishimaki T, Kasukawa R (1997) Suppression of murine collagen-induced arthritis by inoculation of plasmid DNA encoding for interleukin-10. *Arthritis Rheum* 40: S55

6 Czarniecki CW Chiu HH, Wong GHW, McCabe SM, Palladino MA (1988) Transforming growth factor-1 modulates the expression of class II histocompatibility antigens on human cells. *J Immunol* 140: 4217–4223

7 Niemialtowski MG, Rouse BT (1992) Predominance of Th1 cells in ocular tissue during herpetic stromal keratitis. *J Immunol* 149: 3035–3039

8 Hendricks RL, Tumpey TM, Finnegan A (1992) IFG-γ and IL-2 are protective in the skin but pathogenic in the corneas of HSV-1 infected mice. *J Immunol* 149: 3023–3028

9 Tumpey TM, Elner VM, Chen S, Oakes JE, Lausch RN (1994) Interleukin-10 treatment can suppress stromal keratitis induced by herpes simplex virus type 1. *J Immunol* 153: 2258–2265

Animal models of arthritis generated by gene transfer

Steven C. Ghivizzani[1], Eric R. Lechman[2], Daniel Jaffurs[2], Zhibao Mi[2], Richard Kang[2], Thomas S. Muzzonigro[2], Christopher H. Evans[1] and Paul D. Robbins[2]

[1]Center for Molecular Orthopaedics, Harvard Medical School, 221 Longwood Avenue, Boston, MA 02115, USA; [2]Departments of Molecular Genetics and Biochemistry and Orthopaedic Surgery, University of Pittsburgh School of Medicine, Pittsburgh, PA 15261, USA

Introduction

Rheumatoid arthritis (RA) is a crippling autoimmune disease whose primary symptom is chronic inflammation of the joints. Although considered to be a systemic disorder, the most commonly affected sites are the wrist, knees and metacarpophalangeal joints. The debilitating effects of the disease occur progressively over time. The synovium, normally a thin layer of tissue that lines the internal surfaces of the joint capsule, becomes dramatically thickened and hypercellular from infiltrating leukocytes and proliferating synovial cells. The cells within the synovium become activated, giving the hypertrophied tissue an aggressive phenotype. This activated tissue, called pannus, invades and erodes the articular cartilage and subchondral bone. The cumulative degradation of the joint structures often results in severe disfigurement and loss of function. Currently, there is no available treatment that can effectively halt the progression of RA.

Exactly what initiates the progression of RA is largely unknown. Studies of RA patients suggest that exposure to specific infectious agents in concert with a genetic predisposition, likely associated with a particular major histocompatibility complex phenotype, leads to a higher incidence of disease. Although the precise etiology of RA remains unclear, numerous laboratories have demonstrated that certain proteins are found at elevated levels in the joint tissues and fluids of patients with RA. Many of these proteins are known to function as either cytokines or effector molecules that serve to regulate numerous biological processes, including those that drive inflammation. Regardless of the underlying stimulus which initiates the disease, it is thought that within the joint a shift occurs in the balance between anti- and pro-inflammatory proteins, and it is the preponderance of inflammatory proteins that ultimately mediates the pathogenesis of RA. Among the cytokines associated with the inflammatory response are interleukin-1 (IL-1), IL-6, IL-8,

Gene Therapy in Inflammatory Diseases, edited by C. H. Evans and P. D. Robbins

tumor necrosis factor α (TNFα) and transforming growth factor β (TGFβ) [1]. Other factors such as stromelysin [2] and inducible nitric oxide synthase (iNOS) [3] are also thought to contribute to the disease process. Since the intraarticular protein milieu in RA patients is complex, and numerous proteins are elevated within affected joints, the precise contribution that each makes to the disease process is unclear. A better understanding of the specific intraarticular function of each of these arthritis-associated proteins may permit design of treatment strategies with greater therapeutic benefit. Furthermore, an animal model in which a specific human protein associated with RA is overexpressed intraarticularly might also be utilized to evaluate the efficacy of therapeutics designed to target specific inflammatory agents.

Previously, studies of the intraarticular activities of individual biologicals have largely involved direct injection of microgram quantities of purified recombinant protein into the joint space of laboratory animals [4, 5]. While an indication of the biological properties of a particular molecule can be obtained by this method, this type of study is likely to underrepresent the *in vivo* activity of the protein or agent in question. A study by Dingle et al. [6] has shown that following intraarticular injection into the knees of rabbits, human IL-1 can be cleared from the joint space in as little as 30 min. Thus, unlike the chronic presentation of a cytokine to articular tissues found in RA, elevated levels of injected proteins may not persist within the joint capsule. Attempts to overcome this problem have involved the implantation of osmotic pumps into experimental animals [7]. While these pumps can deliver a regulated flow of a soluble agent to the joint space their use, though, is invasive and has been observed to cause a local inflammatory reaction independent of the agent delivered. Finally, recombinant proteins used in experiments such as these may have altered activity since they are often produced by overexpression in bacteria and thus may not be similarly modified post-translationally as when synthesized by a mammalian cell.

We have been exploring the application of gene transfer technology to both the treatment and study of articular pathologies. The idea of gene transfer to the joint was originally conceived as a means to overcome problems with conventional drug delivery in the treatment of diseases like RA. For this procedure, genes encoding therapeutic proteins would be transferred to cells within the synovium; the gene products would then be constitutively expressed and secreted into the joint space and surrounding tissues. In laboratory animals, intraarticular transfer of genes encoding anti-inflammatory proteins such as interleukin-1 receptor antagonist (IL-1Ra) [8] and soluble receptors for IL-1 and TNFα [9] was accompanied by transgene expression sufficient to halt or inhibit the disease process of experimental arthritis. If sufficient expression of anti-arthritic transgene products could be maintained in the joint for extended periods, this type of strategy could be a viable tool for use in the treatment of joint disorders. A clinical trial to assess the safety and feasibility of gene delivery to the joint is nearing completion [10].

Alternatively, gene transfer technology offers a unique method by which to study the contributions of specific cytokines or cytokine combinations to joint disease. By delivering genes encoding proteins associated with RA disease processes to the cells of the synovium and constitutively expressing and secreting the gene products at elevated levels, a situation is established which closely mimics that found in actual disease. Experiments of this nature should lead to changes in joint pathophysiology that reflect the potential contribution of that protein to articular pathology that is perhaps attainable by no other method.

Ex vivo transfer of human IL-1β to the knees of rabbits

To evaluate the utility of the gene delivery approach to the study of arthritis-associated proteins, we initially used an *ex vivo* gene transfer method to deliver and express exogenous genes in the knees of rabbits [11] (Fig. 1). The knee joint of the New Zealand White Rabbit has been the animal model of choice for our experiments concerning intraarticular gene transfer, particularly with respect to determining efficiency of gene delivery vehicles, as well as levels and duration of transgene expression. Since the rabbit knee is approximately the same size as the metacarpophalangeal joints of the human hand and has similar architecture, it offers a reasonable simulation of the process of treating human disease. Additionally, the large size of the rabbit knee permits accurate intraarticular injections and the ability to lavage the joint space. Analyses of recovered knee washings permit quantitation of secretable transgene products as well as certain parameters of arthritis such as leukocytic infiltration and glycosaminoglycan levels.

Human interleukin-1β (hIL-1β) was selected as the first protein to deliver to the joint by gene transfer because it has been studied extensively both *in vitro* and *in vivo* and is considered a principle mediator of the pathophysiology of RA [12]. IL-1β has been attributed with numerous inflammatory activities associated with RA, including induction of leukocytic infiltration, cartilage degradation and depression of cartilage matrix synthesis.

To enable high-level secretion of transgene products by genetically modified cells, prior knowledge of expression pathways of the particular protein is essential. While most proteins are synthesized in the endoplasmic reticulum and secreted via the Golgi complex, IL-1β is not conventional. The immature pro-IL-1β requires processing by IL-1β converting enzyme (ICE) which cleaves the pro-leader sequence and facilitates secretion of the mature protein from the cell [12]. Therefore to allow for efficient secretion of the IL-1β gene product by transduced cells without dependence upon the activity of rabbit IL-1β converting enzyme, or reliance on its ability to correctly process the xenogenic human protein, a leader sequence encoding the secretor oligopeptide from human parathyroid hormone was fused to the coding sequence for mature human IL-1β. This chimeric gene was then inserted into a retro-

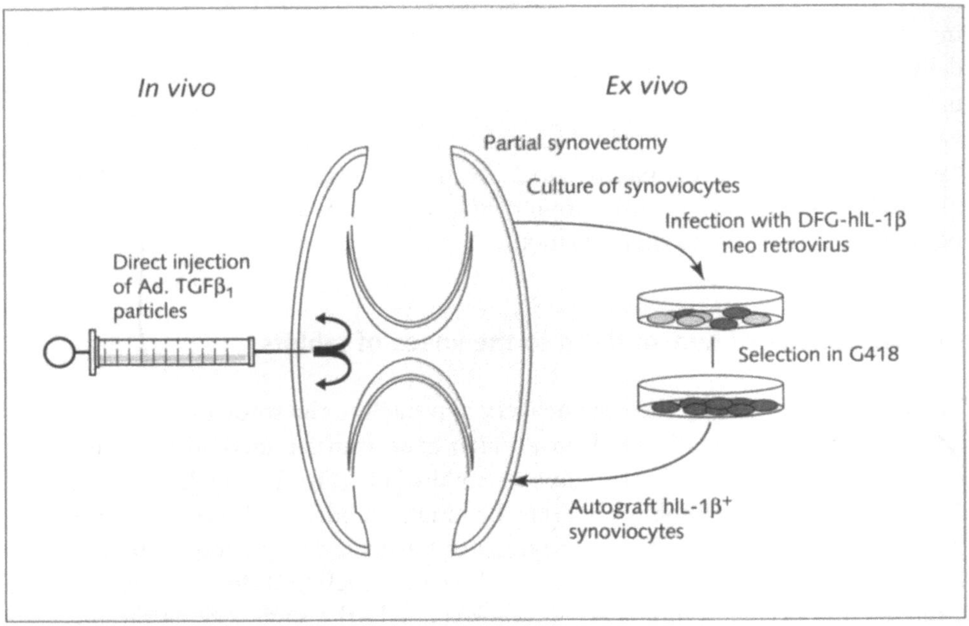

Figure 1
Two routes of adminstration have been used to deliver and express arthritis-associated genes within the rabbit joint. Ex vivo *gene delivery initially involves the surgical isolation of synovial tissue from the joint of the experimental animal and isolation and culture of the synoviocytes. The synovial cultures are then incubated* in vitro *using a retroviral vector, and the transduced cells are positively selected. The genetically modified cells are then harvested and delivered to the joint via intraarticular injection. The cells then engraft into the synovial lining and express the transgene.* In vivo *gene delivery involves direct intraarticular injection of the transfer vector which then infects and transduces the synovial lining cells* in situ.

viral vector, MFG [13]. To allow positive selection of transduced cells, the neomycin phosphotransferase gene (neo) was inserted downstream of the IL-1β coding region. By linking the two coding regions with an internal ribosome entry site [14], a retroviral vector was constructed, DFG-hIL-1-neo, that would permit translation of both genes from a single transcript initiated from the retroviral long terminal repeat. Infection of a rabbit synovial fibroblast cell line, HIG-82 [15], with amphotropic DFG-hIL-1-neo retrovirus was found to enable production of greater than 200 ng of hIL-1β per million cells per 48 h.

In preliminary experiments, HIG-82 cells were used to transfer the hIL-1β gene to the rabbit knee. These cells were infected with the DFG-hIL-1-neo vector and cultured in media containing G418. The hIL-1β$^+$ cells were trypsinized and washed and approximately 1×10^7 were injected directly into the joint capsules of the knees of several New Zealand White rabbits. The response of the joints to the transplantation of the genetically modified cells was clearly apparent within 24 h; the injected knees of each of the animals became dramatically swollen, and remained enlarged for the week-long experiment. Joint lavages at days 3 and 7 showed that the synovial fluid was heavily infiltrated with polymorphonuclear leukocytes. Following sacrifice at 7 days post-injection, gross inspection showed that a thickened synovium had begun to form attachments to the sides of the femoral condyles. Histologically, the synovial lining was fibrotic, and hypercellular with synovial fibroblasts, macrophages and massive numbers of infiltrating polymorphonuclear leukocytes.

These experiments demonstrated the overall feasibility of the gene delivery approach and demonstrated that a genetically modified cell line could express an arthritis-associated transgene product within the joint at levels sufficient to induce a significant biological effect. In subsequent studies it was found that the severity of the inflammatory response could be graded in relation to the number of IL-1β$^+$ cells injected into the joint. Indeed, this type of procedure is used in our laboratory to rapidly generate a model of arthritis driven by IL-1β for short-term evaluation of IL-1 inhibitors. It should be noted that in the experiment described above, *ex vivo* intraarticular transfer of the β-galactosidase gene (lacZ) was used for a negative control to evaluate the inflammatory capacity of injecting an allogenic cell line that expressed a transgene. Injection of HIG-82-lacZ$^+$ cells was observed to induce a drastically reduced but detectable inflammatory response, characterized by a slight increase in the thickness of the synovial cell layer and a modest increase in white blood cell infiltration. This should be a consideration in experiments of this nature involving the use of allogeneic cells, particularly when studying a transgene with subtle activities.

Previous work using marker genes had demonstrated that intraarticular transgene expression from injected HIG-82 cells would only persist for about 10 days and that lack of persistence was likely due to rejection of the allogenic synovial cell line [16]. In an effort to evaluate the effects of longer-term IL-1β expression in the joint, autologous synoviocytes were used for *ex vivo* gene delivery. For this procedure, a small amount of the joint capsule was surgically harvested from one knee joint each of several rabbits. The synovial fibroblasts were then isolated and cultured separately for each animal. Half the cells of each culture were incubated with the DFG-hIL-1-neo retrovirus and the transductants selected by culture in G418. The remaining cells remained untreated and were used as negative controls. The hIL-1β$^+$ synovial cells were then introduced into one knee of the respective donor rabbits while the nontransduced cells were injected into the opposing knee joint. In initial experiments approximately 1×10^7 transduced cells were injected into the joints of three rabbits; however, overexpression of IL-1β proved fatal to two of the animals, and the third had to be sacrificed for health concerns. This result demonstrated the extreme biological potential of overexpressing IL-1β and further, suggested that *ex vivo* gene transfer using autologous primary synoviocytes may result in higher levels of transgene expression.

In subsequent experiments considerably fewer hIL-1β$^+$ synoviocytes were implanted into the respective donors, and IL-1β gene expression was found to persist from between 2 to 4 weeks at levels near 100 pg/ml in recovered lavage fluids. Animals sacrificed periodically during the 4-week period of the experiment showed striking pathophysiological changes in the articular tissues that were remarkably similar to those found in RA patients with advanced disease. As observed previously using allogeneic cells, injection of autologous IL-1β$^+$ cells caused the knees to become swollen by greater than 30% over opposing joints. During the period of the experiment, the synovial fluids of the rabbits were heavily infiltrated, often over 2500-fold greater than controls. At first, the population consisted almost exclusively of polymorphonuclear leukocytes; however, over 7 to 10 days this changed to about equal numbers of mono- and polymorphonuclear cells. Within 3 days of injection of the cells, the synovial lining became massively thickened and hypercellular from polymorphs and fibroblastic cells. Within about 7 days diffuse populations of lymphocytes were also observed which at about 14 days had begun to form foci. A highly aggressive pannus was also seen in almost all of the rabbits that had invaded and eroded the articular cartilages and subchondral bone. At numerous sites, the invading pannus was found to penetrate into the marrow. Numerous systemic effects were also apparent. The rabbits ran elevated body temperatures, often had diarrhea and lost a significant amount of body weight. Analysis of recovered synovial fluids showed that the human IL-1β induced high expression of endogenous rabbit IL-1 and TNFα. Interestingly, when transgenic IL-1 expression was lost at between 2 and 4 weeks post implantation of the genetically modified cells, many of these pathologies quickly resolved. Opposing joints receiving injections of nontransduced synovial cells were virtually indistinguishable from normal naive joints.

Overall, the results of this study provided a remarkable demonstration of the potent biological activity of IL-1β, suggesting that overexpression of IL-1β alone within the joint is sufficient to mediate all major pathologies associated with RA. The potency of IL-1β in this regard is striking. For example, the injection of as few as 10^4 hIL-1β$^+$ HIG-82 cells into a rabbit knee is sufficient to provoke inflammatory and catabolic changes. Moreover, this occurs under conditions where hIL-1β is not detectable by standard ELISA of the lavage fluid. Much research suggests that TNFα resides at the top of the rheumatoid inflammatory cascade and is the primary mediator of the pathogenesis in RA [17]. However, the observation that IL-1β can stimulate production of high levels of endogenous TNFα and IL-1β in the rabbit joint suggests that at least in the rabbit knee joint IL-1β occupies a position alongside TNFα at the top of the cascade, if not by itself.

In vivo gene delivery of TGFβ_1

In early experiments, an *ex vivo* procedure was used to deliver exogenous genes to the joint. Although laborious and time consuming, this technique results in relatively high levels of intraarticular transgene expression with little or no visible alteration in the synovial lining from the procedure itself. Subsequent studies have shown that adenoviral vectors can efficiently deliver genes to the cells of the synovium via a single direct injection of the viral particles into the joint space [9, 18, 19] (Fig. 1). While being highly effective vehicles of *in vivo* gene transfer, caution must be used in the application of adenoviral mediated gene delivery, particularly with respect to studying the effects of arthritis-associated genes. Numerous experiments in our laboratory have shown that injection of certain materials into the joint space can provoke an immediate, nonspecific inflammatory response. To avoid this type of reaction, viral preparations must be highly purified and injected in a minimal working volume of physiologically compatible solution. Furthermore, since first generation adenoviral vectors encode a number of native viral proteins, infected cells will express and present the viral gene products to the immune system of the host [20]. Thus, within about 2 weeks post-injection a local, specific inflammatory response will often occur within the joint. We have found that by delivering an appropriate vector in the opposing joint to serve as a comparative control for responses due solely to the administration of viral vectors, adenoviral-mediated delivery can be used to monitor the effects of intraarticular gene expression for about 10–14 days. This type of gene delivery system was used to evaluate the intraarticular activity of human TGFβ_1 following its transfer and overexpression in the rabbit knee joint.

Originally described as a protein that caused reversible transformation of rat kidney fibroblasts in the presence of epidermal growth factor, TGFβ has since been shown to have numerous biological activities. Contrary to its name, TGFβ does not cause oncogenic transformation and is actually a potent growth inhibitor of many cell types. Members of the TGFβ family are known to inhibit adipogenesis [21], myogenesis [22] and hematopoiesis [23], but promote chondrogenesis [24] and epithelial cell differentiation [25]. That TGFβ is involved in the RA disease process is suggested by several lines of evidence. TGFβ is found at elevated levels in synovial fluids and tissues of afflicted patients [26] and can be detected at cartilage-pannus junctions [27]; however, the specific contribution of TGFβ to RA, whether pathogenic or therapeutic, remains somewhat unclear. *In vitro* analysis of its effects on articular tissues has shown that TGFβ can promote chondrogenesis and is a potent stimulator of collagen and proteoglycan production by fibroblasts [28]. Furthermore it inhibits extracellular matrix degradation and upregulates protease inhibitors. These findings would suggest that TGFβ could serve in tissue reparation, but also could contribute to synovial hypertrophy and fibrosis. Intraarticular injection of TGFβ in naïve animals has been found to stimulate marked swelling and erythema of the joint, accompanied by extensive infiltration of the joint space and synovial fibroblast hyperplasia [29]. Furthermore, TGFβ injection has been found to accelerate the onset of collagen-induced arthritis in rats [30].

TGFβ is a cytokine that is synthesized and secreted in a latent form that is unable to interact with its receptor and must be processed to its smaller mature form to become active. The mature active form of $TGFβ_1$ is a homodimer of two 112-amino acid subunits with a molecular weight of about 25 kDa [31]. Both latent and active forms are found in synovial fluids of RA patients. To study the intraarticular activity of this cytokine, the complete cDNA for human $TGFβ_1$ was inserted into the E1 region of a first generation E1–E3 deleted adenoviral vector, and expression of the gene was placed under control of the human cytomegalovirus promoter. *In vitro*, infection of HIG-82 cells with cesium-chloride gradient purified adenoviral stocks showed the production of high nanogram levels of latent $TGFβ_1$ by ELISA measurments. Infection of primary rabbit chondrocytes with the Ad.TGFβ virus was found to significantly stimulate cartilage matrix synthesis, demonstrating that the gene product synthesized by the transduced cells was secreted, biologically active and recognized by rabbit cells.

To determine the optimal dose with which to evaluate the intraarticular activity of this protein, 10-fold increments of Ad.TGFβ virus, ranging from 1×10^7 to 1×10^{10} particles were directly injected into one knee joint each of four rabbits and the effects monitored periodically over a 2-week period. The opposing knee of each rabbit received a similar dose of an adenoviral vector encoding lacZ. Similar to the *ex vivo* gene transfer experiments with human IL-1β, intraarticular injection of 1×10^{10} particles into the knee of a rabbit resulted in the death of the animal within 3 days. Post-mortem examination of this animal showed that the knee joint as well as the thigh and lower leg of the side injected with the TGFβ virus were enlarged to nearly twice the size of the opposing control limb. Histological analysis of recovered tissue showed that the synovial lining of the joint was significantly hypertrophied and was extremely fibrotic. The increase in size of the leg muscles appeared to be largely attributable to edema. However, muscle tissue near the knee joint showed signs of fibroblast hyperplasia and fibrosis between the muscle fiber bundles. The cause of death was not readily apparent from either gross or histological examination of the major soft organs. Rabbits receiving lower doses of Ad.TGFβ showed similar types of symptoms proportional to the viral dose.

Subsequent studies were conducted where a viral dose of approximately 1×10^9 viral particles was injected into the knee joint of several rabbits which were sacrificed at 3, 7, 14 and 21 days post-injection and analyzed. TGFβ transgene expression was found to peak around day 7 and disappear by day 21. As before, within 3 days of injection, joints and surrounding musculature of knees receiving Ad.TGFβ appeared dramatically swollen. Muscle swelling generally persisted for about two weeks and then abated. During this period serum creatine kinase levels were significantly elevated, suggesting that the swelling was accompanied by considerable muscle damage. Knee joints, though, remained enlarged throughout the 21 days of the experiment. Histological analysis of the longer term animals showed evidence of extreme fibrosis and hyperplasia from synovial fibroblasts in the synovial lining reminiscent of patients with end-stage RA. In some animals, ectopic bone formations could be observed within the thickened synovial mass. Fibrosis was to such an extent that loss of joint extension was observed in each case. Joints were often limited to less than 90° of extension. Interestingly, although the TGFβ joints showed extreme effects of expression including a large increase in joint size, these changes were not associated with a leukocytic infiltrate in the joint space or tissues. In fact, joints injected with the Ad.TGFβ virus had consistently lower numbers of infiltrating white blood cells than opposing joints injected with the Ad.lacZ virus.

These experiments suggest that TGFβ may have antiinflammatory properties, but likely contributes to the cellularity and fibrosis found in the rheumatoid joint. While limited expression of TGFβ may have reparative value to cartilage and damaged tissue, these studies suggest that chronic overexpression of this cytokine within the joint likely contributes to the loss of joint function via the overproduction of fibrous matrices. Thus it is possible that in the rheumatoid joint where numerous cytokines are chronically expressed, persistant elevated TGFβ may actually contribute to joint pathology. Recently, it has been shown that intramuscular delivery of naked DNA encoding TGFβ to rats with experimental arthritis had sytemic therapeutic value [32]. Additionally, injection of splenocytes genetically altered to express $TGF\beta_1$ were found to ameliorate disease in collagen-induced arthritis in DBA/1 mice [33]. While the route of administration, either local or systemic may be critical as to the type of effect observed, the extreme toxicity associated with local overexpression of this protein indicates that caution should be used before transferring this gene into the joints and tissues of humans.

Intraarticular delivery of inducible nitric oxide synthase

Nitric oxide (NO) is a gaseous free radical originally identified as endothelium-derived relaxing factor. As the smallest biologic product of mammalian cells, NO has since been found to be involved in a widely diverse realm of biological processes such as neuronal signaling, platelet function and killing of intracellular pathogens [34]. A number of different cell types have been identified that produce NO, including endothelial cells, hepatocytes, and neurons. Several cells which participate in the RA disease process such as macrophages neutrophils, chondrocytes and synoviocytes also produce measurable levels of NO [3].

NO is synthesized by three distinct nitric oxide synthases (NOS) which remove the terminal guanidino nitrogen from L-arginine to form citrulline and NO (reviewed in [35]). This reaction requires NADPH and tetrahydrobiopterin as cofactors. However, it can be inhibited by guanidino-substituted arginine analogs such as N^G-monomethyl-L-arginine (L-NMA). Two of the synthases are constitutively present (cNOS) and produce NO in small amounts for short periods. NO synthesized by these proteins acts as a neurotransmitter or to relax vascular smooth muscle. Inducible NOS (iNOS), however, is only present following stimulation of certain cells with cytokines, microbes or microbial products, and produces high levels of NO for extended periods of time [34, 36]. Among the cellular signals that stimulate synthesis of iNOS are IFNγ, LPS, TNFα and IL-1, agents associated with inflammation. The activity of cNOS is dependent upon the transient binding of Ca^{2+} and calmodulin, while iNOS, once expressed by a stimulated cell, relies only upon the presence of substrates and cofactors such as tetrahydrobiopterin. It is the inducible NOS that is thought to participate in the inflammatory process [3].

That NO is involved in the pathogenesis of RA and arthritides is suggested by several lines of evidence [3]. Firstly, NO is unstable and quickly converts to nitrate and nitrite, and patients with RA have elevated concentrations of both molecules in synovial fluid, blood and urine [37–39]. The highest levels are found in synovial fluids, which suggests that NO production occurs primarily within the tissues of the joint. Furthermore, correlations have been observed between RA severity and serum nitrate/nitrite levels as well as serum levels of TNFα and IL-6 [38]. Synovium and cartilage harvested from the joints of RA patients express iNOS RNA and protein . In animal models, the onset of arthritis is associated with increases in the synthesis of NO accompanied by increased levels of NO in the blood urine and synovial fluids. Furthermore, inhibitors of NO synthesis have been found to inhibit disease progession in several animal models of arthritis [40, 41]. These findings suggest that NO is involved in the pathogenesis of RA, but are only correlative. The gaseous and unstable nature of this molecule severely limits study of its direct effect on articular tissues. Thus, local delivery and overexpression of iNOS gene may allow for direct evaluation of the *in vivo* properties of NO that is not readily attainable by other methods.

We have employed both indirect and direct gene delivery to study the effects of overexpression of the human iNOS gene on the knees of rabbits. Different from other gene products discussed above, NO generated by expression of iNOS is the same molecule regardless of the species origin of the NOS gene. *Ex vivo* delivery of the iNOS gene by transplantation of genetically modified synoviocytes resulted in no detectable change in joint tissues by either gross inspection or histological analyses. Since direct adenovirus mediated gene transfer has routinely resulted in higher levels of intraarticular transgene expression, we have since introduced the iNOS gene by intraarticular injection of an Ad.iNOS vector. This resulted in high levels of NO production, as determined indirectly by nitrate/nitrite levels in lavage fluids recovered from recipient rabbit joints. The procedure, however, has been associated with only mild inflammatory responses largely indistinguishable from those observed from injection of control adenoviral vectors encoding marker genes. This would suggest two possibilities. One is that within the context of the naïve joint NO has little inflammatory capacity. Any contribution that NO might make to the pathogenesis of RA may rely on the presence and activity of other inflammatory cytokines. The second is that perhaps NO is not a contributor to pathogenesis but simply a byproduct of the process whose levels correlate with disease. To determine how expression of iNOS might influence an arthritic joint experiments are in progress involving the delivery of the iNOS gene to joints of rabbits with antigen-induced arthritis and arthritis generated by intraarticular expression of the human IL-1β gene.

Considerations and future studies

The effects of intraarticular delivery of the human IL-1β and TGFβ genes into the joints of naïve animals proved to be quite dramatic, while the delivery of the iNOS gene to the rabbit joint was met with much less obvious pathology. As might be anticipated, with certain proteins the gene delivery approach to the study of their arthritic potential can be highly informative, but caution must be used in evaluating conclusively the effects of genes whose effects may be subtle or absent in naïve joints. Consideration must be made for those cytokines or proteins that may have different activities depending upon the prevailing cytokine environment. That is, certain receptors may be induced by other proteins that allow responsiveness to the gene product in question, or perhaps two proteins act cooperatively to induce a particular effect. Further, the rabbit, or any other experimental animal may not respond normally, or may fail to respond fully, to certain xenogeneic proteins.

Although there may be hindrances in applying the use of gene delivery to the study of arthritis-associated or other inflammatory proteins, there are several distinct advantages to this approach. The first is that the protein of interest is synthesized constitutively within the joint space and surrounding tissue. This allows persistent, chronic stimulation of cells within the various articular tissues, a situation similar to that which might occur during an inflammatory flare in an RA joint. Secondly, the specific protein of interest is synthesized and secreted by synovial lining cells or cells which have colonized the lining. Since most of the inflammatory and destructive cytokines are produced by macrophage-like and fibroblastic synovial cells within the synovial lining, the cytokine is presented to the articular tissues in a natural fashion. Additionally, the protein of interest is synthesized by eukaryotic cells, allowing post-translational processing to occur. The intraarticular gene delivery procedure is relatively non-invasive. The gene of interest can be transferred directly by injection into the joint of a suitable DNA delivery vector or indirectly by a single injection of genetically modified cells. If a cell line or, for example, autologous skin fibroblasts are used to deliver the transgene then invasion of a joint can be avoided altogether.

We are currently examining the intraarticular effects of overexpression of several other arthritis-associated gene products including TNFα, IL-6, IL-8 and stromelysin. TNFα is thought by many to be the primary mediator of RA pathophysiology inducing such effects as leukocytic infiltration, synovitis and cartilage erosion. IL-6 is present at elevated levels in the synovial fluid and sera of patients with RA, and its levels correlate closely with severity of disease. However, results of various studies disagree on whether this cytokine is pathogenic or protective. IL-8 is associated with acute inflammation and is thought to induce infiltration of neutrophils into the joint space and synovial tissue. Stromelysin is a matrix metalloproteinase that causes degradation of extracellular matrices and is thought to contribute to cartilage degradation. The results of these ongoing studies coupled with those described briefly in the preceeding sections should give a reasonable description of the intraarticular activity of the primary agents associated with RA. To date we have only examined the response of a naïve joint to expression of arthritic gene products. As mentioned above, an individual cytokine or protein may require the presence of other inflammatory cytokines or agents or for its full range of activities to be observable. Thus, it may be informative for these gene products to be evaluated in the presence of the IL-1β gene which has been shown to induce a reasonably complete simulation of human disease. This may prove particularly useful for those genes which have negligible activity when delivered alone into a naïve joint.

References

1 Duff GW (1994) Cytokines and acute phase proteins in rheumatoid arthritis. *Scand J Rheumatol Suppl* 100: 9–19

2 Mauviel A (1993) Cytokine regulation of metalloproteinase gene expression. *J Cell Biochem* 53: 288–295

3 Evans CH, Stefanovic-Racic M, Lancaster J (1995) Nitric oxide and its role in orthopaedic disease. *Clin Orthop* 312: 275–294

4 Henderson B, Pettipher ER (1989) Arthritogenic actions of recombinant IL-1 and tumour necrosis factor in the rabbit: evidence for synergistic interactions between cytokines *in vivo*. *Clin Exp Immunol* 75: 306–310

5 Pettipher ER, Higgs GA, Henderson B (1986) Interleukin-1 induces leukocyte infiltration and cartilage proteoglycan degradation in the synovial joint. *Proc Natl Acad Sci USA* 83: 8749–8753

6 Dingle JT, Thomas DP, King B, Bard DR (1987) *In vivo* studies of articular tissue damage mediated by catabolin/interleukin-1. *Ann Rheum Dis* 46: 527–532

7 Feige U, Karbowski C (1989) Arthritis induced by continuous infusion of hr-interleukin-1 alpha into the rabbit knee-joint. *Int J Tissue React* 11: 225

8 Otani K, Nita I, Macaulay W, Georgescu HI, Robbins PD, Evans CH (1996) Suppres-

sion of antigen-induced arthritis in rabbits by *ex vivo* gene therapy. *J Immunol* 156: 3558–3562
9 Ghivizzani SC, Lechman ER, Kang R, Tio C, Kolls J, Evans CH, Robbins PD (1998) Direct adenoviral-mediated gene transfer of IL-1 and TNF alpha soluble receptors to rabbit knees with experimental arthritis has local and distal anti-arthritis effects. *Proc Natl Acad Sci USA* 95: 4613–4618
10 Evans CH, Robbins PD, Ghivizzani SC, Herndon JH, Kang R (1996) Clinical trial to assess the safety, feasibility, and efficacy of transferring a potentially antiarthritic cytokine gene to human joints with rheumatoid arthritis. *Hum Gene Ther* 7: 1261–1280
11 Ghivizzani SC, Kang R, Georgescu HI, Nita I, Jaffurs D, Engle JM, Watkins SC, Tindal MH, Suchanek MK, McKenzie LR, et al. (1997) Constitutive intraarticular expression of human IL-1B following gene transfer to rabbit synovium produces all major pathologies of human arthritis. *J Immunol* 59: 3604–3612
12 Dinarello CA (1994) The interleukin-1 family: 10 years of discovery. *FASEB J* 8: 1314–1325
13 Robbins PD, Thara H, Mueller GM, Hung G, Bahnson A, Zitvogel L, Galea-Lauri J, Ohashi T, Patrene K, Boggs S et al (1994) Retroviral vectors for use in human gene therapy for cancer, Gaucher disease, and arthritis. *Ann NY Acad Sci* 716: 72–89
14 Ghattas IR, Sanes JR, Majors JE (1991) The encephalomyocarditis virus internal ribosome entry site allows efficient coexpression of two genes from a recombinant provirus in cultured cells and embryos. *Mol Cell Biol* 11: 5848–5859
15 Georgescu HI, Mendelow D, Evans CH (1988) HIG-82: an established cell line from rabbit periarticular soft tissue which retains the "activatable" phenotype. *In Vitro* 24: 1015–1022
16 Bandara G, Mueller GM, Galea-Lauri J, Tindal MH, Georgescu HI, Suchanek MK, Hung GL, Glorioso JC, Robbins PD, Evans CH (1993) Intraarticular expression of biologically active interleukin-1-receptor antagonist protein by *ex vivo* gene transfer. *Proc Natl Acad Sci USA* 90: 10764–10768
17 Feldmann M, Brennan FM, Maini RN (1996) The role of cytokines in rheumatoid arthritis. *Ann Rev Immunol* 14: 397–440
18 Roessler BJ, Allen ED, Wilson JM, Hartman JW, Davidson BL (1993) Adenoviral-mediated gene transfer to rabbit synovium *in vivo*. *J Clin Invest* 92: 1085–1092
19 Nita I, Ghivizzani SC, Galea-Lauri J, Bandara G, Georgescu HI, Robbins PD, Evans CH (1996) Direct gene delivery to synovium: an evaluation of potential vectors *in vitro* and *in vivo*. *Arthritis Rheum* 39: 820–828
20 Yang Y, Nunes FA, Berensci K, Furth EE, Bonczol E, Wilson JM (1994) Cellular immunity to viral antigen limits E1-deleted adenoviruses for gene therapy. *Proc Natl Acad Sci USA* 91: 4407–4411
21 Torti FM, Torti SV, Larrick JW, Ringold GM (1989) Modulation of adipocyte differentiation by tumor necrosis factor and transforming growth factor beta. J Cell Biol 108: 1105–1113

22 Husmann I, Soulet L, Gautron J, Martelly I, Barritault D (1996) Growth factors in skeletal muscle regeneration. *Cytokine Growth Factor Rev* 7: 249–258
23 Hayashi S, Gimble JM, Henley A, Ellingsworth LR, Kincade PW (1989) Differential effects of TGF-beta 1 on lymphohemopoiesis in long-term bone marrow cultures. *Blood* 74: 1711–1717
24 Johnstone B, Hering TM, Caplan AI, Goldberg VM, Yoo JU (1998) *In vitro* chondrogenesis of bone marrow-derived mesenchymal progenitor cells. *Exp Cell Res* 238: 265–272
25 Hall BK, Miyake T (1995) Divide, accumulate, differentiate: cell condensation in skeletal development revisited. *Int J Dev Biol* 39: 881–893
26 Fava RA, Olsen N, Keski-Oja J, Moses HL, Pincus T (1989) Active and latent forms of transforming growth factor beta activity in synovial effusions. *J Exp Med* 169: 291–296
27 Chu CQ, Field M, Abney E, Zheng RQH, Allard S, Feldmann M, Maini RN (1991) Transforming growth factor-beta1 in rheumatoid synovial membrane and cartilage/pannus junction. *Clin Exp Immunol* 86: 380–386
28 Collier S, Ghosh P (1995) Effects of transforming growth factor beta on proteoglycan synthesis by cell and explant cultures derived from the knee joint meniscus. *Osteoarthritis Cartilage* 3: 127–138
29 Allen JB, Manthey CL, Hand AR, Ohura K, Ellingsworth L, Wahl SM (1990) Rapid onset of synovial inflammation and hyperplasia induced by transforming growth factor beta. *J Exp Med* 171: 231–247
30 Cooper WO, Fava RA, Gates CO, Cremer MA, Townes AS (1992) Acceleration of onset of collagen-induced arthritis by intra-articular injection of tumour necrosis factor or transforming growth factor-beta. *Clin Exp Immunol* 89: 244–250
31 Hartsough MT, Mulder KM (1997) Transforming growth factor-beta signaling in epithelial cells. *Pharmacol Ther* 75: 21–41
32 Song XY, Gu M, Jin WW, Klinman DM, Wahl SM (1998) Plasmid DNA encoding transforming growth factor-beta1 suppresses chronic disease in a streptococcal cell wall-induced arthritis model. *J Clin Invest* 101: 2615–2621
33 Chernajovsky Y, Adams G, Triantaphyllopoulos K, Ledda MF, Podhajcer OL (1997) Pathogenic lymphoid cells engineered to express TGF-beta 1 ameliorate disease in a collagen-induced arthritis model. *Gene Ther* 4: 553–559
34 Nussler AK, Billiar TR (1993) Inflammation, immunoregulation, and inducible nitric oxide synthase. *J Leukoc Biol* 54: 171–178
35 Gellar DA, Billiar TR (1998) Molecular biology of nitric oxide synthases. *Cancer Metastasis Rev* 17: 7–23
36 Knowles RG, Moncada S (1994) Nitric oxide synthases in mammals. *Biochem J* 298: 249–258
37 Farrell AJ, Blake DR, Palmer RM, Moncada S (1992) Increased concentrations of nitrite in synovial fluid and serum samples suggest increased nitric oxide synthesis in rheumatic diseases. *Ann Rheum Dis* 51: 1219–1222

38 Ueki Y, Miyake S, Tominaga Y, Eguchi K (1996) Increased nitric oxide levels in patients with rheumatoid arthritis. *J Rheumatol* 23: 230–236

39 Grabowski PS, England AJ, Dykhuizen R, Copland M, Benjamin N, Reid DM, Ralston SH (1996) Elevated nitric oxide production in rheumatoid arthritis. Detection using the fasting urinary nitrate:creatinine ratio. *Arthritis Rheum* 39: 643–647

40 Stefanovic-Racic M, Meyers K, Meschter C, Coffey JW, Hoffman RA, Evans CH (1994) N-monomethylarginine, an inhibitor of nitric-oxide synthase, suppresses the development of adjuvant arthritis in rats. *Arthritis Rheum* 37: 1062–1069

41 McCartney-Francis N, Allen JB, Mizel DE, Albina JE, Xie QW, Nathan CF, Wahl SM (1993) Suppression of arthritis by an inhibitor of nitric oxide synthase. *J Exp Med* 178: 749–754

Index

acinar cell, salivary 85–90
activating protein-1 (AP-1) 21, 23, 24
activation-induced cell death (AICD) 96, 97, 99, 101, 105
adeno-associated virus 4, 5, 6, 85, 165
adenovirus 4–7, 15, 16, 20, 22, 23, 25–27, 84–86, 90, 91, 98, 99, 101–103, 105–109, 120, 139–141, 144–146, 148, 165, 168, 170, 172–181, 183, 216, 247, 248, 250
adhesion molecule 1, 3, 22, 41, 145, 148, 163, 187
adjuvant arthritis (AA) 14, 25, 36, 214
airways hyperreactivity (AHR) 65–69, 72, 74–77
allergic airways disease, mouse model of 65–78
antigen-induced arthritis (AIA) 19, 20, 27, 251
antigen-presenting cell (APC) 1, 66, 97–99, 101, 103, 104, 134, 140, 141, 145, 148, 168, 173, 205, 209, 211–213
anti-sense RNA 3
AP-1; *see* activating protein-1
apoptosis 3, 22–25, 28, 87, 95–97, 100, 101, 103, 105, 107, 109, 140–144, 146, 148
aquaporin 89
arthritis, animal model 14–23, 25–28, 35–47, 54, 56, 84, 214, 238, 241–252
arthritis, osteo- (OA) 38, 40, 41
arthritis, rheumatoid (RA) xi, xii, 4, 13–28, 35–47, 53–61, 241–243, 246–252
asthma xii, 65, 67, 77, 78
autoimmune diabetes; *see* diabetes
basophil 65
B cell; *see* also lymphocyte 17, 28, 36, 38, 100, 123, 133, 141, 163, 168, 212, 215
bone 16, 17, 19, 24, 36, 37, 41, 166, 167, 184, 185, 241, 246, 249

cartilage 16–21, 35–47, 54, 60, 241, 243, 246, 247, 249, 250, 252
catalase 144, 148
cationic lipid; *see* also liposome 139, 141, 175, 183
cathepsin 36, 39, 40, 43, 46, 47
cell cycle 25, 27, 90
chondrocyte 7, 19, 20, 25, 28, 248, 249
clinical trial xii, 4, 14, 18, 28, 53–61, 242
co-stimulatory molecule 97, 101, 103, 123, 137, 142, 146, 170, 176, 210–212
colitis xii, 4, 232, 233, 235
collagen induced arthritis (CIA) 17–21, 24, 25, 27, 36, 232, 237, 238, 248, 249
collagenase; *see* also matrix metalloproteinase 23, 42
complement 146, 147
contralateral effect 18–20, 23, 27,
CTLA4 3, 142, 143, 146, 148, 168, 169, 173, 181, 183, 186
cyclooxygenase 1
cytokines; *see* also individual cytokines 1–3, 9, 16, 18, 21, 22, 26, 36, 39, 42, 45, 46, 65, 66, 68, 72, 77, 87, 90, 96, 101, 119, 121,

128, 136–141, 144, 148, 163, 168, 169, 172–174, 176, 184, 187, 205, 206, 209, 211, 212, 214, 215, 219, 224, 231, 232, 234, 235, 237, 241, 243, 248–252

decoy oligonucleotides 3, 23, 24
dendritic cells 28, 140, 145, 146, 148, 149, 209
DFG; *see* also MFG, retrovirus 244, 245
diabetes xii, 90, 133–149, 167, 168, 180, 186
DNA vaccination; *see* also plasmid DNA xii, 4, 6, 7, 67–70, 74, 77, 205–224
ductal cell, salivary gland 85–89

E2F1 90, 91
E3-19K 169
electroporation 103
endothelium 1, 22, 42, 175, 177, 178, 249
endotoxin; *see* also lipopolysaccharide 22, 26, 58
eosinophils 65, 67, 69, 70, 72, 74–77
epithelium 84, 87, 170, 177, 178, 180
ethics committee 55
ex vivo gene delivery 4, 6, 7, 9, 13–15, 19, 27, 54, 56, 57, 83, 84, 120, 164, 166, 171, 173, 178, 179, 181, 182, 243, 245–247
experimental autoimmune encephalomyelitis (EAE) 119, 121–128, 219

Fas 24, 25, 87, 95–101, 104–107, 109, 111, 143, 144, 148, 169
Fas ligand (fasL) 22, 24, 25, 87, 95, 97–109, 111, 143, 148, 149, 169, 181
fibroblast growth factor 23
fos 16, 23, 24, 46
free radical; *see* also nitric oxide 1, 2

gene expression, regulation of 3, 5, 8, 9, 25, 26, 57
gene gun 5, 120, 139, 142, 181, 209, 216
generalized lymphoproliferative disease (gld) 95–97, 99, 101, 105–109, 111
germ-line cell 57
gld; *see* generalized lymphoproliferative disorder
granulocyte-macrophage colony stimulating factor (GMCSF) 22, 65, 184, 217

heart 141, 165, 166, 175–178
hepatocyte 165–167, 170, 182, 183, 249
herpes simplex virus 4–6, 68, 120, 121, 139, 140, 144, 184
histamine 65, 213, 214
HIV; *see* human immunodeficiency virus
HLA; *see* human leukocyte antigen
HSV; *see* herpes simplex virus
human immunodeficiency virus (HIV) 9, 26, 140, 171, 207
human leukocyte antigen (HLA); *see* also major histocompatibility antigen 121, 133, 137
human trials; *see* clinical trials

ICAM-1; *see* intercellular adhesion molecule-1
IFNγ; *see* interferon
in vivo gene delivery 4, 6, 7, 9, 13, 14, 20, 27, 120, 164, 182
insulin-dependent diabetes mellitus (IDDM); *see* diabetes
insulitis 107, 133–137, 141–144
intercellular adhesion molecule-1 (ICAM-1) 3, 22, 145, 148, 170
interferon (IFN) β 119
interferon (IFN) γ 17, 42, 66, 67, 70–72, 75–77, 100, 119, 122, 134, 136, 137, 141, 142, 144, 148, 168, 170, 171, 174, 183, 205, 206, 210, 212, 214, 219, 221, 250
interleukin (IL)-1 9, 18–23, 36, 42, 54, 134, 143, 144, 148, 171, 241–246, 248, 250–252
interleukin-1 receptor (IL-1R) 20, 27, 42, 143, 148, 170, 242
interleukin-1 receptor antagonist (IL-1Ra) 2, 3, 18, 19, 20, 21, 42–46, 53–61, 143, 148, 173, 242
interleukin (IL)-2 17, 42, 100, 122, 127, 134, 136, 206, 212, 214–216, 219, 231–234, 236, 237

interleukin (IL)-3 65
interleukin (IL)-4 3, 17, 65, 66, 70, 72, 75, 76, 90, 100, 119, 120, 123–125, 136, 140, 141, 168, 206, 212–214, 219, 231, 232
interleukin (IL)-5 17, 65, 66, 70, 72, 75, 76, 206, 212, 214
interleukin (IL)-6 9, 18, 22, 36, 42, 171, 216, 241, 250, 252
interleukin (IL)-7 216
interleukin (IL)-8 18, 22, 170, 241, 252
interleukin (IL)-10; *see* also viral interleukin-10 3, 17, 18, 24, 26, 27, 42, 43–46, 90, 120, 123, 125–128, 136, 137, 140–142, 144, 146, 148, 168, 176, 177, 183, 212, 219, 232, 236–238
interleukin (IL)-12 3, 66–78, 141, 142, 145, 169, 171, 212, 216, 223, 224
interleukin (IL)-13 3, 17
interleukin (IL)-15 212
interleukin (IL)-18 212
intraarticular (i.a.) delivery; *see* joint
intradermal (i.d.) delivery 209, 214
intramuscular (i.m.) delivery; *see* muscle
intravenous (i.v.) delivery 7, 15, 20, 173, 181–183
IRAP; *see* interleukin-1 receptor antagonist
islet of Langerhans 107, 134–136, 138–149, 166–169, 172, 173, 180, 181, 186

joint 8, 13–21, 23–28, 35– 47, 53–61, 238, 241–243, 245, 247–249, 251, 252
joint prosthesis 56, 57
jun 23

keratinocyte growth factor 182
keratitis xii, 4, 232, 233, 236, 237
kidney 39, 40, 138, 166, 178–181

lentivirus 4, 5, 139–141
leukocyte; *see* also individual leukocytes 1, 19, 20, 24, 26, 65, 177, 243, 249, 252
leukotriene 65
lipofectamine 69
lipofectin 175
lipopolysaccharide (LPS); *see* also endotoxin 22, 26, 250
liposome; *see* also cationic lipid 4, 5, 23, 24, 84, 85, 120, 175–177, 179
liver 7, 15, 25–27, 84, 105, 143, 165, 166, 166, 169, 178, 182–184
local gene delivery 7, 8, 13–15, 18–21, 25–28, 83, 105, 119, 123, 165, 167, 173
lpr-lymphoproliferation, lpr/lpr; *see* also MRL/lpr mouse 95–97, 99, 103–105, 107, 109, 111
lung 27, 66–72, 75–77, 84, 105, 109, 110, 165, 177–179
lupus erythematosus; *see* systemic lupus erythematosus (SLE)
lupus; *see* systemic lupus erythematosus (SLE)
lymphocyte; *see* also Th1, Th2 xii, 1, 3, 4, 15–17, 20, 24, 25, 27, 28, 35–38, 41, 43, 65, 66, 69–72, 75, 76, 87, 90, 95–101, 103, 105–109, 122–128, 133–137, 140–146, 148, 163, 164, 168–174, 176, 177, 183–185, 205, 206, 209–217, 219, 221, 222, 224, 233, 246
lysozyme 96, 101

macrophage 15, 18, 22, 25, 28, 36, 37, 41–43, 65, 101, 103–105, 133, 134, 136, 163, 168, 170, 209, 245, 249, 251
major histocompatibility complex (MHC) 100, 108, 134, 141, 142, 145–148, 163, 165, 167–170, 172, 174, 184, 185, 187, 205, 209–212, 233, 241
MAP kinase; *see* mitogen activated kinase
mast cell 65, 75, 76, 176, 213
matrix degradation 37, 40–42, 44, 45, 247, 252
matrix-metalloproteinase (MMP) 24, 36, 39, 40, 42, 46, 47, 60, 252
metacarpophalangeal (MCP) joint 57–60, 241, 243
MFG; *see* also retrovirus 39, 43, 45, 57–59, 244

MHC; *see* major histocompatibility complex
mitogen activated kinase 6, 23, 29, 46, 172
Moloney murine leukemia virus; *see* also retrovirus, MFG, DFG 4–6, 14, 43, 54, 139
monocyte 22, 134, 185
MRL-lpr/lpr mouse 36, 96, 99, 100, 104, 219, 220, 233
multiple sclerosis xii, 119–128
murine cytomegalovirus (mCMV) 105–108
muscle 4, 7, 84, 141, 142, 175, 178, 185, 186, 207, 209, 212–214, 217, 222, 231, 232, 235– 237, 248–250
myc 16
myoblast 143, 165, 166, 181, 184–187
myocyte 168, 175, 177

naked DNA; *see* plasmid DNA, DNA vaccination
natural killer (NK) cell 66, 141, 148, 170, 171
neuron 6, 135, 249
neutrophil; *see* also polymorphonuclear leukocyte 101, 143, 148, 168, 170, 184, 249, 252
NFκB; *see* nuclear factor κB
nitric oxide (NO) 22, 143, 242, 249–251
NOD mice 90, 107, 133, 135–137, 140–145
nuclear factor κB (NFκB) 6, 21–24, 27, 171

organ transplantation; *see* transplantation
organoid 7
orthopaedic surgery 55–59
osteoblast 24

p53 17, 216
PAF; *see* platelet activating factor
PAI; *see* plasminogen activator inhibitor
pancreas; *see* also islet of Langerhans, diabetes 131, 138, 139, 141, 180, 181
parotid gland 85, 108
particle bombardment; *see* gene gun
patient, safety and welfare of 56
PDGF; *see* platelet-derived growth factor
phospholipase 76
plasminogen activator inhibitor (PAI) 3, 171
platelet activating factor (PAF) 3, 65
platelet-derived growth factor (PDGF) 22, 23
plasmid DNA; *see* also DNA vaccination xii, 3–5, 13, 75, 84, 120, 139, 141, 142, 165, 168, 171, 173–176, 181, 186, 206–208, 210, 212, 214, 220, 221, 231–237, 249
polymorphonuclear leukocyte; *see* also neutrophil 1, 245, 246
promoter 6, 8, 9, 26, 27, 68, 85, 101, 107, 127, 141, 164, 166, 174, 176, 183, 187, 207, 208, 216, 218, 219, 248
proteinase; *see* also matrix metalloproteinase 1–3, 76
proto-oncogene 16, 46
poxvirus 66

raf 46, 47
rapamycin 9
ras 16, 39, 43, 46
recombinant vaccinia virus (VV) vector 66
retrovirus; *see* also Moloney murine leukemia virus, MFG, DFG 4–6, 14, 15, 19, 54, 57, 58, 83, 84, 96, 120, 121, 125, 128, 139, 140, 144, 146, 147, 165, 167, 171, 174, 176, 179, 184–186, 243, 244
rheumatoid arthritis (RA); *see* arthritis, rheumatoid
ribozyme 3, 47
RU486 9

safety testing 57
salivary gland xii, 83–91, 106–108
SCID mouse; *see* severe combined immunodeficiency mouse
SCW arthritis; *see* streptococcal cell wall arthritis
septic shock xii
severe combined immunodeficiency (SCID) mouse 17, 20, 25, 35–47, 97, 141, 186
Sjögren's syndrome xii, 87, 88, 90, 105–108

skin 4, 7, 39, 40, 216, 251
soluble IL-1 receptor (sIL-1R); *see* interleukin-1 receptor
soluble TNF receptor (sTNF-R); *see* tumor necrosis α receptor
stem cell 7, 90, 166, 167, 169, 180, 184
streptococcal cell wall (SCW)-induced arthritis 14, 16, 18, 19, 21–23, 26, 27
stromelysin; *see* also metalloproteinase 42, 244, 252
sublingual gland 85
submandibular gland 85, 86
superoxide dismutase 3, 148
surgical joint replacement 59
synovial cell 14–23, 25, 28, 35–47, 56–61, 238, 241–246, 248, 249, 251
synovium 13–26, 28, 36, 42, 44, 45, 54, 56–61, 241–245, 247, 250–252
systemic gene delivery 7, 8, 17–20, 26–28
systemic lupus erythematosis (SLE) xii, 4, 95–111, 214, 215, 232–234

T cell; *see* lymphocyte, Th1, Th2
tetracycline 9, 26
TGFβ; *see* transforming growth factor β
Th1 3, 17, 66, 75–78, 90, 100, 122, 123, 136, 140, 141, 144, 148, 168, 170, 176, 177, 206, 212–214, 217, 219, 232, 233, 237, 238
Th2 3, 17, 65, 66, 72, 75, 77, 78, 90, 100, 122, 123, 125, 136, 140, 146, 148, 168, 177, 206, 212–214, 232, 237, 238
tissue inhibitor of metalloproteinases (TIMP) 3
TNF-R; *see* tumour necrosis factor α receptor
TNFbp; *see* tumor necrosis factor binding

transcription factor; *see* also individual transcription factors, proto-oncogenes 3, 21–25, 27, 46, 95
transforming growth factor β (TGFβ) 27, 119, 123, 126, 136, 137, 141, 142, 144, 146, 148, 168, 176, 177, 179, 183, 214, 231–235, 242, 247–249, 251
transgenic mice 17, 22, 24, 25, 99, 100, 142
transplantation xii, 138, 142–147, 163–187
tumor necrosis factor α (TNFα) 9, 18, 20–23, 26, 36, 42, 53, 96, 100, 108, 109, 122, 134, 137, 144, 148, 168, 171, 172, 174, 183, 184, 219, 242, 246, 250, 252
tumor necrosis factor binding protein (TNFbp) 109
tumor necrosis factor soluble receptor (sTNF-R) 20, 27, 43, 44, 53, 108, 109, 148, 168, 242

vaccinia virus 66–77
vascular adhesion molecule 1 (VCAM-1) 22, 41, 148, 169
vector; *see* also individual vectors xii, 3–7, 9, 24, 25, 27
viral interleukin 10 (vIL-10) 17, 18, 27, 140, 141, 146, 148, 172, 173, 176, 177, 181, 183

xerostomia (dry mouth) 87

MIX
Papier aus verantwortungsvollen Quellen
Paper from responsible sources
FSC® C105338

If you have any concerns about our products,
you can contact us on
ProductSafety@springernature.com

In case Publisher is established outside the EU,
the EU authorized representative is:
Springer Nature Customer Service Center GmbH
Europaplatz 3, 69115 Heidelberg, Germany

Printed by Libri Plureos GmbH
in Hamburg, Germany